ATLAS OF DISEASE DISTRIBUTIONS

ATLAS

OF

DISEASE DISTRIBUTIONS

ANALYTIC APPROACHES

TO

EPIDEMIOLOGICAL DATA

ANDREW D. CLIFF AND PETER HAGGETT

BLACKWELL REFERENCE

First published 1988
First published in paperback 1992
Reprinted 1993

Blackwell Publishers
108 Cowley Road, Oxford, OX4 1JF, UK

238 Main Street
Cambridge, Massachusetts 02142, USA

British Library Cataloguing in Publication Data
Cliff, A.D. (Andrew David), *1943–*
  Atlas of disease distributions.
  1. Man. Diseases. Epidemiology
  I. Title II. Haggett, Peter
  616.4

Library of Congress Cataloging-in-Publication Data
Cliff, A.D. (Andrew David)
  Atlas of disease distributions: analytic approaches to
  epidemiological data.
  Bibliography: Includes indexes.
1. Medical geography–Maps. 2. Cartography–
Statistical methods. 3. Epidemiology–Statistical
methods. 4. Epidemiology–Mathematical models.
1. Haggett, Peter. II. Title. [DNLM: 1. Epidemiology
–atlases. WA 17 C637a]
G1046.E51C5 1988   912′.16144′2   88–675321

ISBN 0–631–13149–3 hb.
ISBN 0–631–18529–1 pb.

Typeset in 10½/12 pt Plantin
Printed in Great Britain by Redwood Books, Trowbridge, Wiltshire

CONTENTS

PREFACE

Atlases of disease

In the medical literature, the term 'atlas' has at least two distinct meanings. First, and most commonly, it denotes a volume with plates which show parts of the human body or its pathology. Titles such as 'Atlas of anatomy', 'Atlas of orthopaedic surgery', 'Atlas of tumour pathology' or 'Atlas of skin diseases' illustrate this genre. Second, and less commonly, 'atlas' is used in its conventional geographical sense to show the distribution of some medical condition, either for the world as a whole or some part of it. The *World Atlas of Epidemic Diseases* (Rodenwaldt and Jusatz, 1952–61)), the *Seuchen Atlas* (Zeiss, 1941–5) or the *Atlas of Cancer Mortality in England and Wales* 1968–1978 (Gardner, Winter, Taylor and Acheson, 1983) are good examples. The number of volumes in this second category is much smaller than in the first but it is growing rapidly as the environmental and geographical setting of diseases becomes more sharply defined. We provide a selected list of such atlases in the references section at the end of this volume.

This Atlas is conventional in the second sense because it shows maps of the distribution of various diseases in specific parts of the world. It is, however, unconventional in that its aim is also methodological. It sets out to illustrate a range of approaches to the mapping of medical data, both as static cross-sections and over time, by outlining and critically examining the methods used. Our central argument is that, since maps are being increasingly used in the medical literature (especially computer-produced maps), it is essential to evaluate their effectiveness. This is important because, while maps are sometimes used to good effect, in other instances they tend to obscure evidence, to suggest false concentrations and to start false trails. By combining cartographic and statistical arguments, appreciation of the value of maps can be sharpened and errors of interpretation reduced.

The Atlas can therefore be seen as an exercise in bridge-building. First, it demonstrates the strengthening links between statistical and cartographic methods, thus encouraging that unified approach to spatial data analysis which contemporary computing power now allows. Second, it acts as a handy reference volume for those in environmental and public health who are charged with reporting disease data which are collected on a geographical basis, and including those who use maps as part of an epidemiological investigation. Third, it illustrates for cartographers, demographers, geographers and other regional scientists the potential of one set of statistical sources for spatial analysis, one that is particularly rich in both its historical timespan and in its geographical range.

History of medical mapping

In the early history of the mapping of disease, the distribution maps of yellow fever in 1798 are often given pride of place (Robinson, 1982). But these were predated by maps of topics as diverse as hospital capacities and the distribution of dressing stations on a battlefield, through to maps of pestilential swamps and other hostile medical environments. With the start of the nineteenth century the number of medical maps rose sharply. By the 1820s the spread of cholera from India over Eurasia and North America saw the production of a spate of cholera maps with plates showing routes of spread, and dates and regions of occurrence. Some, such as Rothenburg's 1836 map of Hamburg, showed variations in cholera intensity in a more sophisticated manner and were reprinted by the British General Board of Health when cholera appeared in Britain again in 1948–49.

But such maps were usually of secondary importance and incidental rather than central to the epidemiological report. Thus although Dr Robert Perry, senior physician to the Glasgow Royal Infirmary, included a map in his report on the major influenza epidemic which affected the city in 1832, he admitted that its printing and colouring were 'wholly the work of the inmates of the Gartnavel Lunatic Asylum' (Robinson, 1982, p.174). But by the 1830s the potential of such maps for hypothesis testing began to be explored. Thus J.F. Malgaigne's map of hernia amongst military recruits in France, published in 1839, was critically compared with maps showing the levels of ingestion of olive oil and regions where cider drinking predominated over wine, both currently fashionable as supposed causes of high hernia rates. Superimposed regional boundaries were duly drawn on the hernia map and Malgaigne was forced to discard both hypotheses.

The breakthrough in disease mapping occurred mid-century with the cholera map produced by Dr John Snow to accompany the second edition of his prize-winning essay on the communication of cholera. What set Snow's work apart was not the cartography (dot maps, which were a well-established cartographic device, to show the geographical distribution of individual cholera deaths), but his inductive reasoning from the map. By showing what he termed the 'topography of the outbreak', Snow was able to draw inferences about the central source of infection. In tribute to Snow's work, we devote the opening chapter of this book to maps of cholera in general and to Snow's map in particular; they form a common starting point for the cartography and the statistical analysis of this Atlas.

Cartographic and statistical methods

The handling of maps and of statistical data are closely intertwined. It was no accident that early geographical societies were sometimes founded jointly with statistical societies; the American Geographical and Statistical Society of New York (founded in 1854) provides a nineteenth-century example. Today, Brazil's government agency, the Instituto Geográfica e Estatística, provides a latter-day equivalent. The current wide availability of high-speed computers has rebuilt that close relationship.

For the cartographic methods used here we generally refer readers to a single source rather than a range of literature which may not be readily available in a medical library. The latest edition of Robinson's *Elements of Cartography* (Robinson, Sale, Morrison and Muehrcke, 1984) is a good, readable introduction. The statistical methods introduced in this volume range from simple techniques that need scarcely more than a slide-rule or a hand calculator to more complex mapping techniques that demand high-speed computing. Where mathematical ideas occur, these are set to one side as technical appendices which can be explored or bypassed; where space

does not permit a full explanation, follow-up reading is suggested.

Our approach is to mix theory and application and to make cross-reference to appropriate computer software where this is widely available. The general purpose MINITAB statistical system developed at the Pennsylvania State University is now extensively implemented in the western world on various micro, mini, and mainframe computers. It is supported by a good graphics package which can be simply adapted for many cartographic purposes; spatial statistics are readily added by using its macro facilities and some are available on request from the authors. We therefore refer to statistical methods which are easily used with MINITAB and we make appropriate cross reference to those textbooks which are written around the MINITAB package; the MINITAB manual (Ryan, Joiner and Ryan, 1985) and Cryer's *Time Series Analysis* (1986) are good examples.

Range of diseases

An Atlas of this size can only cover some of the vast range of recognizable diseases. We restrict ourselves (except for one figure) to human diseases but, as Chapter 2 shows, there are more than one thousand categories and sub-categories in the Ninth Revision of the International Classification of Diseases. Nine of the seventeen main groups are sampled, with a heavy emphasis on infectious diseases (Group I). To some extent this reflects the pattern of medical mapping itself and to some degree it reflects our own work which has largely been confined to one infectious disease (measles). Inevitably there are fascinating areas which we have not included, such as river blindness in West Africa (Hunter, 1956) or kuru in the Pacific which we would hope to include in

future editions. Thus our prime purpose has been to illustrate the methodological range of mapping rather than to attempt a complete coverage.

Geographical and historical coverage

Likewise the geographical range of the Atlas is illustrative rather than exhaustive. Most of the maps are of northwest Europe and of Iceland in particular, the country where we have both worked longest. But we go outside that area to include maps of disease distribution in the United States, in the southwest Pacific, in India, and in central Africa. The scale focus also ranges from the global level in our treatment of the Asian influenza epidemic of 1957 (section 6.4), down to the detail of individual accidents on London's streets (Figure 3.17).

Although most of the maps are of disease patterns in the late twentieth century, the Atlas spans more than a century. We use Snow's classic area of concern, the London cholera outbreaks in 1849 and 1855, to illustrate many methods (see Chapter 1). We look at maps of the closing stages of one great pandemic disease (smallpox; section 6.3) and the start of a new pandemic (AIDS; section 6.2). We also include maps of the fallout from the 1986 Chernobyl accident (Figure 5.3) and the potential new radon gas hazards whose geographical distribution is only being mapped in detail as this Atlas goes to press (Figure 3.9).

Thus the spatial distribution of disease remains one of the oldest of puzzles and yet one of the most contemporary. For example, the concentration of AIDS cases in central Africa or the argument over clusters (or non-clusters) of leukaemia cases adjacent to nuclear power stations (Figure 3.8) raise many of the same questions as puzzled the map makers of disease distributions a centry ago. But it is essential to ensure that apparent geographical patterns are not merely artifacts of the mapping process which set off wild goose chases that consume scarce resources. If disease maps are to be a serious aid to the epidemiologist, then they need to be handled with as much care and critical attention as any other source of evidence. We hope that the methods surveyed and illustrated here will help towards that goal.

Atlas structure

The Atlas begins with a consideration of the wide variety of cartographic methods available for the mapping and analysis of medical data. For reasons already given, these are all illustrated by examples drawn from the cholera epidemics which affected Britain in 1849 and 1854. In Chapter 2, the data gathering problems which affect the interpretability of medical data are examined. Thus we discuss the headings under which diseases are grouped in the International Classification of Diseases, the reliability and coverage of morbidity and mortality data, missing data problems and the difficulties caused by changes in the definitions of collecting units.

The majority of the statistical material is contained in Chapters 3–5. The incidence of disease varies not only from one part of the globe to another but also over time. So we begin in Chapter 3 by examining techniques for the analysis of geographical variability at a single point in time before outlining, in Chapter 4, methods for studying the time-series behaviour of single regions. In Chapter 5, time and space are reunited and a series of methods are described to isolate space–time interactions.

The material presented in the first five chapters has, with the exception of section 1.1, been carefully structured so that each provides, at the expense of a small amount of repetition, a relatively self-contained account of a single cartographic or statistical technique. While there is a clear logical structure to the ordering of the material so that each chapter can be easily read from beginning to end, it is also possible to treat each section in isolation as a reference source for that technique. Each section includes almost a full page of illustrative material and, where appropriate, a technical appendix which explains the statistical analysis employed.

In Chapter 6, the layout is different. Here the full range of methods described in the previous chapters is drawn upon to provide integrated accounts of the epidemiology of four diseases, namely AIDS, smallpox, influenza and measles.

The proper use of cartographic and statistical methods can greatly enhance our understanding of the epidemiology of many diseases. As epidemological knowledge improves, so will an ability to predict the likely paths in time and space which will be followed by these diseases. Although the prospect is still a distant one, it may be possible to forecast maps and so be in a position to provide early warning of disease events and their public-health consequences. We therefore conclude the Atlas in Chapter 7 by considering future mapping technologies and the different ways of forecasting such maps.

Acknowledgements

Our principle debt is to the Wellcome Trust for providing a grant to allow us to continue our work in Iceland and for underwriting, with Christ's College Cambridge, the high cost of preparing more than 300 maps and diagrams for the Atlas.

The Atlas forms a third in a trilogy of volumes that make heavy use of the exceptional demographic and epidemiological records available for Iceland. Like its predecessors, *Spatial Diffusion: An Historical Geography of Epidemics in an Island Community* (Cliff, Haggett, Ord and Versey, 1981) and *Spatial Aspects of Influenza Epidemics* (Cliff, Haggett and Ord, 1986), it could not have been written without the active help of the Icelandic medical and demographic authorities. We are grateful to Dr Ólafur Ólafsson (Director General of Public Health in Iceland), to successive directors of the Statistical Bureau of Iceland for their continuing help over more than a decade of work in Reykjavík, to Professor Frank Fenner, John Curtin School of Medicine, Australian National University for comments on the smallpox maps, and to Dr Clare Tait and Dr T.I. Haggett for reviewing our use of medical terms. Such errors of interpretation as remain, are our own.

The specific sources for the maps in the Atlas which are not our own original work appear in the Sources and Further Reading attached to each figure. We are grateful to those named individuals and institutions who have given permission to draw on their work. We are particularly indebted to Ian Gulley and to Stella Gutteridge in the Drawing Office and Department of Geography, University of Cambridge, who drew the maps, working up our very rough roughs into finished drawings.

John Davey, one of Blackwell's senior editors, took an active interest in the project from its early days and worked hard to produce a volume which would be reasonably easy both to use and to shelve, always a problem in atlas design.

Finally to both our families we owe a debt for drastically shortened or cancelled summer holidays and month after month of unsociable evenings. Computer output was checked at the edge of tennis courts or bowling greens (according to the age of the author) and it is left to the reader to decide whether the sheets which threatened to blow away into neighbouring fields should or should not have been rescued.

Christ's College,
Cambridge.

ADC and PH
September 1987.

ACKNOWLEDGEMENTS

The Authors and Publisher are grateful to the following persons and institutions for permission to reproduce the figures specified below. (Publication details of sources not cited in full below will be found in DATA SOURCES, ATLASES AND REFERENCES.)

Figure 1.1 (C) Reprinted from *The Economist* 6 (1848) p.1436.

Figures 1.1 (H) and **(I)** Reprinted from *Punch* 17 (1849) pp.144–5, and 22 (1852) p.139.

Figure 1.15 (E) A.H. Robinson and The University of Chicago Press. (From Arthur H. Robinson (1982) p.178, Figure 88.)

Figure 1.18 (E) *Annals of the Association of American Geographers.* (Redrawn from J.M. Hunter and J.C. Young (1971) p.641, Figure 3.)

Figure 2.2 (A) A.S. Evans and Plenum Press. (Redrawn from A.S. Evans, ed. (1982, 2nd edn 1984) p.20, Figure 2.)

Figure 2.3 (A) Churchill Livingstone. (Redrawn from F. Brockington (1975) p.247, Figure 24.1.)

Figure 2.4 (A) J.W.G. Smith and the Public Health Laboratory Service. (Redrawn from J.W.G. Smith (1976).)

Figure 2.4 (C) *American Journal of Epidemiology.* (Redrawn from K. Choi and S.B. Thacker (1981) pp.215–26 and 227–35, Figures 1 and 2.)

Figure 3.2 (A)–(F) G.M. Howe and the Royal Geographical Society. (Redrawn from G.M. Howe, ed. (1970) pp.56–7 and 66–9.)

Figure 3.3 (C) K.B. Fraser, Ballindalloch.

Figures 3.5 (B) and **(C)** A.T.A. Learmonth and the Royal Geographical Society. (Redrawn from A.T.A. Learmonth (1957), Figures 13–16.)

Figures 3.6 (A) and **(B)** M.J. Gardner and John Wiley & Sons Limited. (Redrawn from M.J. Gardner *et al.* (1983) pp.28–9, 32–3 and 46, 48.)

Figures 3.7 (A) and **(B)** China Map Press. (Redrawn from Chinese Academy of Medical Sciences (1981) pp.77–8 and 85–6.)

Figure 3.7 (C) G. de Thé and Plenum Press. (Redrawn from G. de Thé *et al.* (1984) p.542, Figure 1.)

Figures 3.9 (B) and **(C)** M.C. O'Riordan and © National Radiological Protection Board. (Redrawn from M.C. O'Riordan *et al.* (1987) pp.14–15, Data Tables and Figure 2.)

Figure 3.9 (D) Collins Publishers. (Photograph by Humphrey and Vera Joel, reproduced in L.A. Harvey and D. St.Leger-Gordon (1953) p.15, Plate IVa.)

Figure 3.11 (A) G.M. Howe and the Royal Geographical Society. (Redrawn from G.M. Howe, ed. (1970) pp.58–61.)

Figure 3.12 (C) The Keystone Collection, London.

Figures 3.16 (A) and **(B)** H. Moellering. (Redrawn from H. Moellering (1974) pp.31, 46, 56 and 65.)

Figure 5.1 (B) H.J. Jusatz and Falk Verlag. (From E. Rodenwaldt (1961). 'Cholera in Asia 1931–1955'. In E. Rodenwaldt and H.J. Jusatz, ed. (1952–61) pp.4–7, Map 81.)

Figure 5.3 (A) © Her Majesty's Stationery Office and reprinted by permission from *Nature* 322, pp. 690–1/Copyright © 1986 Macmillan Magazines Ltd. (From F.B. Smith and M.J. Clark (1986).)

Figure 5.3 (B) H. ApSimon and *New Scientist*, London, the weekly review of science and technology. (From H. ApSimon and J. Wilson (1986).)

Figure 5.3 (C) D. Horrell, Institute of Terrestrial Ecology and the *Guardian*, 25 July, 1986.

Figure 5.3 (D) P. Orlando and reprinted by permission from *Nature* 323, p.23/Copyright © 1986 Macmillan Magazines Ltd. (From P. Orlando *et al.* (1986).)

Figure 5.4 (E) The National Maritime Museum, London.

Figures 5.6 (C) and **(D)** A.W. Gilg and the Royal Geographical Society. (Redrawn from A.W. Gilg (1973).)

Figure 5.7 (A) B.McA. Sayers and Taylor & Francis Ltd. for *Medical Informatics* (Redrawn from B.McA. Sayers *et al.* (1977).)

Figures 5.7 (C) and **(D)** J.D. Murray and Academic Press Inc. (London) Ltd. for the *Journal of Theoretical Biology.* (From A. Källen *et al.* (1985).)

Figure 5.16 (B) G. de Thé and reprinted by permission from *Nature* 274, pp.756–51/ Copyright © 1978 Macmillan Magazines Ltd. (From G. de Thé (1978).)

Figure 5.16 (C) J. Siematycki and the *International Journal of Cancer.* (From J. Siematycki *et al.* (1980).)

Figure 6.2 (A) Hans Gelderblom, Robert Koch Institut, Berlin.

Figure 6.2 (F) © *The Daily Telegraph* 1987.

Figure 6.2 (H) (*upper*). T.A. Peterman and *Epidemiologic Review.* (Redrawn from T.A. Peterman *et al.* (1985) p.7, Figure 2.)

Figure 6.2 (L) E.G. Knox and the *European Journal of Epidemiology.* (Redrawn from E.G. Knox (1986).)

Figure 6.3 (E) World Health Organization. (From F. Fenner *et al.* (1988) p.1067.)

Figures 6.4 (F) and **(G)** *Annals of the Association of American Geographers.* (Redrawn from J.M. Hunter and J.C. Young (1971). **(A)** from p.643, Figure 5; p.644, Figure 6; p.647, Figure 9, and (**B**) from p.650, Figure 11.)

Figures 7.1 (A)–(D) D.R.F. Taylor and John Wiley & Sons Limited. (From D.R.F. Taylor, ed. (1980). (**A**) p.203, Figure 9.9 by courtesy of the Minister of Supply and Services, Canada; (**B**) p.204, Figure 9.10 (*upper*) by courtesy of *The Canadian Cartographer* 14 (1977) pp.21–34; (**C**) p.210, Figure 9.13 (*upper*) by courtesy of the Minister of Supply and Services, Canada; and (**D**) p.215, Figure 9.15 by courtesy of the Census Research Unit, Department of Geography, University of Durham.)

Figure 7.2 (B) P. Forer, University of Canterbury, Christchurch, New Zealand.

Figure 7.3 (C) M. Taylor and *Regional Studies*. (Redrawn from M. Taylor and C.C. Kissling (1983).)

Figures 7.5 (A)–(F) P.R. Gould and *Tijdschrift voor Economische en Sociale Geografie*. (Redrawn from P.R. Gould and T.R. Leinbach (1966).)

Every effort has been made by the Publisher to trace the copyright-holder of all figures in this publication. If copyright has been infringed, we will be pleased to make proper acknowledgement, on being satisfied as to the owner's title, in future editions.

CHAPTER ONE
MAPPING PROBLEMS

Figure over   East London slum life, 1899
Source   The British Library. *Photograph*: Local History Library, Bancroft Library/Godfrey New Photographics.

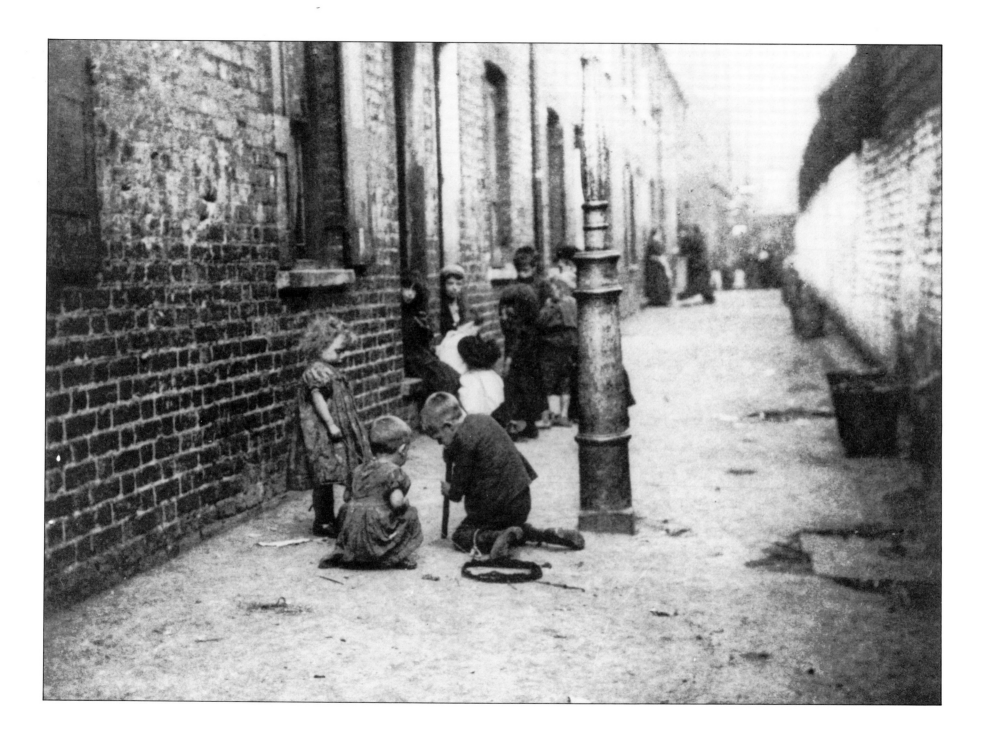

MAPPING PROBLEMS

INTRODUCTION

In this opening chapter, we focus upon the various cartographic techniques available for the display and analysis of those medical data which have a geographical basis to them. In order to emphasize the different techniques we have chosen to keep three things constant, first the *geographical area* covered by the maps, second the *time period* for the medical data, and third the *disease* itself. For the area we have chosen the 10 mile by 8 mile rectangle covering metropolitan London illustrated in diagram (A); for the time period we have chosen the middle years of the nineteenth century; for the disease we have chosen cholera.

The clue to all three selections is one of the most famous early maps of epidemiological data, that of John Snow showing the geographical distribution of cholera deaths in the Soho area of London in 1854. A portion of Snow's map is reproduced later in Figure 1.15(D), and its location is also shown in diagram (A). All the maps in this chapter are prepared from data relating to the great epidemics of Asiatic cholera which affected London in 1848–9 and 1854.

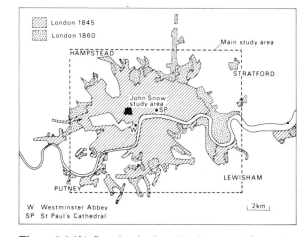

Figure 1.1 (A) London in the mid-nineteenth century

1.1 CHOLERA IN LONDON, 1848–1854

Cholera

The selection of cholera from the range of diseases available for study brings several advantages. As Rosenberg (1962, p.1) remarks in his book, *The Cholera Years*, 'cholera was the classic epidemic disease of the nineteenth century as plague had been in the fourteenth'. It was fear of the consequences of epidemic cholera in the middle of the nineteenth century which, more than anything else, stimulated the growth of the sanitary reform and public health movements in the cities of Europe. The disease has therefore attracted a great deal of attention from medical workers. For example, Koch himself, in one of his letters, referred to cholera as 'our old ally' in recognition of the impetus it provided to research in preventive medicine (Ackerknecht, 1965, p.23). As a result of this interest, a wealth of data and literature are available about it.

The aetiology of cholera Many of the patterns shown in the figures contained in this chapter can be readily related to the aetiology of cholera and so, before proceeding to the cartographic methods, we consider briefly the main features of the disease. The German bacteriologist, Robert Koch (1843–1910), is usually credited with the isolation of the comma-shaped bacterium, *Vibrio cholerae*, which is the causative agent of Asiatic cholera. Koch discovered the bacterium when examining the intestines of a cholera victim. Nevertheless, it does appear that Koch may have been preceded by the Italian investigator, Filippo Pacini, in 1854. As a result the judicial committee of the International Commis-

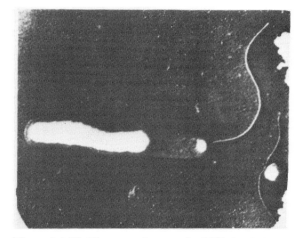

Figure 1.1 (B) Electron micrograph of *Vibrio cholerae*

sion on Bacterial Nomenclature designated the vibrio as *Vibrio cholerae Pacini, 1854* (Spink, 1978, p.162). An electron micrograph of the vibrio at a magnification of 50,000 times appears in diagram (B).

CHOLERA (ICD 001) has a very short incubation period and attacks man with such speed that serious symptoms may occur within a few hours and, in any case, within days of infection by *vibrio cholerae*. The symptoms include the abrupt onset of watery bowel movements (the so-called rice water stools) which may recur with increasing frequency, leading to rapid dehydration from massive water and electrolyte loss. At the same time, there may be severe acidosis, a fall in body temperature and symptoms of vomiting, shock and collapse. Without appropriate treatment the illness may last from 12 hours to seven days. Loss of body fluid causes death in 40–60 percent of untreated cases, and often within 24 hours of the onset of disease.

In the nineteenth century epidemics, it was the high and rapid mortality in infected individuals and the frequent lack of discrimination between social classes that contributed to a sense

of crisis when the visitations occurred. As diagram (C) shows, anything which gave hope was sold. Social disruption was common and, as Kearns (1985, p.43) has noted, the sense of crisis was heightened by the Eastern origins of the disease. The authorities saw a steep rise in the death rate from diarrhoeal disease and feared a possible breakdown in law and order within the cities. The anticipation of such a collapse called forth the crisis mentality attending these epidemics.

Figure 1.1 (C) Advertisement for cholera cure

The pattern of epidemic cholera

Several factors may be identified which create conditions favourable for epidemic cholera (Jusatz, 1977). The vibrio enters the body via the mouth, sometimes on infected food, but most usually in contaminated water. So dominant is the latter as a source of infection that vibrio-carrying water is generally regarded as a prerequisite for any large-scale diffusion; it is the most frequent transport medium of the vibrios

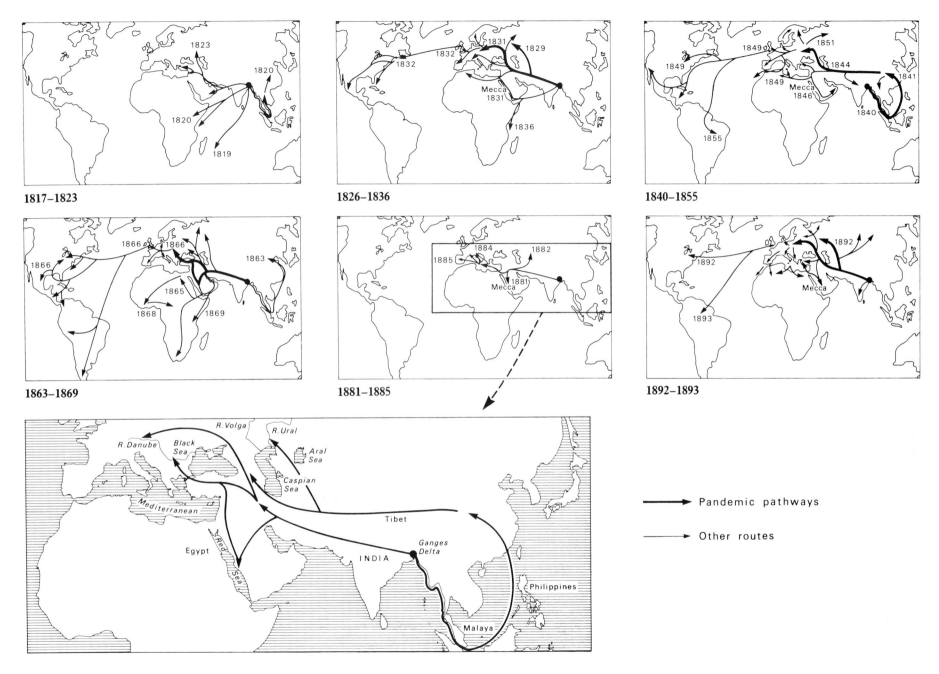

1817–1823

1826–1836

1840–1855

1863–1869

1881–1885

1892–1893

Pandemic pathways

Other routes

Figure 1.1 (D) World maps of six cholera pandemics in the nineteenth century showing the main pathways followed

outside the human body. Contaminated rivers and water courses are the most common originating sites. Water velocity is important and there is a strong inverse correlation between the possibility of persistent cholera and velocity.

The pH of the water also appears to play a role. It is well-known that the cholera vibrios multiply better and remain viable for longer periods of time in alkaline rather than acid conditions. Where tanks are used for the supply of drinking water, algal infestation greatly increases the alkalinity of the resulting stagnant water, thereby enhancing the living and breeding conditions of cholera vibrios once the tanks become infected.

The disease is strongly seasonal. Cold acts as an inhibiting factor and the cholera epidemics in Europe over the last 150 years all collapsed at the start of winter.

The nineteenth century pandemics

In the western world, Asiatic or Indian cholera has been known as an acute intestinal disease since the early years of the nineteenth century. Its natural locus was in the alkaline soils and water of the delta region of the rivers Ganges and Brahmaputra. It is likely that the disease in its endemic and epidemic forms occurred in India, as it still does today, for centuries before that, causing great loss of life (Jusatz, 1977). While on a map showing the distribution of cholera today, cholera appears as endemic in only India and China, in the last century it spread out across the globe in a series of pandemics causing huge mortality wherever it went.

The reasons why these outpourings occurred are not known for certain, but they have been linked to the steady improvements throughout the nineteenth century in travel and transport facilities. Cholera became in this way one of the

most important modern pandemics and, apart from influenza, it has covered larger areas of the globe than any other infectious disease (Acker-knecht, 1965, p.23).

The disease began to assume global significance between 1817 and 1823 when it spread out of its natural heartland by both sea and overland routes to affect large parts of Southeast Asia, East Africa, Persia, Arabia, and Astrakhan in non-European Russia. It was checked there by the actions of the authorities and so failed to reach Europe. The corridors followed are shown by vectors on the first map of diagram (D). Since 1823, there have been six occasions on which pandemic Asiatic cholera has left its traditional home in the Ganges and Brahmaputra valleys to sweep across large areas of the globe. Each pandemic lasted for several years. Five occurred in the nineteenth century and the corridors followed are mapped in diagram (D). As noted in Clemow (1903, pp.94–99), Ackerknecht (1965, pp.24–29) and Spink (1978, pp.163–64), these nineteenth century pandemics travelled on each occasion from India into Asia and Europe via the great trade routes to create the pandemic pathways plotted on the final map of diagram (D).

The 1848–1849 cholera epidemic in Britain

The third of the nineteenth century pandemics, that of the 1840s, has been selected from those available as the data base for the figures presented in the main part of this chapter. It was the impact of this pandemic upon Great Britain in general, and London in particular, which first provided John Snow with clues to the water-borne nature of the disease. As we shall see later in Figures 1.15 and 1.16, it led eventually in 1854 to one of medical history's most fascinating detective stories, one which determined the structure of this opening chapter.

Britain had been heavily affected by the pandemic of 1826 which reached these shores in October 1831. The devastation wrought led to the Cholera Acts, but to no avail, for in 1848 the disease returned. It began with a brief but very severe epidemic in southern Scotland in October 1848, entering Leith Docks and Edinburgh by boat from Hamburg. Nearly 8000 deaths occurred in Scotland by the early part of 1849, when the epidemic abated. In May of 1849 cholera reappeared, but this time in England; the first cases were reported in London. By the end of December, when the epidemic disappeared, it had spread over almost all of Great Britain causing 52,293 deaths (Howe, 1972, p.175).

The geographical centroid of new outbreaks (calculated by a method described later in the Atlas in Figure 5.10) is shown for the months of 1849 in diagram (E). From May to the end of August, the disease was concentrated in the southern half of the country. Rapid northward movement then ensued, with the epidemic terminating in Scotland at the end of the year. The associated graph, above diagram (F), shows both the number and the cumulative percentage of new outbreaks against time. Some 492 places were affected over the course of the epidemic, and the cumulative distribution takes the classic logistic shape of wave-like diffusion processes discussed later in Figure 5.9.

Cholera in London

The effect of cholera on London itself was dramatic. The graph in diagram (F) plots the number of cholera deaths recorded on a weekly basis in the 34 registration districts of the metropolis between 5 May and 24 November, 1849. The level of mortality began to build up in the early part of June and rose steeply from the second week in July, almost without respite, to a

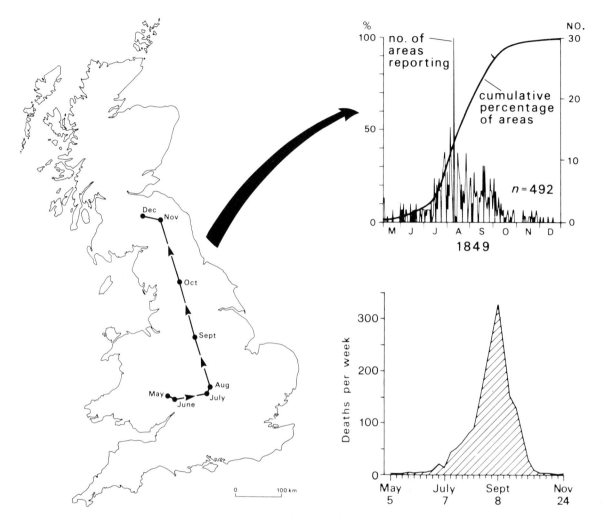

Figure 1.1 (E) Shifts in the centre of gravity of the cholera outbreak in Britain, May–December 1849

Figure 1.1 (F) Weekly deaths from cholera in London, May–November 1849

Dr John Snow (1813–1858) was a London anaesthetist and Queen Victoria's obstetrician. It was during the visitation of cholera to the United Kingdom in 1848–9 that Snow formulated his ideas that cholera might be spread by contaminated water supplies. It was 'since the latter part of 1848, when I first arrived at my present conclusions respecting the mode of communication of cholera' (Snow, 1854, p.125). These ideas were published in 1849 in a relatively slim book entitled *On the Mode of the Communication of Cholera*. His work led on to a much enlarged second edition, published in 1854, containing his celebrated map and account of the Broad Street Pump affair.

Snow demonstrated that most of the cholera deaths in a restricted area of London near Golden Square, Soho, occurred among people who had drunk water from a single pump in Broad Street which had become contaminated by seepage from a leaking cesspool or drain. A map of this central area of London appears in Figure 1.15(D), while its location in the metropolis is delimited on diagram (A). As Pelling (1978, chapter 6) has noted, although some writers have sought to reduce both Snow, and the procedures by which he arrived at this conclusion about cholera transmission, from their status as a 'tutelary deity to teachers and pupils alike' (p.203), most accept the priority of his discovery. 'He is also commonly regarded as a voice crying in the wilderness for the germ theory' (Pelling, 1978, p.203).

The role of the water companies Snow (1854, pp.56–7) comments:

> Each epidemic of cholera in London has borne a strict relation to the nature of the water supply of its different districts, being

peak in the week of September 8. Thereafter the epidemic collapsed and it had effectively disappeared from the city by mid October. It thus displayed the typical summer peak for *Vibrio cholerae*. The number of deaths from Asiatic cholera registered in this period totalled 13,194. This contrasts with a total of 388 cholera deaths

in London in the three years preceding the epidemic and 502 in the three years following.

The geographical incidence of cholera deaths in the registration districts of London is mapped in a variety of ways in the rest of this chapter. All show excess mortality rates in areas adjacent to and south of the River Thames.

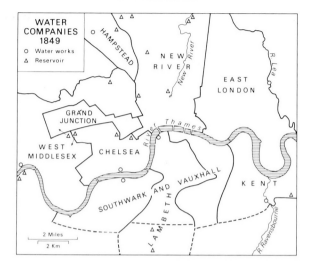

Figure 1.1 (G) Boundaries of the main water companies supplying London in 1849

modified only by poverty, and the crowding and want of cleanliness which always attend it.

Diagram (G) maps the parts of the main study area shown in diagram (A) served by each of the metropolitan water companies; the sources of water and reservoirs of the companies also appear. Four companies, namely the Southwark and Vauxhall, the Lambeth, the West Middlesex and the Chelsea, drew their water directly from the Thames; the Southwark and Vauxhall at Battersea Fields, the Lambeth opposite Hungerford Market, the West Middlesex from the Thames at Hammersmith, and the Chelsea from the Thames at Chelsea.

The remaining companies drew their supplies from sources away from the Thames; the New River from the River Lea above Ware, having 'entirely ceased to employ the steam-engine for obtaining water from the Thames' (Snow, 1854, p.61), the Kent from the River Ravensbourne

below Lewisham, the East London from the Lea above Lea Bridge 'out of the influence of the tide and free from sewage, except that from some part of Upper Clapton' (Snow, 1854, p.61) and the Hampstead from springs and artesian wells at Hampstead.

The Thames at the time was, in effect, an open sewer into which excrement was discharged. Snow notes (1854, pp.136–37):

In 1849 . . . the sewers of London were frequently flushed with water, – a measure which was calculated to increase the disease in two ways: first, by driving the cholera evacuations into the river before there was time for the poison to be rendered inert by decomposition; and second, by making increased calls on the various companies for water to flush the sewers with, – so that the water which they sent to their customers remained for a shorter time in the reservoirs before being distributed. It should be remarked, also, that the contents of the sewers were driven into the Thames by flushing, at low water, and remained flow-

ing up the stream for four or five hours afterwards.

and (p.96)

. . . the river becomes a kind of prolonged lake, the same water passing twice a day to and fro through London, and receiving the excrement of its two millions and more inhabitants, which keeps accumulating till there is a fall of rain.

The Thames therefore approximated a well-mixed cesspool from which the four companies with riverside water sources drew their supplies. Using data given in Snow (1854, p.64) the deaths from cholera per 10,000 population in each of the water company areas may be determined and appear in Table 1.1.1.

The particularly close association of cholera deaths with the Southwark and Vauxhall and Lambeth Companies is evident. A chemical analysis of their waters undertaken by Dr Hassell in 1850 showed them to be 'in a most impure condition', containing 'the hairs of animals and

Table 1.1.1 *Population, deaths from cholera and rate per 10,000 population in the areas served by the metropolitan water companies in the epidemic of 1849*

Water Company	Population	Deaths	Deaths/10,000 population
Southwark & Vauxhall	338,820	4,668	138
Lambeth	118,691	1,479	125
Kent	136,857	990	72
East London	443,915	2,312	52
Chelsea	192,236	876	46
New River	652,865	2,432	37
Hampstead	59,160	123	21
West Middlesex	249,950	473	19
Grand Junction	129,506	177	14

THE WATER THAT JOHN DRINKS.

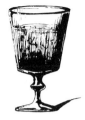

This is the water that JOHN drinks.

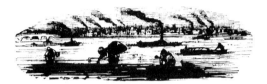

This is the Thames with its cento of stink,
That supplies the water that JOHN drinks.

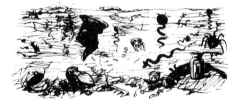

These are the fish that float in the ink-
-y stream of the Thames with its cento of stink,
That supplies the water that JOHN drinks.

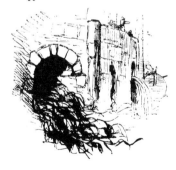

This is the sewer, from cesspool and sink,
That feeds the fish that float in the ink-
-y stream of the Thames with its cento of stink,
That supplies the water that JOHN drinks.

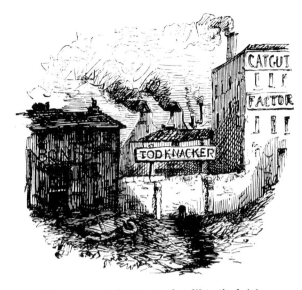

These are vested int'rests, that fill to the brink,
The network of sewers from cesspool and sink,
That feed the fish that float in the ink-
-y stream of the Thames, with its cento of stink,
That supplies the water that JOHN drinks.

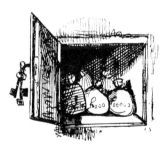

This is the price that we pay to wink
At the vested int'rests that fill to the brink,
The network of sewers from cesspool and sink,
That feed the fish that float in the ink-
-y stream of the Thames with its cento of stink,
That supplies the water that JOHN drinks.

Figure 1.1 (H) Contemporary description of London's water supply problems from *Punch*

numerous substances which had passed through the alimentary canal' (Snow, 1854, p.64). Conversely, the other two companies drawing water directly from the Thames 'took great pains to filter it' (p.64) in the case of the Chelsea, and had 'large settling reservoirs' (p.65) in the case of the West Middlesex. In contrast to the companies which drew their water directly from the Thames, the remainder (Kent, Grand Junction, Hampstead, New River and East London) not only had cleaner sources but also had settling reservoirs which provided some measure of protection.

An 1849 cartoon from *Punch* appears in diagram (H) and shows what the popular press thought of the quality of the Thames water and the vested interests which prevented its improvement. By 1858, diagram (I) indicates that *Punch* had become completely explicit.

In the discussion of the epidemiology of cholera at the beginning of this chapter, it was noted that the viability of the *Vibrio cholerae* is enhanced as the basicity of the water in which it finds itself increases. The chemical composition of the waters supplied by the various companies was determined by the General Board of Health at the time of the 1854 epidemic. A modern interpretation of their data enables the water companies to be ranked in Table 1.1.2 in order of increasing alkalinity [as measured by the calcium carbonate ($CaCO_3$) content of their water in milligrams per litre]. This shows that three of the companies with high death rates from cholera in their areas, the Lambeth, Southwark and Vauxhall and East London, had among the most alkaline waters in London.

The role of elevation The relationship between cholera incidence and elevation of the land is also discussed in Snow's monograph, and is mapped later in this chapter in Figures 1.13 and 1.14.

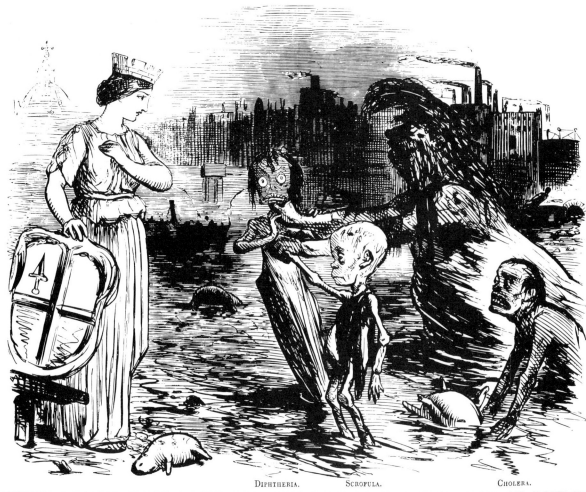

DIPHTHERIA.   SCROPULA.   CHOLERA.

FATHER THAMES INTRODUCING HIS OFFSPRING TO THE FAIR CITY OF LONDON.

Figure 1.1 (I) *Punch* **cartoon of links between cholera and River Thames**

Dr Farr [the Registrar General's Office] discovered a remarkable coincidence between the mortality from cholera in the different districts of London in 1849, and the elevation of the ground; the connection being of an inverse kind, the higher districts suffering least, and the lowest suffering most from this malady. Dr Farr was inclined to think that the level of the soil had some direct influence over the prevalence of cholera. . .

But Snow was less convinced:

I expressed the opinion in 1849, that the increased prevalence of cholera in the low-lying districts of London depended entirely on the greater contamination of the water in these districts. . . (Snow, 1854, pp.97–98).

Current knowledge on the epidemiology of cholera suggests both were right. The poor drainage found in low-lying areas is more likely to result in contamination of fresh water by foul, especially at times of flood, while stagnant water provides better breeding conditions for the vibrios. The consequences will be seen in Figures 1.13 and 1.14.

Conclusion

The 1848–9 epidemic of *Vibrio cholerae* at the restricted geographical scale of a single city displays many of the features classically associated with the disease on the international stage. The epidemic peaked in the warmer half of the year and collapsed when the colder days of autumn arrived. The disease favours areas with contaminated, sluggish water supplies of high basicity, and this association is to be seen in the

Table 1.1.2 *Calcium Carbonate (CaCO₃) content of the waters of the metropolitan water companies, 1854, in milligrams per litre.*

Company	mg/1 CaCO$_3$	Company	mg/1 CaCO$_3$
Grand Junction	197	Lambeth	220
Kent	198	Southwark & Vauxhall	229
Chelsea	204	East London	261
West Middlesex	210	New River	263

Note:
We are indebted to R.D. Heath, Senior Chemist, Anglian Water Authority, for providing this reinterpretation of the original data of the General Board of Health.

London data. The initial focus of the disease was in the districts served by the Southwark and Vauxhall Water Company. It may be traced to the Company's foul water supply, with vibrio survival enhanced by its alkaline character.

As we shall see from the figures in this chapter, these associations result in some striking geographical distributions, and it is to the mapping and cartographic pattern recognition methods which may be used to characterize these distributions that we now turn. We look first in Figures 1.2–1.6 at several different ways of mapping the cholera incidence data. This leads on to a consideration in Figures 1.7–1.9 of how to interpret the spatial patterns produced when medical data are mapped. For example, some areas on a map may appear to have 'particularly high' or 'particularly low' occurrence of a disease. Ways of converting these qualitative notions into precise statistical definitions which can be used for practical epidemiological purposes are discussed. This need to isolate the significant 'signals' on a map from background 'noise' is pursued further in the latter half of the chapter, where we outline in Figures 1.10–1.12 a series of techniques which can be used to separate the main trends on a map from local detail. Once the characteristics of a mapped distribution have been described, it is natural to want to test hypotheses about them, and so we conclude the chapter in Figures 1.13–1.18 with a consideration of mapping methods which can be used for this task.

Sources and Further Reading

The sources of the illustrations are as follows: (C) *The Economist*, 6 (1848), p.1436; (H) *Punch*, 17 (1849), pp.144–5; and (I) *Punch*, 22 (1852), p.139. The source material on the 1848–9 and 1854 cholera epidemics used in drawing the remainder of the figures is contained in the following British Parliamentary Papers: *Great Britain Parliamentary Papers 1850*, XXI: *Report of the General Board of Health on the Epidemic Cholera of 1848 and 1849*; *Great Britain Parliamentary Papers 1850*, XXII: *Report by the General Board of Health on the Supply of Water to the Metropolis*; and *Great Britain Parliamentary Papers 1854–5*, XXI: *Report and Appendix to Report of the Committee for Scientific Inquiries in Relation to the Cholera Epidemic of 1854*.

General accounts relating to the geography of cholera at the global scale (see map D) are included in: E.H. Ackerknecht (1965), *History and Geography of the Most Important Diseases*, New York: Hafner; F.G. Clemow (1903), *The Geography of Disease*, Cambridge: Cambridge University Press; H. Jusatz (1977), 'Cholera', in *A World Geography of Human Diseases*, edited by G.M. Howe, London: Academic Press, pp.131–43; and W.W. Spink (1978), *Infectious Diseases: Prevention and Treatment in the Nineteenth and Twentieth Centuries*, Folkestone, Kent: Dawson for the University of Minnesota Press.

The social upheaval accompanying the epidemics is discussed in G. Kearns (1985), *Urban Epidemics and Historical Geography: Cholera in London, 1848–9*, Publication number 16, Research Paper Series of the Historical Geography Research Group of the Institute of British Geographers (editors I. Whyte, E. McIntire), Norwich: Geo Books.

The classic account of the epidemiology of the disease is, of course, J. Snow (1854), *On the Mode of Communication of Cholera*, second edition, London: Churchill Livingstone. See also C. Creighton (1894, 1965), *History of Epidemics in Britain, vol. 2, 1666–1893*, second edition with additional material by D.E.C. Eversley, E.A. Underwood, and L. Overrall, London: Cass.

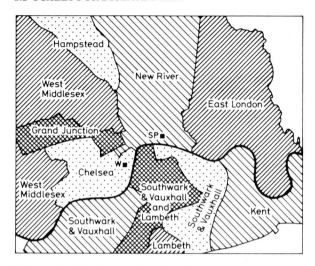

Figure 1.2 (A) Nominal level: the London water companies in 1849

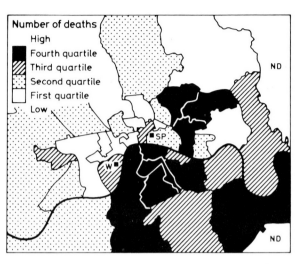

Figure 1.2 (B) Ordinal level: cholera deaths by district, 1849

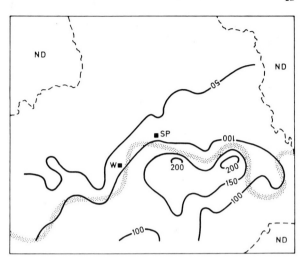

Figure 1.2 (C) Ratio level: cholera death rate contours, 1849

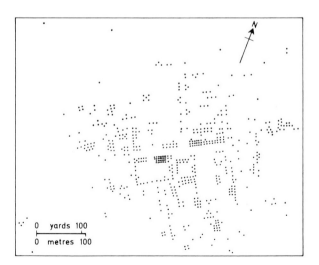

Figure 1.2 (D) Point data: deaths from cholera in the Soho district of London, 1854

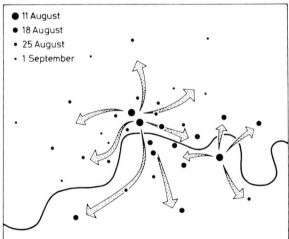

Figure 1.2 (E) Vector data: sequence of cholera epidemic peaks in 1849

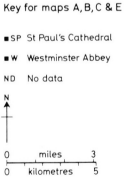

1.2 SCALES FOR DISEASE DATA

Levels of measurement

Before a mapping process can begin, it is necessary to recognize the characteristics of the data being mapped since these characteristics will, in large part, determine the method of representation. The theory of measurement states that there are four different scales, each with radically different properties (see Siegel, 1956).

Measurement is at its weakest at the *nominal* (or classificatory) level, where numbers or symbols are used to identify an object. Thus, in attempting to account for the geographical distribution of deaths from cholera in the registration districts of London during the epidemic of 1849, we begin by recording which of the metropolitan water companies of the time served which districts; as discussed in Figure 1.1, cholera is a water-borne disease. There were nine such companies, the West Middlesex, the Hampstead, the Chelsea, the Southwark and Vauxhall, the Lambeth, the New River, the East London and the Kent. A particular symbol (for example, *1*) might be used to denote the districts served by the Grand Junction, a *2* to denote the districts served by the West Middlesex, and so on. Clearly which number is assigned to which district is arbitrary and any sequence could be substituted. Thus the only formal property of members of the classes is *equivalence* ($\equiv$) and the range of cartographic operations we can perform is very limited.

The nominal map is commonly only a mosaic of differently coloured or shaded areas in which the shadings are used simply to distinguish the various classes or categories, here, as shown in map (A), the districts of London served by each of the water companies. For clarity, the registration district boundaries have been drawn on map (B).

At the *ordinal* (or ranking) scale of measurement, numbers or symbols are used both to identify objects and to describe their relationship to other objects. When we say that a certain registration district had a greater incidence of cholera deaths than some other registration district in the 1849 epidemic, we are using a symbol not only to identify the district, but we are also putting it in some kind of relationship to other districts which were higher or lower on the scale.

The formal difference between the ordinal and the nominal scale is that it not only has (a) equivalence but also (b) the relation 'greater than' or 'less than' ($>$ or $<$). Ordinal scales are common in mapping conventions and we use symbols of different sizes, or shadings of varying density, to represent variations in disease intensity from area to area. The data used to construct map (B) are ordinal scaled. Four shading intensities, ranging from white (for low levels of deaths) through black (for high levels of deaths) have been used to represent cholera severity in four ranked categories. The categories have been defined by the quartiles of the frequency distribution of number of deaths from cholera in London between April and November, 1849. We know not only whether cholera was present or absent in a particular registration district, but also the size sequence for deaths.

The difference between the two highest scales, the *interval* scale and the *ratio* scale, is important in certain statistical operations, but since most medical data are measured on ratio scales, it has less direct significance for mapping. The fundamental difference between the two scales is that on the interval scale there is no natural origin, whereas ratio scales do have a natural origin. In formal terms, both scales have the property of (a) equivalence, (b) rank, and (c) the known ratio of any two intervals. Only the ratio scale has the additional property of (d) the known ratio of any two point values on the scale. A wide variety of cartographic techniques may be used to map interval- and ratio-scaled data. Many are illustrated in this chapter. In the example given in map (C), isarithms have been drawn linking areas of London with the same death rate from cholera per 10,000 population in the 1849 epidemic.

Kinds of maps

Maps can be used to display three main sorts of information. Most commonly, the value of a variable will have been collected at a series of geographical locations. Whether this variable has been measured on nominal, ordinal, interval or ratio scales, we may call such maps *real-valued* maps. All the maps in diagrams (A) – (C) provide examples. In diagram (A), an *indicator variable* has been mapped that indicates which water companies served each of the registration districts of the metropolis in 1849. The variable is also *discrete*, in that it can only take on a limited number of values (between *1* and *9*, representing each of the nine water companies). A discrete variable is formally defined as one which can only assume values which are whole numbers; counting, rather than measuring, is generally involved. The variable mapped in (B) is also discrete. In contrast, the variable mapped in (C) is continuous. Showing, as it does, the number of cholera deaths per 10,000 population in the registration districts, it can potentially take on any value between zero and the upper limit of the data. Thus the formal definition of a *continuous* variable is that it can potentially assume any value in some interval of values.

The second kind of information is point data. In this case, no variable values are collected for the locations, but interest focuses upon the pattern formed by the locations themselves. An example is provided in map (D). This shows, as a series of points, the geographical locations of each of the deaths from cholera mapped by Dr John Snow in the Golden Square area of Soho in the cholera epidemic of 1854. Here, it is the peculiar geographical pattern formed by the points that draws our attention and for which explanations may be sought.

The third kind of information relates to the operation of the networks which link point or area distributions. An example is given in map (E). The week in which the peak number of deaths from cholera was recorded in each of the registration districts is shown as a point. There is some evidence to suggest a time-ordering of events. Those registration districts which peaked in the weeks ending on 11 and 18 August, 1849, are located along the margins of the River Thames in the central part of the map; registration districts which peaked in the weeks ending on 25 August and 1 September are located outside this zone towards the margins of the map. Such a pattern raises the question of the nature of the network, shown schematically by the vectors, by which this kind of centrifugal transmission could occur.

Chapter examples

Examples of maps based upon data measured on all the scales (nominal, ordinal, interval and ratio) and relating to real-valued, point and network information, are given in this chapter. However, since most medical data relates to interval- and ratio-scaled, real-valued maps, it is these which are stressed and to which most of the subsequent figures in this chapter are addressed.

Sources and Further Reading

Levels of measurement and their significance for the appropriate type of statistical analysis are set out in S. Siegel (1956), *Nonparametric Statistics for the Behavioral Sciences*, New York: McGraw Hill. See also K.-T. Chang (1978), 'Measurement scales in cartography', *American Cartographer*, 5, pp.57–64.

The main reference work on cartographic methods used in Chapter 1 is A.H. Robinson, R.D. Sale, J.L. Morrison and P.C. Muehrcke (1984), *Elements of Cartography*, fifth edition, New York: John Wiley. This is regularly updated and includes material on computer mapping as described in Chapter 7 of this Atlas.

Other valuable reference works on cartography are J.S. Keates (1982), *Understanding Maps*, London: Longman; G.C. Dickinson (1963), *Statistical Mapping and the Presentation of Statistics*, London, Edward Arnold; F.J. Monkhouse and H.R. Wilkinson (1971), *Maps and Diagrams: Their Compilation and Construction*, third edition, London: Methuen; and H.T. Fisher (1982), *Mapping Information: the Graphic Display of Quantitative Information*, Cambridge, Mass.: Abt Books. The best short book on the concepts behind map design is probably A.H. Robinson and B.B. Petchenik (1976), *The Nature of Maps: Essays Towards Understanding Maps and Mapping*, Chicago: Chicago University Press.

A useful review of medical maps is given in G.F. Pyle (1979), *Applied Medical Geography*, New York: John Wiley, and by G.M. Howe (1986), 'Disease mapping', in *Medical Geography: Progress and Prospect*, edited by M. Pacione, London: Croom Helm.

1.3 POINT MAP DISTRIBUTIONS

Irregular collecting units

Most area-based data used in geographical analysis are available only for irregularly shaped collecting units, and these pose major problems for mapping methods. For example, the cholera data from which Figure 1.2(C) was prepared were recorded for the system of registration districts illustrated in map (A). This shows the number of deaths from cholera occurring in each of the 34 registration districts of the metropolis between 28 April and 24 November 1849. The registration districts vary greatly in area, becoming progressively smaller towards the central part of the city. The inset map shows part of this central area at a larger scale, with the pecked lines demarcating the boundaries of the parishes which made up each registration district. The data were compiled at the parish level and then aggregated by registration officers to obtain a return for their district. The course of the Thames is shown as a meandering ribbon, and the principal bridges in 1849 are also marked.

The range of cartographic problems arising when there is such great variety in the areas of the collecting units may be illustrated using the various dot, circle and sphere methods available for mapping.

Dot maps

Diagram (B) is a dot map of the spatial distribution of deaths given in (A); one dot represents ten deaths. The locations of the dots do not show actual places of death. Instead, the correct number of dots for each registration district is distributed over the district in a way which reflects the broad geographical distribution of the population. Thus the main parks and open spaces (Battersea Fields, Hyde Park, Regent's Park, Victoria Park and the Isle of Dogs) have no dots located within them.

The first problem created by irregularly sized collecting units is in choosing an appropriate ratio of number of deaths to be represented by a single dot (here, ten to one). This ratio, or the *unit value*, is determined by the relationship between the scale of the map and the number of deaths. Thus, if one dot had been chosen to represent five deaths, dots would have coalesced in the central part of the map in the small registration districts with large numbers of deaths. A very 'heavy' looking map, with geographically extensive black areas, would have resulted. Conversely, if one dot had been used to represent twenty deaths, the dots in the larger and peripheral districts would have been so few that the varying geographical distribution would not have been shown accurately, the map would have looked barren and open, and its visual impact would have been reduced. A good working rule to follow in choosing both the unit value and the drawing size of the dots is that, in the denser parts of a distribution, the dots should just coalesce to form a dark area. This is beginning to occur in the central areas of (B).

Proportional circles

The scale problem is also present when the technique of *proportional circles* is used to map the spatial distribution of deaths recorded in (A). One circle appears in each of the 34 registration districts of the metropolis. The name of the method comes from the fact that the size of the circles is chosen in such a way that the *area of* each circle is proportional to the number of deaths; that is, the radii of the circles are some function of the square root of the number of deaths. This function (called the unit radius value), whereby the square roots are scaled into convenient plotting units such as millimetres, is chosen so that overlap between circles is kept to a minimum, while at the same time producing sufficient contrast to shown up the spatial variability in the data. As in (B), the choice is a compromise between the conflicting objectives of accuracy and visual appearance.

A difficulty with the proportional circle method as given is that the reader's perceptual response to circle sizes is not linear, so that the ordinary observer tends to underestimate the sizes of the larger circles in relation to the smaller ones. It is possible to compensate for this effect by the following steps. Instead of making the radii of the circles proportional to the square roots, (a) take logarithms of the data, (b) multiply the logarithms by 0.57, (c) antilog the result and finally, (d) divide the antilogs by the unit radius value chosen for the circles.

It frequently happens that the data comprising the distribution to be mapped are not regularly spread over the range of the values collected. Often the data are bimodal, with some very large values, some small values, and little in between. In such instances, it is advisable to combine the dot and proportional circle methods, using dots to represent the smaller data values and proportional circles to represent the larger. This approach enables the problem of excessive dot coalescence, noted above, to be by-passed.

Proportional spheres

If the large values are substantially greater than the small values, it may be necessary to represent them using *proportional spheres*. Diagram (D)

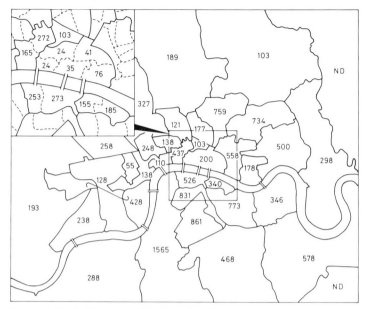

Figure 1.3 (A) Number of cholera deaths

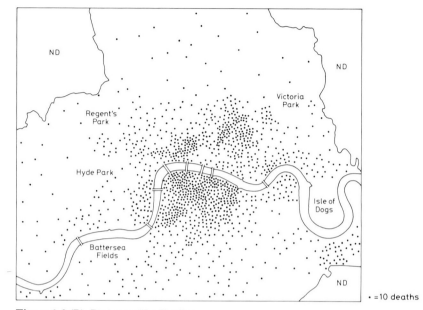

Figure 1.3 (B) Dot map distribution

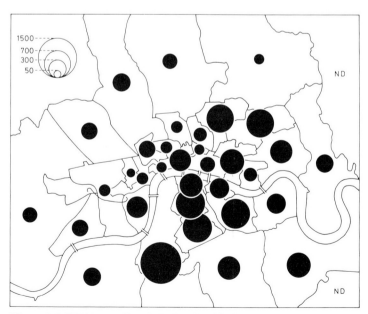

Figure 1.3 (C) Proportional circles distribution

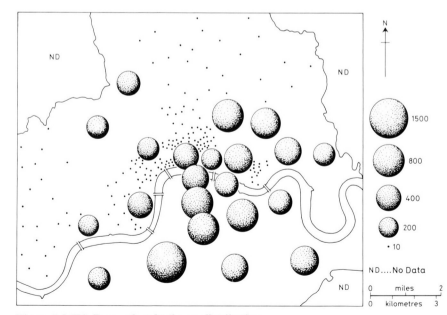

Figure 1.3 (D) Proportional spheres distribution

illustrates this method by plotting the spatial distribution of deaths shown in (A). One sphere appears in each of the 22 registration districts with the largest number of deaths. In the other twelve districts, deaths are plotted as in diagram (B), with one dot representing ten deaths. Proportional spheres are constructed so that the volume of each sphere is directly proportional to the number of deaths. The volume of a sphere is given by the formula, $4/3\pi r^3$, so that, using the mortality data shown in (A), the radii of the spheres are drawn a suitable plotting function of the cube root of the number of deaths in a given registration district. As with proportional circles, the precise functional form is chosen to minimize overlap between the spheres, while at the same time representing spatial variability as accurately as map scale allows. The problem of visual underestimation noted with proportional circles occurs also with proportional spheres, and to a greater degree.

The choice between the three methods shown in (B) – (D) depends on the degree of spatial contrast in the phenomenon being mapped. Dot maps, such as (B), are highly effective when the contrasts are relatively slight; conversely, proportional spheres can cope with extreme variations in the data. In many cases it is useful to combine methods as in (D). The particular advantage of proportional circles is that they can be combined with *pie-charts* (see Figure 2.5) to enable more information about the data to be represented on a map.

Sources and Further Reading

The source material for the dot maps of the 1848–9 cholera epidemics is contained in the following British Parliamentary Papers: *Great Britain Parliamentary Papers 1850*, XXI: *Report of the General Board of Health on the Epidemic Cholera of 1848 and 1849*; *Great Britain Parliamentary Papers 1850*, XXII: *Report by the General Board of Health on the Supply of Water to the Metropolis*; and *Great Britain Parliamentary Papers 1854–5*, XXI. These sources are used throughout the remainder of this chapter.

The various cartographic methods for producing point maps are described in A.H. Robinson, R.D. Sale, J.L. Morrison and P.C. Muehrcke (1984), 'Symbolization: mapping with point symbols', in *Elements of Cartography*, fifth edition, New York: John Wiley, pp.276–306. See also J.J. Flannery (1971), 'The relative effectiveness of some graduated point symbols in the presentation of quantitative data', *The Canadian Cartographer*, 8, pp.96–109, and H.W. Castner and A.H. Robinson (1969), *Dot Area Symbols in Cartography: The Influence of Pattern on their Perception*, Technical Monograph No. CA-4, Washington, DC: American Congress on Surveying and Mapping.

1.4 TRANSLATING DISTRICT VALUES TO A REGULAR GRID

Spatial frameworks

The maps shown in Figure 1.3 are based upon data relating to the geographical distribution of cholera deaths in London in 1849, and were gathered for the irregular set of collecting areas comprising the registration districts of the metropolis. These form a framework somewhat like a jigsaw. We have seen in Figure 1.3 that such irregular spatial frameworks may cause severe cartographic problems, especially if the range of data values is large. In contrast, regular systems of grid cells make mapping much more straightforward. Since the area of each cell is the same, they possess the important property that the data are automatically standardized for the size of the individual collecting units. It is also necessary for other reasons, which are discussed below, to establish procedures that permit data to be moved between one spatial framework and another. This set of diagrams illustrates one approach to the problem.

Methods for translating between frameworks

Diagram (A) shows a hypothetical set of nine areas, labelled *a* through *i*, all of which are highly irregular in shape. The ticks around the margin of the map define a set of geographical units which comprise a regular lattice of square cells, onto which it is proposed to map data originally collected for the set of areas, *a–i*. This regular lattice is shown fully drawn in diagram (D).

In diagram (B), the irregular areas, *a–i*, are

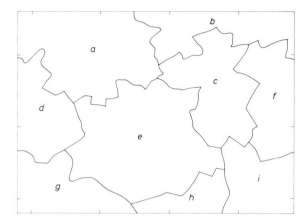

Figure 1.4 (A) Original district boundaries

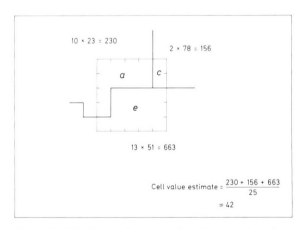

Figure 1.4 (C) Estimation procedure for a single cell

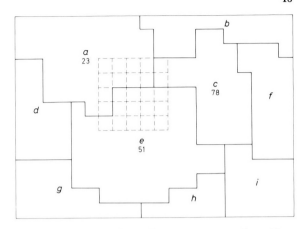

Figure 1.4 (B) Boundary adjustment to a regular grid

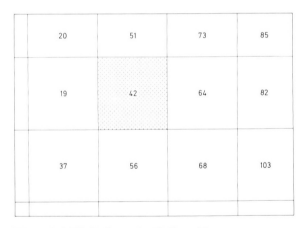

Figure 1.4 (D) Estimated cells for grid

illustrated after conversion into grid-like shapes. The transformation used eliminates the irregularities in the original boundaries by replacing them with boundaries which consist entirely of straight-line sections which preserve the basic shapes and areas of the original units, but in a generalized, rectangular form. The minimum length of a single straight-line section is fixed by the user; it must, however, be an integer divisor

(here, five) of the length of the cell sides of the units comprising the regular lattice into which the irregular areas are to be translated. The minimum length selected represents a trade-off between the competing criteria of accurate representation of the original boundaries, and acceptable spatial generalization. All other boundary segments are multiples of this minimum length. The data values attached to areas *a*, *c*, and *e* are as illustrated, namely 23, 78 and 51 respectively, and it is assumed that these values apply uniformly throughout the designated area.

Diagram (C) summarizes the procedure by which an estimated value is obtained for the stippled cell shown on diagram (D). The marginal ticks around the perimeter of the cell in diagram (C) permit this cell to be divided into 25 sub-cells, each with a side-length equal to the minimum straight-line length fixed in (B). The estimated value for the stippled cell is then calculated as a weighted sum of the values of the three regions, a, c and e, and which contribute part of their areas to it. The weightings are in exact proportion to their areal contributions to the grid cell. Thus area a makes up 10 of the 25 units of the cell to be estimated, and so we take (10/25) of its value of 23 as the contribution of a to the final cell value. Area c which provides only two of the 25 units, contributes (2/25) of its value of 78, while area e contributes (13/25) of its value of 51.

Diagram (C) shows these calculations in a computationally equivalent, but slightly different form. The values of each of the areas a, c and e are first multiplied by their cell-overlap counts of 10, 2 and 13, respectively, before dividing through by the common denominator of 25. A general computational formula is given in the technical appendix to this section.

Diagram (D) gives the matrix of all cell values estimated by this area-weighting method; the stippled cell contains the value of 42 carried over from (C).

Importance of framework translation

It is important in cartography to be able to move data between different lattice systems. Most medical data reflect the administrative areas for which they are collected, such as nations, states, counties, local health districts, and so on. These units have boundaries which are usually historically determined and vary greatly both over time and within and between countries. A regular grid system offers particular advantages for statistical and cartographic analysis, most notably in computer mapping (see Figure 7.1). The various computer-based methods which produce *isopleth maps* and *block diagrams* like those to be illustrated both in the next figure and Figure 7.1 all either require regularly gridded data as input, or else translate irregularly located data points onto a regular lattice using procedures like those outlined here.

The particular conversion employed in the present diagram (from an irregular to a regular lattice) is but a special case of the general problem of translation between different collecting areas. The technique provides one way in which changes over time in the boundary systems of collecting areas may be brought to a common base, a problem which is discussed further in Figures 2.9 and 2.11. Because regular collecting areas like those shown in (D) also result in automatic standardization of the data for the sizes of the areal units, any distortions due to this source are rendered constant across the map.

Sources and Further Reading

The problem of compiling maps from various base maps is described in A.H. Robinson, R.D. Sale, J.L. Morrison and P.C. Muehrcke (1984), *Elements of Cartography*, fifth edition, New York: John Wiley, pp. 400–30. More advanced problems in map transfer are discussed in D.H. Maling (1973), *Coordinate Systems and Map Projections*, London: George Philip.

Technical appendix

Let p_i be the proportion of the area of the regular grid cell, whose value is to be estimated, which is contributed by the irregular area i, and let x_i be the value associated with i. Then the grid cell value, g_j say, for the j-th cell is given by

$$g_j = \sum_{i=1}^{k} p_i x_i. \qquad (1.4.1)$$

The summation is over the k irregular areas overlapping the grid cell.

1.5 AREA-BASED MAP DISTRIBUTIONS

Maps of cholera deaths

The major epidemic of Asiatic cholera which struck London between 28 April and 24 November 1849 was the most severe to have affected the capital since the outbreak of 1832. That epidemic resulted in the passage of the Cholera Acts through the British Parliament in a vain attempt to control the repeated visitations of the disease. Despite these Acts, the disease returned again and again, culminating in the epidemic of 1849 which caused over 52,000 deaths in England and Wales. In London, over 14,000 died between April and November.

All four maps shown here cover metropolitan London. To give a point of reference the course of the River Thames is shown by the line meandering across the southern half of the map; the locations of St Paul's Cathedral (SP) and Westminster Abbey (W) are also marked. The area covered by the maps extends as far as Hendon and Tottenham in the north, Dulwich and Balham in the south, Putney in the west and Woolwich in the east. If the geographical distribution of cholera deaths in London is mapped onto a regular grid using the technique described in Figure 1.4, then map (A) is obtained. This shows the number of deaths per 10,000 population in a series of grid squares each approximately one mile square. In terms of Figure 1.2, the variable is continuous and ratio-scaled. Cells without data are coded as ND (no data). The values on this map range from a maximum death rate of 235 per 10,000 population in part of southeast London, to a minimum of twelve northwest of Westminster Abbey.

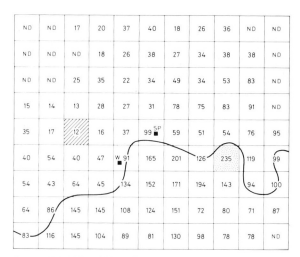

Figure 1.5 (A) Original data

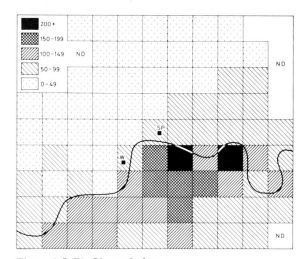

Figure 1.5 (B) Choropleth map

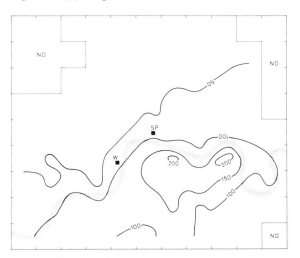

Figure 1.5 (C) Isopleth map

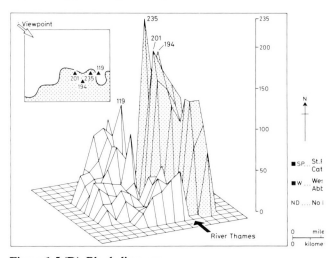

Figure 1.5 (D) Block diagram

Choropleth maps

One of the commonest ways of representing such information cartographically is by drawing a *choropleth map*. The name comes from the Greek words, *choros* (meaning place) and *plethos* (mean-

ing quantity). Such a map uses shading, graded in intensity from light to dark, to represent the variability in the data mapped. Thus map (B) is a choropleth map of the values given in (A) obtained by, first, dividing the range of the data into five equal classes and then, second, by assigning to each class shading which increases in intensity from a light stipple for the lowest category (0–49 deaths per 10,000 population) to black for the highest category (200 deaths or more per 10,000 population). It is usual practice to allocate the darkest category of shading to the data class which it is desired most to emphasize (here high mortality). The division of the data into equal classes is arbitrary; ways of choosing the most appropriate class divisions are examined in Figure 1.6. In the same way, the number of classes into which the data are split is at choice. However, it is worth noting that it is difficult to obtain visual discrimination between more than eight categories of shading, while less than three will rarely do justice to the variability in the data unless, of course, they fall into two 'natural' classes, such as presence and absence.

The choropleth map is thus a visual representation of data which are tied to areal units and it will highlight any spatial organization that may be present.

Isopleth maps

An alternative way of representing the data shown in (A) is to draw *isopleths* (Greek *isos*, equal), as in map (C). Isopleths therefore link locations which are of equal value on the variable mapped. The most familiar isopleth is the contour, which joins places of equal height. Four isopleths are shown on (C), drawn at intervals of fifty deaths per 10,000 population, starting at fifty (that is, at 50, 100, 150 and 200). Note the contrast in cartographic technique between maps (B) and (C) for representing the same data. Choropleth methods are best used for data which fall into well-defined groups or classes. Conversely, isopleths run continuously across a map and therefore imply that the data upon which they are based also vary continuously over the map surface.

The locations on a map at which data are available are referred to as *control points*, while the contours themselves are drawn by linear *interpolation* at the desired 'height' between the control points (cf. Figure 1.10). It is therefore important that a relatively even and dense scatter of control points exists on any map for which isopleths are to be drawn. Otherwise interpolation will occur across areas about which little information exists, and a sense of accuracy will be imparted to parts of the map for which there is no justification in reality.

Block diagrams

A pictorially dramatic way of representing any three-dimensional distribution is by drawing a perspective block diagram. The data mapped in (A) comprise, in fact, a three-dimensional distribution, in which the position of each cell on the base plane axes defines two dimensions (x and y), while the death rate defines the third dimension on an imaginary z-axis rising vertically out of the book page. This implies that we can regard (A) as a 'surface' of deaths per 10,000 population. Diagram (D) shows (A) as a perspective block diagram, with the height of the surface proportional to the number of deaths per 10,000 population in each cell. The viewpoint taken is from the northwest corner of (A), looking towards the southeast. The area south of the Thames is stippled. The course of the Thames itself is obscured by the high death rates on the northern and southern banks of the river. It thus appears to run in a 'canyon' of zero cholera death rates.

There is almost infinite variety in the way a basic block diagram like that shown in (D) may be enhanced by shading to emphasize the undulations in the surface. In the same way, the vertical scale chosen for the z-axis can dramati-

cally affect the visual appearance of the surface. But, while block diagrams are exceedingly useful as devices for obtaining a rapid impression of the characteristics of any surface, they are weak analytically. It is extremely difficult to scale off exact values on the z-axis, as diagram (D) shows for the death rates from cholera in London.

All three methods of representation shown in diagrams (B) – (D) confirm that the areas of excess deaths lie primarily to the south of the Thames.

Sources and Further Reading

The sources for the cholera maps of London in 1849 are as set out in Figure 1.3 of this Atlas.

The cartographic methods for choropleth maps are given in A.H. Robinson, R.D. Sale, J.L. Morrison and P.C. Muehrcke (1984), 'Cartographic gerneralization and symbolization', in *Elements of Cartography*, fifth edition, New York: John Wiley, pp.276–306. See also D.J. Cuff and M.T. Mattson (1982), *Thematic Maps: Their Design and Production*, New York: Methuen.

1.6 CRITICAL INTERVALS ON CHOROPLETH MAPS

Number of shading classes

In drawing any choropleth map, two basic problems have to be resolved. First, we must decide upon the number of classes of shading that are to be used. Second, once this has been fixed, it is necessary to determine which areas are to be allocated to which classes. Preservation of information contained in the data argues for a large number of classes. However, as we have seen in Figure 1.5(B), on a choropleth map areas are shaded according to the data class into which they fall. The shadings employed are generally graded in terms of visual value from light to dark. The human eye is capable of distinguishing only a limited number of shading steps, at most eight between black and white and usually less in any colour. This places a strict limitation on the number of classes which can, in practice, be portrayed. As a result, increasing the number of classes simultaneously reduces the visual impact of the map.

Thus, for the data set being mapped, choosing the number of classes involves resolving the conflict between the competing criteria of (a) preservation of information in the data and (b) visual impact. In practice, four or five classes is the compromise usually adopted. If the patches of shading belonging to each of the classes are geographically compact, more classes can sometimes be used. Conversely, if the patches are spatially very intermixed, fewer classes should be chosen if the visual information is to be preserved.

The set of choropleth maps drawn as diagrams (B) – (D) use either four or five classes to show

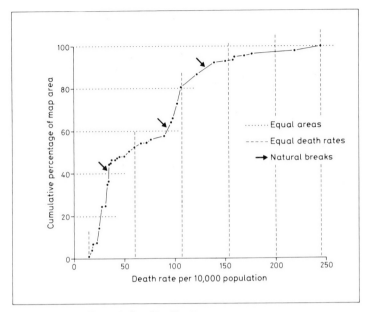

Figure 1.6 (A) Cumulative distribution

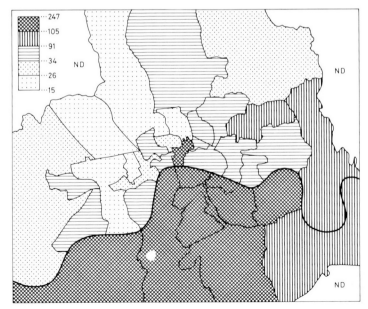

Figure 1.6 (B) Equal area divisions on the vertical axis of (A)

the geographical distribution of deaths from cholera per 10,000 population in the 34 registration districts of London in the epidemic of 1849. They present very different visual images because of the way that the range of the data has been divided into classes. The classes are referred to as *critical intervals*, and it is to their selection that we now turn.

Critical interval construction

We begin in diagram (A) by plotting the cumulative frequency curve of the death rates in the 34 registration districts. The vertical axis of the graph shows the cumulative percentage of the total map area taken up by all the districts which have been added to the curve up to a given point. It thus ranges from 0–100 percent. The horizontal axis records the death rate per 10,000 population, ranging from a minimum of 15.0 to a maximum of 247.0. Both axes are scaled arithmetically. Note that the differences between the minimum and maximum in this diagram and the minimum and maximum quoted in Figure 1.5(A) arise because Figure 1.5 uses a regular grid of cells, as opposed to the framework of registration districts employed here.

The curve is constructed by finding the registration district with the lowest death rate first. This is plotted on the horizontal axis against, on the vertical axis, the percentage of the total map area occupied by the district. Then the district with the next lowest death rate is located and added to the curve; the death rate is located on the horizontal axis as before, while the position on the vertical axis is fixed by adding the percentage of the total map area occupied by the district to the cumulative percentage of all districts already added to the curve. The process is repeated until all districts have been allocated. The resulting curve must, therefore, by

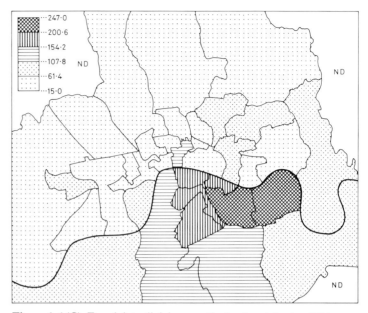

Figure 1.6 (C) Equal data divisions on the horizontal axis of (A)

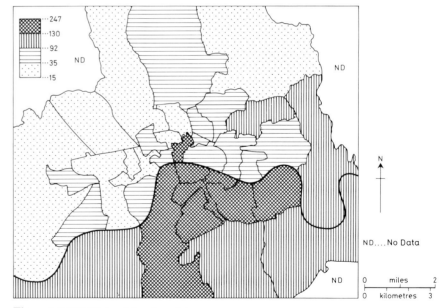

Figure 1.6 (D) Natural break points

construction rise continuously from the origin of the graph to the top right-hand corner, when the last point is plotted and the value on the vertical axis will equal 100 percent.

Equal area divisions Using such a cumulative frequency curve, three main ways of defining critical intervals may be established. Map (B) has been constructed by focusing upon the information provided by the vertical axis of (A). In (B), each of the five categories of death rates occupies an approximately equal area of the map. The divisions between the classes are shown by the dotted lines on the vertical axis of the graph in (A); that is at the 20, 40, 60, 80, and 100 percent points. The advantage of this scheme is that it produces a spatially balanced picture.

Equal data divisions If attention is turned to the horizontal axis, a similar strategy produces map (C) by dividing the range of death rates into five equal classes. Since this range is 232.0 (that is, 247.0–15.0), the width of each interval is 46.4 (that is, 232.0/5). Hence the first band runs from 15.0 to 61.4. These divisions are shown by the pecked lines rising from the horizontal axis. The advantage of this map is that the geographical zones defined are directly interpretable in terms of the variable of interest, here death rates from cholera. There are, however, two important disadvantages. First, a very unequal proportion of the total map area may be in one class. An example is provided by the lowest category on (C), which covers most of the area to the north of the River Thames, whose course is shown by the bold line running east to west across the map. The second is that it is possible for some categories either to be poorly represented on the map [the top two categories on (C)] or, in extreme cases, not at all.

Natural breaks If the information provided by both the horizontal and vertical axes of the graph in (A) is used simultaneously, map (D) is produced as a compromise between (B) and (C). On (D), the 'natural breaks' in the cumulative distribution curve of (A) have been used to locate the class boundaries. These are marked by the arrows on (A); they represent the points where the slope of the curve changes. The critical intervals defined by dropping perpendiculars, called *ordinates*, from the arrow heads to the horizontal axis indicate the variable values separating regions of different gradient provided, of course, that the data adjacently plotted on the graph are reasonably contiguous geographically. The registration districts in each class have then been appropriately shaded to produce map (D). The great advantage of this approach is that it maximizes information about both map area and death rates to give a very efficient picture. The disadvantage of the 'natural breaks' map is that the class boundaries defined are specific to each problem and therefore comparisons between maps showing different variables are made extremely difficult.

Sources and Further Reading

The sources for the cholera maps of London in 1849 are as set out in Figure 1.3 of this Atlas.

The problem of critical intervals on choropleth maps is discussed in A.H. Robinson, R.D. Sale, J.L. Morrison and P.C. Muehrcke (1984), 'Mapping with area symbols', in *Elements of Cartography*, fifth edition, New York: John Wiley, pp.338–66. See also G.F. Jenks and M.R. Coulson (1963), 'Class intervals for statistical maps', *International Yearbook of Cartography*, 3, pp.119–34; R.W. Armstrong (1969), 'Standardized class intervals and rate computation in statistical maps of mortality', *Annals of the Association of American Geographers*, 59, pp.382–90; and M. Monmonier (1974), 'Measures of pattern complexity for choropleth maps', *American Cartographer*, 1, pp.56–69. An alternative approach to choropleth mapping is given in W.R. Tobler (1973), 'Choropleth maps without class intervals', *Geographical Analysis*, 5, pp.262–5, 358–60.

1.7 PROBABILITY MAPS I: DETECTING EXTREME VALUES

Significance of high and low cells

When a map showing the geographical distribution of a disease is studied, it is important to be able to decide which areas display either particularly high or particularly low incidence, since the geographical locations of such extrema may shed some light on the aetiology of the disease. Some of the methods which can be used to delimit these extrema are illustrated in this figure. The variable mapped is the death rate from cholera per 10,000 population in 86 subdivisions of London, each approximately one square mile in area, in the great epidemic of 1849. The raw data are shown in Figure 1.5(A), the subdivisions forming a regular grid or lattice of cells. The rates were originally gathered for a set of 34 irregularly shaped registration districts which comprised the collecting units for mortality data at the time. They have been translated onto the regular lattice of cells shown in (B) – (D) using the methods described in Figure 1.4.

Diagram (A) shows the frequency distribution obtained by plotting the number of cells in this regular lattice (on the vertical axis) against death rate (on the horizontal axis). The mean death rate of 73.3 cholera deaths per 10,000 population is marked with an arrow.

The use of quantiles

The most straightforward way of deciding which cells have particularly high or particularly low death rates from cholera is to partition the total *frequency* of the frequency distribution into a number of equal proportions; the number is at the choice of the researcher. The partition values are known as *quantiles*. The cells which lie beyond the largest quantile, in the upper tail of the frequency distribution, may then be mapped as 'significantly high'. The cells which lie below the smallest quantile, in the lower tail of the frequency distribution, may be similarly mapped as 'significantly low'.

Map (B) was produced by dividing the frequency distribution given in diagram (A) into eight parts, or *octiles*. Data are available for 86 cells of the lattice. The arithmetical problem caused by the fact that 86 is not exactly divisible by eight was overcome by assigning the first and eighth octiles ten cells, and the remainder eleven. The cells comprising the first and eighth octiles were then shaded in map (B) to define, respectively, significantly low and significantly high areas of disease incidence. As in Figure 1.5, it is evident that the cells with the greatest death rates from cholera are concentrated south of the River Thames, while the cells least affected are in the northwest part of the study area in the vicinity of the great parks and Hampstead Heath; the river has been drawn with a heavy line.

The Normal probability distribution

A more sophisticated approach to the problem is to compare the frequency distribution shown in diagram (A) with that expected under some theoretical model of the disease process. In map (C) the significantly high areas have been identified by assuming that death rates from cholera have been drawn from a *Normal distribution*. As discussed and illustrated in the technical appendix to this Figure, this has a symmetric, bell-shaped frequency distribution, and it is not an unreasonable model for this purpose. Diagram (F) in the appendix shows that death rates conform roughly to this shape. For any disease, only a few areas are likely to record very high or very low rates, while most will be close to the mean.

The probability of obtaining, by chance, values which are greater than or equal to any particular death rate can be readily calculated for a Normal distribution; computational details are given in the technical appendix. On map (C), cells in the upper tail of the distribution (that is, those which are 'significantly high') have been shaded if they fell into one of the four categories which correspond to a likelihood of occurring by chance in a Normal distribution of only 10, 5, 2.5, and 0.5 percent. The cells which are least likely to have arisen by chance are closest to the south bank of the Thames, while those which are more likely to have occurred by chance are located further away from the river, albeit still on the south bank.

The Poisson distribution

In map (D), the ideas of 'significantly high' and 'significantly low' cells are articulated by determining the chance of obtaining a level of deaths from cholera at least as big or at least as small as that recorded if the process generating cholera deaths in 1849 was spatially random. Such a random generating process may be characterized by the statistical model known as the *Poisson*. The important assumptions underlying the Poisson are that (a) there are no interactions between subareas [lattice cells in map (D)], (b) there is no possibility of point clusters of deaths within subareas and (c) there is no tendency for neighbouring subareas to display similar traits. Subareas are therefore assumed to act independently of each other, and each subarea is taken to have an equal and independent chance of having an event occur in it. The main role of the Poisson is therefore to act as a 'no dependence' or spatially random benchmark against which data

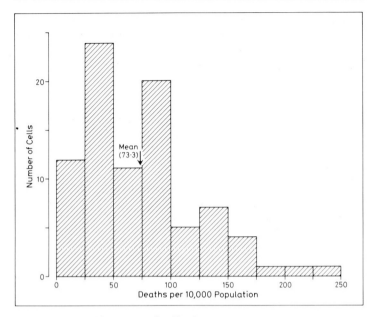

Figure 1.7 (A) Histogram of cell values

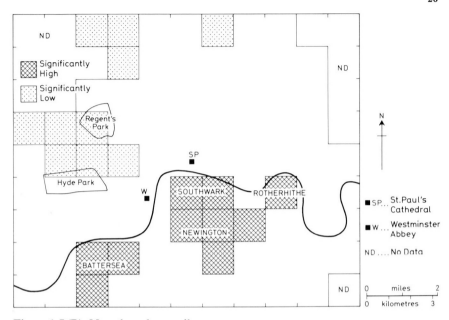

Figure 1.7 (B) Maps based on octiles

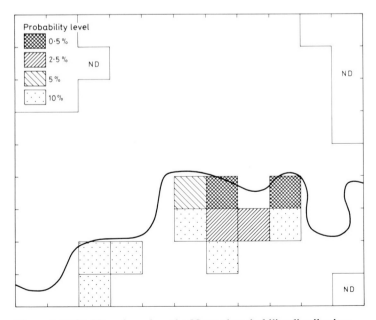

Figure 1.7 (C) Maps based on the Normal probability distribution

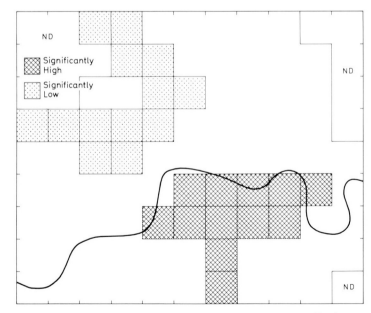

Figure 1.7 (D) Maps based on the Poisson probability distribution

may be tested for departures from the three assumptions listed. Statistical details are given in the technical appendix.

Map (D) has been produced by shading only those cells whose chance of occurrence under a Poisson process is less than five times in a hundred. The map tells a similar story to map (B), with the high incidence areas concentrated south of the Thames and the low incidence areas located in the northwest part of the study area. Given the water-borne nature of the disease (see Figure 1.1), it is highly likely that assumptions (1) and (3) of the Poisson model have been broken. There is likely to have been *interaction* between subareas because the homes and workplaces of the population would frequently be located in different lattice cells. Contiguous cells may be expected to display *similar traits* if they drew their water supply from the same source.

Sources and Further Reading

The sources for the cholera maps of London in 1849 are as set out in Figure 1.3 of this Atlas.

The statistical properties of the Normal and Poisson distributions are set out in most standard statistical texts; see for example G.W. Snedecor and W.G. Cochran (1980), *Statistical Methods*, seventh edition, Ames, Iowa: State University Press, pp.39–63, 130–5. An elementary introduction in a medical context is given in T.D.V. Swinscow (1983), *Statistics at Square One* (articles published in the British Medical Journal), eighth edition, London: British Medical Journal.

The fitting of Normal and Poisson probability distributions can be simply done on a desktop microcomputer; see B.F. Ryan, B.L. Joiner and T.A. Ryan (1985), *Minitab Handbook*, second edition, Boston: Duxbury Press, pp.120–57.

For a medical application of the Poisson distribution see M. Choynowski (1959), 'Maps based upon probabilities', *Journal of the American Statistical Association*, 54, pp.385–8, and the discussion of the probability distribution of leukaemia deaths in Figure 3.8 of this Atlas.

Technical appendix

The Normal distribution
The graph of a general Normal distribution is shown in diagram (E). The equation for the curve is given by

$$f_N(x) = (1/\sqrt{2\pi}\sigma)\exp\left[-(x-\mu)^2/2\sigma^2\right] \qquad (1.7.1)$$

where $f_N(x)$ denotes the proportion of the variate values [plotted on the vertical axis in diagram (E)] at x [plotted on the horizontal axis in diagram (E)]. The mean and standard deviation of the distribution are denoted by μ and σ respectively. The Normal distribution is continuous, contains an infinite number of observations, and runs between $-\infty$ and $+\infty$ on the x-axis. Thus any empirical frequency distribution such as that shown in diagram (A) can, at best, only approximate a Normal distribution which may be regarded as a theoretical limiting shape. Diagram (F) shows diagram (A) with a fitted Normal distribution. The natural origin of zero on death rates accounts for the poor fit of the lower tail.

Equation (1.7.1) implies that the Normal distribution is a two-parameter (μ and σ) curve whose location is fixed by the mean and whose shape is fixed by the standard deviation. Diagram (G) shows three Normal distributions with the same standard deviations (1.0) but different means (4.0, 8.0 and 12.0), while diagram (H) shows three Normal distributions with the same mean (0.0) but different standard deviations (0.4, 1.0 and 2.5).

The fact that the shape of a Normal distribution is completely determined by its standard deviation means that it is possible to reduce the family of Normal curves, each of which has its own particular mean and standard deviation, to a single *standard Normal distribution* by a simple change of variable. This is achieved by working with the quantities

$$z = (x-\mu)/\sigma \qquad (1.7.2)$$

instead of the original variable values, x, in equation (1.7.1), so that

$$x = \mu + z\,\sigma. \qquad (1.7.3)$$

Table 1.7.1 *The Normal distribution*

The tabulated function is defined as

$$f_N(z) = \frac{1}{\sigma\sqrt{2\pi}}\,e^{-(z^2/2)}$$

with $z = (x-\mu)/\sigma$. In the figure, the probability density is represented by the ordinate of the graph, while the lower and upper tail probabilities, Q and P, are represented by the areas under the curve.

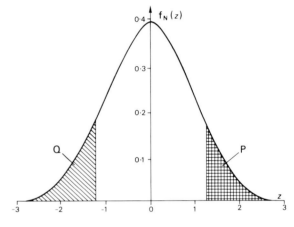

Lower tail		Upper tail		Lower tail		Upper tail	
z	Q	z	P	z	Q	z	P
−3.0	0.0013	0.0	0.5000	−1.4	0.0808	1.6	0.0548
−2.9	0.0019	0.1	0.4602	−1.3	0.0968	1.7	0.0446
−2.8	0.0026	0.2	0.4207	−1.2	0.1151	1.8	0.0359
−2.7	0.0035	0.3	0.3821	−1.1	0.1357	1.9	0.0287
−2.6	0.0047	0.4	0.3446	−1.0	0.1587	2.0	0.0228
−2.5	0.0062	0.5	0.3085	−0.9	0.1841	2.1	0.0179
−2.4	0.0082	0.6	0.2743	−0.8	0.2119	2.2	0.0139
−2.3	0.0107	0.7	0.2420	−0.7	0.2420	2.3	0.0107
−2.2	0.0139	0.8	0.2119	−0.6	0.2743	2.4	0.0082
−2.1	0.0179	0.9	0.1841	−0.5	0.3085	2.5	0.0062
−2.0	0.0228	1.0	0.1587	−0.4	0.3446	2.6	0.0047
−1.9	0.0287	1.1	0.1357	−0.3	0.3821	2.7	0.0035
−1.8	0.0359	1.2	0.1151	−0.2	0.4207	2.8	0.0026
−1.7	0.0446	1.3	0.0968	−0.1	0.4602	2.9	0.0019
−1.6	0.0548	1.4	0.0808	0.0	0.5000	3.0	0.0013
−1.5	0.0668	1.5	0.0668				

The standard Normal curve is illustrated in diagram (I). Since any variable which has been transformed using equation (1.7.2) has a mean of zero and unit variance, the standard Normal distribution also has this property.

The area, and therefore the number of observations, under the standard Normal curve between any pair of values of z may be calculated from equations (1.7.1) and (1.7.2). As diagram (I) shows, approximately 68 percent of the area lies within one standard deviation either side of the mean, and 95 percent within two standard deviations. To enable the Normal distribution to be used in a staightforward fashion as a model for calculating the probability of obtaining, by chance, either very small or very large values of some variable, Table 1.7.1 has been prepared. Based on equations (1.7.1) and (1.7.2), it gives the lower and upper tail probabilities, denoted by Q and P respectively, of obtaining values less than or equal to selected values of z (in the case of the lower tail), and greater than or equal to z (in the case of the upper tail).

To illustrate the use of Table 1.7.1, consider diagram (C) in which cells were shaded different intensities if the death rate from cholera observed in them in the 1849 epidemic was so large that the likelihood of their arising by chance in a Normal distribution was less than 10, 5, 2.5 and 0.5 percent. The death rates per 10,000 population (x) corresponding to these probability levels may be calculated from equation (1.7.3) and Table 1.7.1 as 136.3, 154.2, 169.7 and 200.2 repectively. For example, for the 10 percent probability level (P = 0.10), Table 1.7.1 shows that, in a standard Normal distribution, such an area is delimited by the ordinate, $z = 1.28$. Linear interpolation between tabulated values is usually sufficient for most purposes. The frequency distribution in diagram (A) has a mean of 73.3 and a standard deviation of 49.2 which may be used as estimates of μ and σ respectively in equations (1.7.1) – (1.7.3). Substitution of these values and $z = 1.28$ into equation (1.7.3) yields $x = 136.3$.

The Poisson distribution

Under the assumptions stated for the Poisson process in the discussion of diagram (D), the probability, $P(X = x)$, of observing, say, a certain number, x, of deaths from cholera in a particular subarea is given by

$$P(X = x) = [\exp(-\lambda)\lambda^x]/x! \ , \ x = 0, 1, 2, \ldots \ (1.7.4)$$

where the parameter, λ, is the expected, or mean, number of deaths in that subarea. It is thus possible to

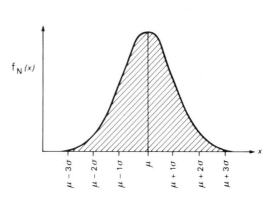

Figure 1.7 (E) The Normal distribution

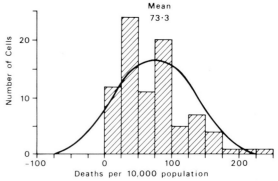

Figure 1.7 (F) A Normal distribution fitted to the cholera data

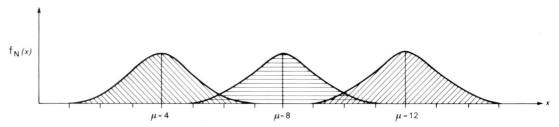

Figure 1.7 (G) Three Normal distributions with different means and fixed standard deviations

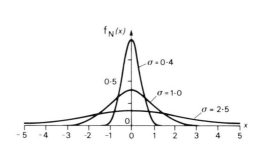

Figure 1.7 (H) Three Normal distributions with fixed means and different standard deviations

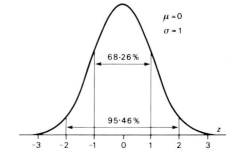

Figure 1.7 (I) Areas under the Normal curve

determine the probability of observing by chance, in a Poisson process with a given mean, at least as many deaths as those recorded by solving equation (1.7.4) from $(X = x)$ to $(X = \infty)$, and summing all the terms. The parameter may be estimated by the mean, m, of the observed data. Diagram (J) shows the probability distributions obtained from equation (1.7.4) with $m = 0.7$ and $m = 3.3$.

The computational labour is reduced if the chart shown in diagram (K) is used. This plots the probability, P, on the vertical axis of obtaining a value of x or more in a Poisson distribution whose mean is estimated by m. The probability, Q, of a value of m or less is given by $Q = [1.0 - P(x + 1)]$. The probability, P, is read off at the point at which the curved lines (values of x) intersect the straight vertical lines (values of λ).

To illustrate the use of chart (K), we return to map (D). In the 1849 epidemic, the crude death rate from cholera in London as a whole was 73.3 per 10,000 population. This figure was multiplied by the population (in ten thousands) of each of the grid cells in turn to give an expected number of deaths, m for each grid cell based upon the 'no dependence' assumption of the Poisson model; i.e., that the disease process operated at uniform spatial intensity across the city at a rate fixed by the average for the city as a whole. These expected values were used as the estimates for λ in chart (K). To obtain the observed number of deaths in each grid cell, the death rates per 10,000 population mapped in Figure 1.5(A) were multiplied by the cell populations (in ten thousands). These defined the quantities, x in (K). The probabilities were then read off.

Normal approximation to the Poisson
For $\lambda > 30$, a Poisson distribution approximates to a Normal distribution with the same mean and variance. The upper tail probability, $P(X \geq x)$, in a Poisson process with parameter λ is approximately equal to the corresponding upper tail probability for the standard Normal distribution given in Table 1.7.1 with $z = (x - \lambda - 0.5)/\sqrt{\lambda}$ [cf. equation (1.7.2)]; the value of 0.5 is a correction for continuity. For example, in a Poisson process with $\lambda = 36$, the probability of a value of 40 or more is, from chart (K), 0.28. The Normal approximation yields $z = 3.5/6.0 = 0.58$, which, from Table 1.7.1, corresponds to $P = 0.28$ by linear interpolation. Table 1.7.1 may therefore be used to obtain the upper tail probabilities for the Poisson when the value for λ is off the Poisson chart.

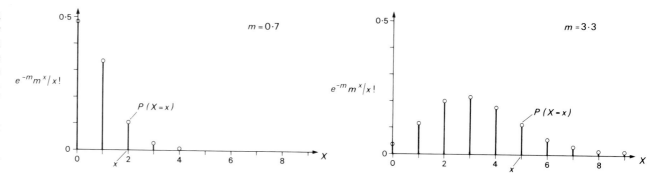

Figure 1.7 (J) Poisson probability distributions with different means

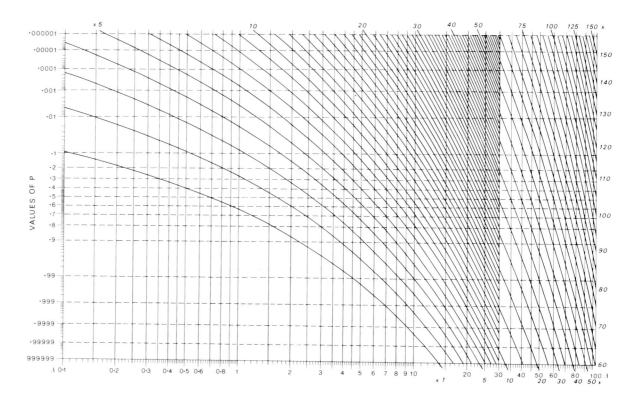

Figure 1.7 (K) Poisson probability chart

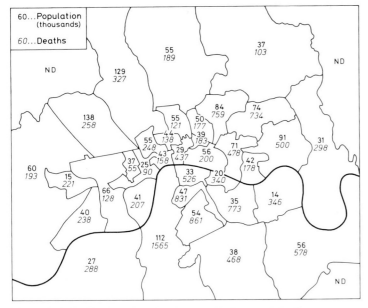

Figure 1.8 (A) Registration district populations and deaths

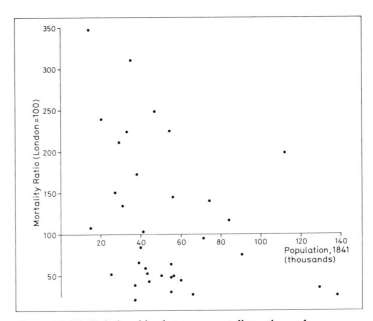

Figure 1.8 (B) Relationships between mortality ratios and population size of districts

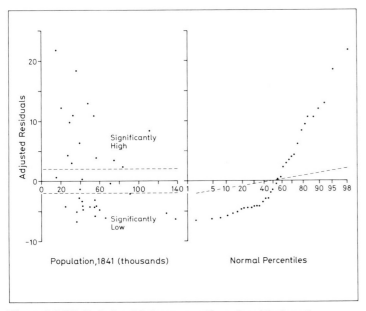

Figure 1.8 (C) Relationship between adjusted residuals and population size of districts

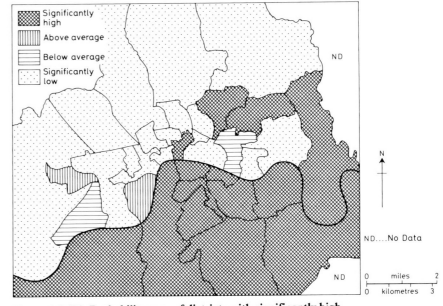

Figure 1.8 (D) Probability map of districts with significantly high and low cholera death levels

1.8 PROBABILITY MAPS II: ADJUSTED RESIDUALS

Rates of mortality

So far in this chapter, the geographical distribution of deaths from cholera in London in the epidemic of 1849 has been examined primarily by mapping, in various ways, the death *rate* per 10,000 population. However, the use of rates alone tells only part of the story and may sometimes even be misleading. This is because the same rate will be generated by five deaths in the small population of 100 as is generated by 500 deaths in the much larger population of 10,000. Therefore, as in Figure 1.3, the investigator will also need to study the absolute magnitude or number of deaths in each area when assessing the significance or otherwise of any spatial pattern.

Levels of mortality

The use of levels rather than rates presents its own problems in that they are not independent of the sizes of the areal units for which they are collected. A large number of deaths may be recorded simply because an area is geographically large and populous. The problem is particularly acute in the case of London in 1849, where there was great variety in the sizes of the data collecting units, namely the 34 registration districts.

A geographical example

Map (A) illustrates these points by showing, for each of the 34 registration districts, their geo-graphical extent, their population in thousands, and the number of cholera deaths recorded in the 1849 epidemic. The smallest districts in the centre of the map are less than one twentieth of the area of the largest; the smallest population count is 29,000, the largest is 138,000; and the deaths range from 55 to 1565. Many of the high levels of deaths are in the smallest districts, and so the geographical significance of this central area concentration may be underestimated if the size of the collecting units is not taken into account.

The variability is shown in a slightly different way in diagram (B) by plotting (a) on the vertical axis, the death rate from cholera per 10,000 population in each registration district as a ratio of the death rate for London as a whole (multiplied by 100 so that London = 100) against (b) on the horizontal axis, the population of each registration district recorded at the Census of 1841. Some areas of low population experienced huge mortality, while some high population districts experienced low mortality.

Standardized residuals

Thus neither plotting rates nor levels is entirely satisfactory. The problem was taken a stage further in Figure 1.7(D), where the level of deaths in each area was compared with that expected under the assumption of a geographically random disease process, characterized by the Poisson distribution. Even this is not wholly appropriate since the *residual* difference between observed and expected numbers can never be large for areas with small populations. A further modification which meets this difficulty is to scale the difference between observed and expected values by some function of the expected values, producing a *standardized residual*. As was seen in the technical appendix to Figure 1.7, the values expected under the Poisson model can be generated in a way which reflects the population sizes of the collecting units. Dividing by these quantities will inflate the differences between observed and expected values in small populations.

Adjusted residuals

This is basically the approach adopted in diagram (C). For reasons which are given in the technical appendix to this figure, the residuals defined by the difference between the observed number of deaths from cholera in each registration district, and those expected under Poisson or multinomial sampling, are scaled in a slightly different manner to that described above to produce *adjusted residuals*. These adjusted residuals have been plotted against the district populations in 1841, and also on a Normal probability graph. It is indicated in the technical appendix that individual adjusted residuals are Normally distributed. Thus adjusted residuals bigger than or equal to 1.96 denote registration districts with significantly high numbers of deaths from cholera, while those with adjusted residuals less than or equal to −1.96 denote districts with significantly low levels of deaths; these critical cut-off levels are shown by the horizontal pecked lines on the left-hand graph of diagram (C).

The Normal distribution for the residuals also implies that, when the residuals have been ranked from smallest to largest and plotted against Normal percentiles, a good fit of the Poisson model is indicated if the residuals are approximately scattered along the pecked line of the right-hand graph of diagram (C). It is readily seen that there are marked departures from Poissonian randomness.

Map (D) was formed by shading the registration districts according to their position in one of the four categories, significantly high (adjusted residual $\geq$ 1.96), above average (adjusted residual between 0 and 1.96), below average (adjusted residual between 0 and -1.96) and significantly low (adjusted residual ≤ -1.96), on the left-hand graph of (C). These divisions split the distribution of deaths by registration districts rather precisely along the line of the River Thames, with only a few areas of high deaths lying to the north of the river.

Sources and Further Reading

The sources for the maps of cholera data are as set out in Figure 1.3 of this Atlas.

The use of residuals is discussed in J.W. Tukey (1962), 'The future of data analysis', *Annals of Mathematical Statistics*, 33, pp.1–67, while an application to stroke patients is given in S.J. Haberman (1973), 'The analysis of residuals in cross-classified tables', *Biometrics*, 29, pp.205–20.

Technical appendix

The central idea behind diagrams (C) and (D) is that, in a contingency table consisting of r rows and c columns, the quantities,

$$d_{ij}^{(2)} = \frac{O_{ij} - E_{ij}}{\sqrt{E_{ij}}} \qquad (1.8.1)$$

are, in large samples, approximately Normally distributed with mean zero and unit variance (Haberman, 1973). In equation (1.8.1), O_{ij} is the observed frequency in cell i, j of the contingency table, E_{ij} is the expected frequency, and the $\{d_{ij}^{(2)}\}$ are referred to as standardized residuals. The Normal distribution for the $\{d_{ij}^{(2)}\}$ implies that

$$\chi^2 = \sum_i \sum_j \left[d_{ij}^{(2)} \right]^2 \qquad (1.8.2)$$

A rather better approximation is provided if the adjusted residuals

$$d_{ij}^{(3)} = \frac{O_{ij} - E_{ij}}{\sqrt{E_{ij}(1 - \frac{R_i}{N})(1 - \frac{C_j}{N})}} \qquad (1.8.3)$$

are used, where R_i is the sum of the observed frequencies in row i, C_j is the sum of the observed frequencies in column j and $N = \sum_i \sum_j O_{ij}$.

Although the $\{d_{ij}\}$ are correlated, the correlations are generally small in relatively large tables so that individual coefficients may be examined, as in the left-hand graph of diagram (C), to see if they lie outside a 95 percent confidence interval (that is $\pm$ 1.96). In fact,

$$d_{ij}^{(2)} = \sqrt{\chi^2_{ij}} \qquad (1.8.4)$$

plus the sign.

A further test, as in the right-hand graph of diagram (C), is to order the $\{d_{ij}\}$ as

$$d_{(1)} \leq d_{(2)} \leq \ldots \leq d_{(M)}, \qquad (1.8.5)$$

where $M = rc$, and to plot these against Normal percentiles. Following Tukey (1962), the k-th smallest (adjusted) residual d_k is assigned to the probability coordinate, $(3k - 1)/(3rc + 1) = (3k - 1)/37$. Ideally, the residuals should lie near the straight pecked line on the right-hand graph of diagram (C), which represents percentiles for the standard Normal distribution.

1.9 MAP PATTERN AND SPATIAL AUTOCORRELATION

Spatial patterns on maps

So far we have addressed the question of significance simply in terms of identifying the few data collecting areas on a map with exceptionally high and exceptionally low values (see Figures 1.7 and 1.8). The methods outlined there treat these areas in isolation and do not permit the geographical interrelationships between them to be examined. But to analyse maps in this fashion is unrealistic. The geographical location of any area on a map is unique to it as is its locational relationship to other areas, and it is the interactions between areas which create the distinctive patterns of disease incidence frequently seen on maps.

It is therefore important to have available methods of pattern analysis which permit the spatial characteristics of a map as a whole to be examined, and which preserve the positional information about areas with respect to each other. For example, we may wish to establish not just whether a data collecting unit has significantly high incidence of some disease, as in Figures 1.7 and 1.8, but also whether all high incidence units cluster together in a specific part of the map, or whether they form a regular pattern as do the black cells over the surface of a chessboard. Such systematic patterning may yield clues about the aetiology of a disease. In this figure, we look at the most basic techniques of *spatial autocorrelation* analysis which enable the issues outlined above to be addressed.

Maps as graphs

Map (A) shows the distribution of cholera deaths in the 34 registration districts of London in the epidemic of 1849, with the seventeen areas above the median level of deaths shaded; the remaining seventeen below the median have been left white. A point node has been located at the geographical centre of each district and each node has been coded black, B, or white, W, depending upon whether the district was, respectively, above or below the median. Links have been drawn between nodes where two registration districts share a common boundary.

The combined structure of nodes and links forms what is known as a *graph*, where the term is used in its topological sense and not to describe the form of chart typified by Figure 1.8(C). Once a map has been reduced to a graph, and the value of some variable has been recorded at each of the nodes, a variety of spatial autocorrelation techniques may be applied to the analysis of the resulting geographical distribution. The 86 links can be divided into three types namely (a) those connecting two black nodes and which are termed *BB joins*; (b) those connecting two white nodes (*WW joins*); and (c) those connecting a black node and a white node (*BW joins*).

Join count statistics

If we focus upon the BW joins in map (A), it can be seen that these are relatively few in number because the registration districts above the median are clustered in the southern half of the map. Hence BW joins only occur along the frontier between the two colours. We can make use of this intuitive association between the number of BW joins and the geographical pattern formed by the B and W nodes in a formal statistical test. The technical details are given in the appendix to this figure, but the quantity

$$z = [BW - \text{E}(BW)] / \sigma(BW) \qquad (1.9.1)$$

may be treated as a standard Normal score and tested for significance using Table 1.7.1 and the approach outlined in the technical appendix to Figure 1.7. In equation (1.9.1), BW is used to denote the observed number of BW joins, E(BW) to denote the expected number under the null hypothesis of no systematic spatial variation in the location of nodes of a particular colour on the graph, and $\sigma(BW)$ to denote the standard deviation. Thus the z-value of -3.02 implies a significant deficit of BW joins with, from Table 1.7.1, a probability of only about one in one thousand occurring by chance. The spatial pattern of nodes of each colour displays a very high degree of clustering.

Spatial clustering and dispersion

The remaining diagrams in this figure show hypothetical arrangements of B and W nodes to illustrate the variety of spatial patterns which might occur. In diagram (B), maximum spatial clustering of B and W nodes results in only 17 BW joins and a z-value of -6.22, with a probability of occurring by chance of about one in 1,000 million. An indeterminate or random pattern of B and W nodes appears in map (C), yielding 46 BW joins and a z-value of 0.41; such a value of z occurs by chance about 50 percent of the time. A uniform spatial arrangement of B and W nodes is illustrated in map (D), in which the B and W nodes are regularly intermixed on the graph. This results in a high BW count of 60 joins and a z-value of 3.62; such a value has a probability of about one in one thousand of

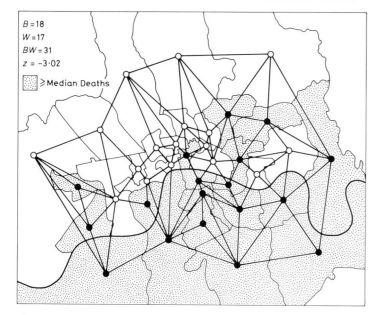

Figure 1.9 (A) Observed pattern on graph

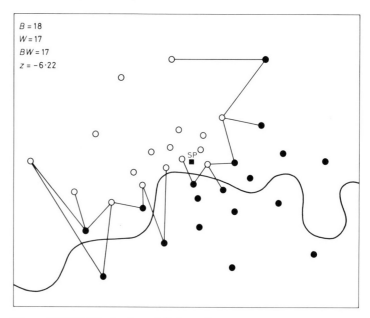

Figure 1.9 (B) Maximal spatial clustering

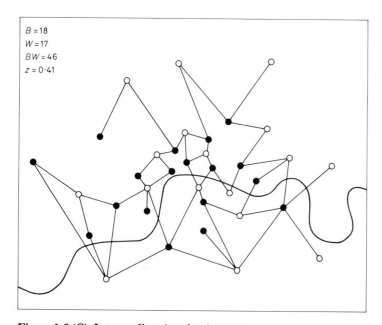

Figure 1.9 (C) Intermediate (random) pattern

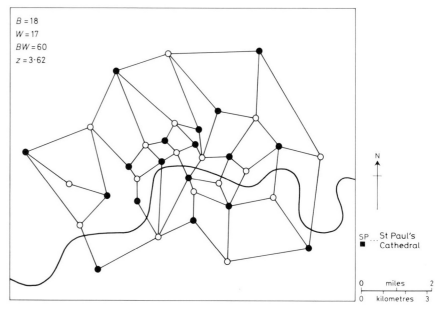

Figure 1.9 (D) Minimum spatial clustering (uniform pattern)

occurring by chance. Note that in all three diagrams, (B) – (D), only the BW links on the graph have been drawn.

Together the maps illustrate how a relatively simple statistical test allows the spatial pattern of cholera deaths to be accurately described and related to other map patterns. The relationship between the sign of BW and the type of spatial pattern may be summarized as follows:

Sign of BW

negative
- (1) disease spread from few sources
- (2) large areas favouring similar disease levels
- (3) gradient or trend in disease intensity across map

positive
- (1) heterogeneous study area
- (2) small areas favouring similar disease levels

More advanced spatial autocorrelation techniques are discussed in diagrams 5.13–5.15.

Sources and Further Reading

The sources for the maps of cholera data are as set out in Figure 1.3 of this Atlas.

The conversion of maps to graphs is discussed by A.D. Cliff and P. Haggett (1981), 'Graph theory', *Quantitative Geography*, edited by N. Wrigley and R.J. Bennett, London: Routledge and Kegan Paul, pp.225–34. The join-count statistics for spatial autocorrelation tests on graphs are given in A.D. Cliff and J.K. Ord (1973), *Spatial Autocorrelation*, London: Pion, pp.1–21, and A.D. Cliff and J.K. Ord (1981), *Spatial Processes: Models and Applications*, London: Pion, pp. 1–33. See also P.A.P. Moran (1948), 'The interpretation of statistical maps', *Journal of the Royal Statistical Society B*, 10, pp.243–51.

Technical appendix

In the following discussion, the term 'unit' is used to refer to any arbitrary data collecting unit, such as nodes on a graph counties, countries, and so on. We assume that there are n units on the map. Let $\{\delta_{ij}\}$ be a connection matrix in which $\delta_{ij} = 1$ if the ith and jth units are joined, and $\delta_{ij} = 0$ otherwise. Let $x_i = 1$ if the ith unit is B and $x_i = 0$ if the ith unit is W. The observed number of BW joins on the map is then given by

$$BW = \frac{1}{2} \sum_{(2)} (x_i - x_j)^2, \qquad (1.9.2)$$

where

$$\sum_{(2)} = \sum_{\substack{i=1 \\ i \neq j}}^{n} \sum_{j=1}^{n} . \qquad (1.9.3)$$

The usual method employed to determine whether BW departs significantly from random expectation is to use the fact that BW is asymptotically Normally distributed and to assume that this holds approximately for moderate n. The first two moments of BW are then used to specify the location [$E(BW)$] and scale [$\sigma^2(BW)$] parameters of the Normal distribution. Using this approach, the moments of BW may be evaluated under either of two assumptions:

(a) free sampling (or sampling with replacement), where we suppose that the individual units are independently coded B or W with probabilities p and $q = (1 - p)$ respectively;

(b) nonfree sampling (or sampling without replacement), where we assume that each unit has the same probability, *a priori*, of being B or W, but coding is subject to the overall constraint that there are n_1 units coloured B, n_2 coloured W and that $n_1 + n_2 = n$.

The first two moments are given by the following equations.

Free sampling

$$E(BW) = 2Apq, \qquad (1.9.4)$$

$$\sigma^2(BW) = 2(A+2D)pq - 4(A+2D)p^2q^2. \qquad (1.9.5)$$

Nonfree sampling

$$E(BW) = \frac{2An_1n_2}{n^{(2)}}, \qquad (1.9.6)$$

$$\sigma^2(BW) = \frac{2An_1n_2}{n^{(2)}} + \frac{4[A(A-1)-2D]n_1^{(2)}n_2^{(2)}}{n^{(4)}}$$
$$+ \frac{2Dn_1n_2(n_1+n_2-2)}{n^{(3)}} - 4\left[\frac{An_1n_2}{n^{(2)}}\right]^2. \qquad (1.9.7)$$

In these equations, A is the total number of joins on the map. Denote the number of units joined to the ith unit by L_i. A is then given by

$$A = \frac{1}{2} \sum_{i=1}^{n} L_i, \quad \text{while} \quad D = \frac{1}{2} \sum_{i=1}^{n} L_i (L_i - 1). \qquad (1.9.8)$$

In addition, $n^{(b)} = n(n-1) \cdots (n-b+1)$.

1.10 MAP GENERALIZATION I: LOCAL OPERATORS

Signal and noise on maps

When the geographical distribution of any disease is mapped, the resulting spatial pattern may be very complex so that the broad features of the distribution become lost in local detail. In such cases, interpretation may be made more straightforward if the main features of the data are separated from local variability. A simple physical parallel is provided by a radio operator who faces the problem of isolating the signal of the station to which he or she wishes to listen from the background noise. In this case, the tuning knob is used to 'filter out' signal from noise. In the geographical case *local operators* or *smoothing filters* constitute one spatial equivalent of the tuning knob on a radio set, and may be similarly used to separate signal (broad trends across a map) from noise (local variability).

This notion of signal versus noise introduces another important geographical idea, namely that spatial processes work at different geographical scales, and the spatial scale of operation will be reflected in our ability to separate out signal from noise. Some disease processes will undoubtedly result in distributions which vary only slowly across a map; these will produce a readily identifiable signal. Others will vary rapidly over short geographical distances and may produce very noisy or dirty spatial patterns which are extremely difficult to interpret or to generalize. Thus if we can split the total variation in a mapped pattern into the two components of broad signal and local noise, we may simultaneously learn a great deal about the spatial scale of the generating mechanism producing the

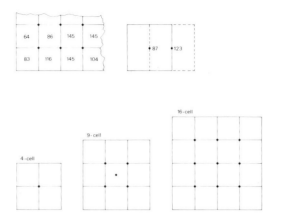

Figure 1.10 (A) Smoothing operators applied to maps

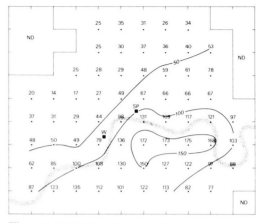

Figure 1.10 (B) 4-cell smoothed map

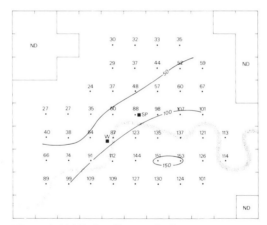

Figure 1.10 (C) 9-cell smoothed map

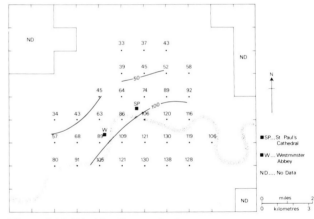

Figure 1.10 (D) 16-cell smoothed map

map. This issue is addressed further in Figures 1.11 and 1.12.

Smoothing filters

Diagram (A) shows the principle by which a smoothing filter is applied to a map. The first diagram in (A) shows the set of eight cells taken from the southwest corner of Figure 1.5(A) and gives the number of deaths from cholera per 10,000 population in subareas of London in the epidemic of 1849. The first four cells (with values of 64, 86, 83 and 116) have an average death rate of 87 [i.e., (64 + 86 + 83 + 116)/4] which we may allocate to the common corner point of the four cells and use to replace the four separate cell values. In the same way, we may progress over the entire surface of the map. Each block of four cells is taken in turn and replaced, along with their separate values, by the single value given by the average of the four separate cells. Thus the next four have values of 86, 145, 116 and 145, yielding a smoothed or average value of 123 to be located at the next common corner point.

Several names are used interchangeably to describe the procedure outlined. Statistically, the generated value is a four-cell *moving average*, and it has been obtained by *spatial filtering*, *spatial averaging*, *spatial smoothing* or by applying a four-cell *local operator*.

Smoothed maps

Diagram (B) shows the map obtained by applying the four-cell operator to the full set of death rates from cholera given in Figure 1.5(A). The resulting surface has been contoured in the manner of Figure 1.5(C) at intervals of fifty deaths per 10,000 population. The operator produces a ridge of high death rates, with an east–west axis, lying south of the River Thames. Death rates decline smoothly away from this ridge, both to the north and to the south.

Other sizes of operator may be applied to maps, and nine- and sixteen-cell versions are illustrated in the remainder of diagram (A). In the case of the nine-cell operator the smoothed value is calculated as the average of the nine cells falling within the operator, and it is assigned to the central point of the centre cell. The same principle applies to the sixteen-cell operator and to all larger sizes. As with the four-cell operator, the filter is applied to the map by moving the operator cell by cell over the entire map. Maps (C) and (D) show the application of the nine- and sixteen-cell operators respectively to the same data set used to generate diagram (B). Note that,

as the operator increases in size, the resulting map displays a progressively greater degree of generalization and becomes smoother and smoother in outline. Thus by map (D) the ridge shown in map (B) has entirely disappeared, to be replaced by a simple surface sloping from southeast (high) to northwest (low).

Comparison of the maps (B) to (D) shows one of the disadvantages of the filter method, namely loss of information for the buffer zone around the edge of the map. This becomes larger as the filter size increases.

Sources and Further Reading

The sources for the maps of cholera data are as set out in Figure 1.3 in this Atlas.

The technical issues in using local operators are described at an advanced level in A.D. Cliff and J.K. Ord (1981), *Spatial Processes: Models and Applications*, London: Pion, pp.141–83; P. Whittle (1954), 'On stationary processes in the place', *Biometrika*, 41, pp.434–49; and B.D. Ripley (1981), *Spatial Statistics*, New York: John Wiley, pp.28–77.

The question of generalization on isarithmic maps and its effect on the accuracy of isopleths is studied in M.L. Hsu and A.H. Robinson (1970), *The Fidelity of Isopleth Maps: An Experimental Study*, Minneapolis: University of Minnesota Press, and in N.S.Lam (1983), 'Spatial interpolation methods: a review', *American Cartographer*, 10, pp.129–49. See also D.I. Blumenstock (1953), 'The reliability factor in the drawing of isarithms', *Annals of the Association of American Geographers* 43, pp.289–304; J.R. Mackay (1953), 'The alternative choice in isopleth interpolation', *Professional Geographer* 5, pp.2–4, and A.T.A. Learmonth and M.N. Pal (1959), 'A method for plotting two variables on the same map using isopleths', *Erdkunde*, 13, pp.145–50.

Computer methods for spatial data handling are set out in E.B. MacDougall (1976), *Computer Programming for Spatial Problems*, London: Edward Arnold, and in D.F. Marble, editor (1980), *Computer Software for Spatial Data Handling*, Washington, DC: US Geological Survey.

Technical appendix

The spatial smoothing procedure described is a member of a general class of linear spatial transfer functions defined as follows. Let Z_{ij} denote the random variable on the map in cell (i, j) of a regular lattice. Then we may formulate the linear operator as

$$E(Z_{ij}) = a + \sum_{p=-k}^{k} \sum_{q=-k}^{k} b_{pq} z_{i+p, j+q} + e_{ij}, \quad (1.10.1)$$

where $E(Z_{ij})$ is the expected value in cell (i, j), the $\{e_{ij}\}$ are uncorrelated error terms and a $(2k + 1) \times (2k + 1)$ or K-cell operator is postulated. In the example used above, we have arbitrarily set $a = e_{ij} = 0$, and each of the $\{b_{pq}\}$ equal to $1/K$. However, more generally, these quantities may be estimated. Note that the ordinary least squares estimators are inconsistent (Whittle, 1954), and there is no viable alternative to maximum likelihood.

ND	ND	17	20	37	40	18	26	36	ND	ND
ND	ND	ND	18	26	38	27	34	38	38	ND
ND	ND	25	35	22	34	49	34	53	83	ND
15	14	13	28	27	31	78	75	83	91	ND
35	17	12	16	37	99 SP	59	51	54	76	95
40	54	40	47	W 91	165	201	126	235	119	99
54	43	64	45	134	152	171	194	143	94	100
64	86	145	145	108	124	151	72	80	71	87
83	116	145	104	89	81	130	98	78	78	ND

Figure 1.11 (A) Original cell values

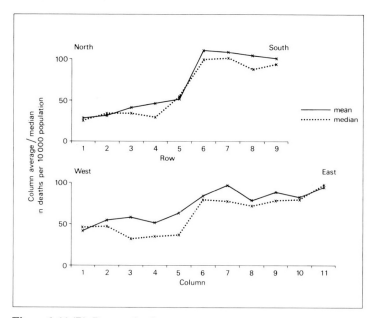

Figure 1.11 (B) Row and column averages

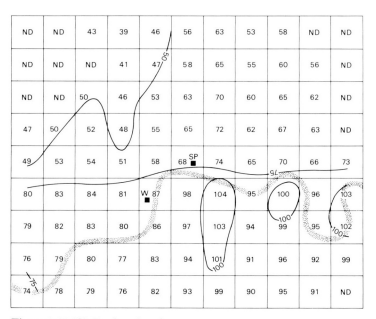

Figure 1.11 (C) Regional surface

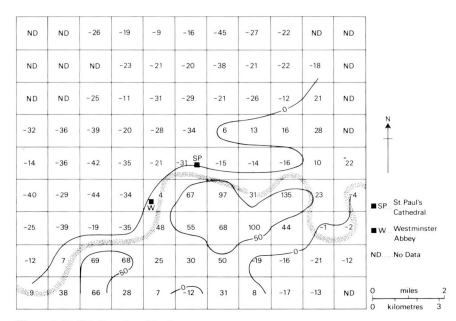

Figure 1.11 (D) Local residuals

1.11 MAP GENERALIZATION II: REGIONAL TRENDS AND LOCAL RESIDUALS

Row-column averaging

When confronted with a map showing the geographical distribution of some disease, it is not always straightforward to appreciate the main trends in the data displayed. The eye is often drawn to the local detail of highs and lows on the map, thus deflecting attention from broader patterns. In Figure 1.10, a moving average method for isolating trend from local detail was described. An alternative approach is to employ a smoothing procedure based upon the average values in the rows and columns of the lattice used to partition the study area. This technique is very much quicker than the filter method described earlier but it is more wasteful of local detail.

The technique is illustrated by an application to the death rate per 10,000 population in the cholera epidemic of 1849 in various subareas of London. The data are given in map (A) and the course of the River Thames is shown by the solid west to east meandering line. The technique begins, as shown in diagram (B), by calculating some measure of centrality for every row and column of the lattice. Commonly this measure is the arithmetic mean, although the median is sometimes used. So, for example, column three in diagram (A) contains the values 17, 25, 13, 12, 40, 64, 145 and 145. The column average is 57.6 (that is, 461 divided by 8) and this value is plotted on the lower graph of diagram (B). The median of column three is 32.5. This is the midpoint of the two central values when the data values in the column are ranked from smallest to largest. The ranked values are 12, 13, 17, 25, 40, 64, 145 and 145. The advantage of the median over the mean is that it is less affected by one or two extreme values. In this example, the extrema are the high death rates south of the Thames.

Regional trend

The regionally smoothed map shown in (C) is then formed by defining the cell value in a given row and column as the average of the corresponding row and column means or medians calculated in (B). In the example considered here, diagram (C) has been formed on the basis of the arithmetic means. Thus row one in diagram (A) has an average of 27.7 (i.e., 194 divided by 7) while, as we have already seen, column three has an average of 57.6. The smoothed value appearing in (row one, column three) is 43, the rounded average of 27.7 and 57.6.

In contrast to the approach based upon linear operators described in Figure 1.10, there is no loss of information around the margins of the map using the smoothing method described here. It also generates an 'expected' map, in that statisticians define the average of any distribution as its expected value; that is, it is the value which is most likely to occur. The regionally smoothed map illustrated in (C) shows a surface of death rates from cholera which slopes broadly from high levels in the southeast to low levels in the northwest. As in diagram 1.10, the surface has been contoured. The details of the contours differ slightly from those shown on the maps of Figure 1.10, emphasizing that each method produces its own distinctive map.

Local residuals

The loss of local detail in a map resulting from the application of any smoothing method can be determined by computing the residual differences between the actual observations, as shown in diagram (A), and the regional trend constructed in (C). The residuals are conventionally defined as (observed–expected) values. Thus the residual for (row one, column three) is given by (17 − 43); that is −26.

The map of residuals shown in diagram (D) emphasizes the local departures from the broad regional trend of declining death rates from southeast to northwest which are to be found in the cholera mortality data. There is a large excess of deaths, denoted by positive residuals, along the southern bank of the Thames and this excess mortality forms a ridge sandwiched between relatively low mortality areas to the northwest and southeast (denoted by the negative residuals).

The causative mechanism generating cholera deaths thus appears to have operated at two distinct spatial scales in 1849. Locally very high levels of mortality were experienced in the southern floodplain area of the Thames, while at a coarser spatial scale the whole of the area to the south of the Thames was more badly affected than the area to the north. A full explanation of events would need to encompass both these features of the data.

Sources and Further Reading

The sources for the maps of cholera data are as set out in Figure 1.3 of this Atlas.

The technical issues are described by A.D. Cliff and J.K. Ord (1981), *Spatial Processes: Models and Applications*, London: Pion, pp.118–140; B.D. Ripley (1981), *Spatial Statistics*, New York: John Wiley, pp. 28–77; and by H. Moellering and W.R. Tobler (1972), 'Geographical variances', *Geographical Analysis*, 4, pp.34–50.

Technical appendix

It is possible to establish the relative importance of different geographical scales in any spatial process using the hierarchical (Model II) analysis of variance. Suppose that the lattice has 2^{2m} cells and is square ($2^m \times 2^m$). We can define ($m + 1$) levels by taking square blocks of cells one, four, sixteen . . . at a time. See diagram (E). If X_i denotes the random variable corresponding to the ith cell, we may postulate a hierarchical model for the m levels as

$$X_i = \mu + \epsilon_1(i) + \ldots + \epsilon_m(i), \quad (1.\ 11.\ 1)$$

where

(a) the means of the $\{X_i\}$ are taken to be equal to μ;
(b) the random variables $\epsilon_j(i)$ have zero means and variances $\sigma_\epsilon^2(j)$ denoting the variance attributable to the jth level of the hierarchy.

The magnitudes of the variances $\sigma_\epsilon^2(j)$ indicate the importance to be attached to the jth level of the hierarchy. These variances may be estimated as follows. If s cells are combined at each stage of the hierarchy, write

$$X_i(j) = \sum_{r \in A_{ij}} X_r(j - 1) \quad (1.\ 11.\ 2)$$

where A_{ij} denotes the set of s cells at level ($j - 1$) which are combined into one cell (the ith) at level j. The jth sum of squares, SS_j, corresponding to the jth row of the analysis of variance table may be written as

$$SS_j = \sum_i [X_i(j) - s^{-1}X_i(j + 1)]^2, \quad (1.\ 11.\ 3)$$

whence the mean square at level j, MS_j, is

$$MS_j = SS_j/(n_j - n_{j+1}), \quad (1.\ 11.\ 4)$$

where $n_j = sn_{j+1}$. Finally the jth component variance may be estimated as

$$\sigma_\epsilon^2(j) = (sMS_j - MS_{j-1})/(s - 1), j = 1, 2, \ldots, m.$$

$$(1.\ 11.\ 5)$$

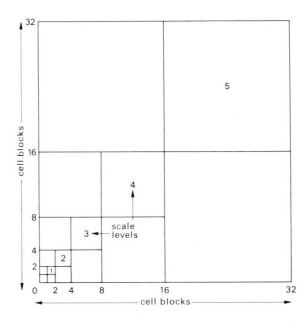

Figure 1.11 (E) Scale levels in the Model II analysis of variance

1.12 MAP GENERALIZATION III: TREND SURFACES

The third and most advanced approach to the identification of spatial trends in a mapped data set is mathematically to fit different surface shapes to the data and then to decide which of the fitted surfaces best describes the mapped distribution. Of the wide range of surface fitting techniques available, we choose to illustrate the use of a polynomial method which can be readily programmed for a small computer.

Map (A) shows the data to which the method is to be applied; these give the number of deaths per 10,000 population from cholera in 86 sub-areas of London in the epidemic of 1849. As demonstrated in the technical appendix to this figure, the method defines the height of the surface, denoted by Y (the number of cholera deaths per 10,000 population), at each location on the map as a polynomial function of the cartesian coordinates of the locations. We use x_1 to denote positions on the horizontal axis of the coordinate system, and x_2 to denote positions on the vertical axis.

Linear surface

The simplest surface which can be constructed is described by an equation with three coefficients (β_{00}, β_{10} and β_{01}), namely

$$Y = \beta_{00} + \beta_{10}x_1 + \beta_{01}x_2 + \epsilon. \qquad (1.12\ 1)$$

Here ϵ is an error term. Values of the coefficients are estimated from the data using the methods outlined in the technical appendix, where computational details are also given.

The resulting map, illustrated in diagram (B), forms a simple shed-roof surface sloping from high death rates in the southeast to low death rates in the northwest. It accounts for 47 percent of the total geographical variability in the original data of diagram (A). The course of the River Thames is stippled. Map (B) confirms the general pattern of deaths shown on earlier maps in this chapter.

Quadratic surface

By adding powers of x_1 and x_2 to the right-hand side of the basic equation given in (1.12.1), it is possible to produce inflections in the modelled surface. Diagram (C) shows the surface resulting from the use of both linear and quadratic terms in x_1 and x_2. This is conventionally referred to as the quadratic surface although it contains both linear and quadratic elements. In the technical appendix, it is shown that the number of coefficients to be estimated goes up to five and that a single inflection can be modelled. The resulting surface accounts for 53 percent of the variability in the original data and, while it still displays the basic southeast to northwest decline in death rates of the linear surface, it models a little more accurately the area of high rates to the south of the River Thames.

Higher order surfaces

By generating even higher order polynomial equations in the coordinate variables, x_1 and x_2, to describe Y, progressively more complex shapes can be produced capable of handling more and more inflections, and therefore local detail, in the original data. Map (D) illustrates the surface resulting from the use of linear, quadratic and cubic terms in x_1 and x_2. This is conventionally called the cubic surface. The number of coefficients to be estimated rises to ten, but two inflection points in the original data can be handled. It accounts for 68 percent of the variability in the raw data, a 15 percent increase on the previous surface. The map shows a 'high' in cholera deaths over the southeast and a 'low' over the northwest of the study area.

While it is possible to increase the complexity of the surface still further by fitting to the data yet higher-order polynomials of the locational coordinates, the number of coefficients to be estimated increases rapidly. The following general relationships may be noted: (a) the number of inflections able to be modelled is one less than the order of the polynomial fitted, and (b) the number of terms in the polynomial is given by the binomial coefficient, $\binom{n+2}{2}$ where n is the order of the polynomial.

Scale and spatial processes

Apart from general surface fitting, a particularly important application of the model is to identify which spatial scale accounts for most of the point-to-point variation on a map. Regional scale processes should be well fitted by low-order surfaces. Conversely, local scale processes will produce small-scale features and will generally only be able to be modelled by high order polynomials.

The results obtained for the London cholera data suggest, as did Figure 1.11, that both regional and local scale processes were operative in the 1849 epidemic. Hence the linear and cubic terms account for large amounts of the variability in the data across the map, whereas the quadratic terms only contribute six percent over and above those of the linear surface.

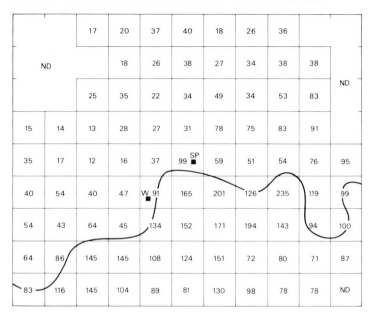

Figure 1.12 (A) Original cell values

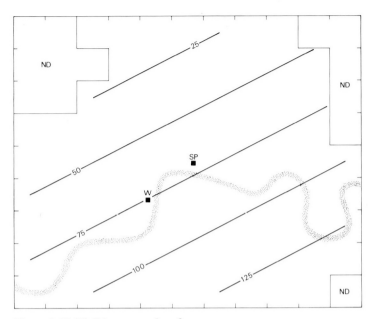

Figure 1.12 (B) Linear trend surface

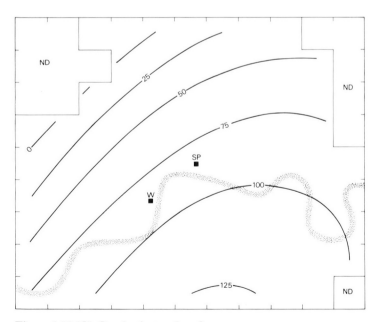

Figure 1.12 (C) Quadratic trend surface

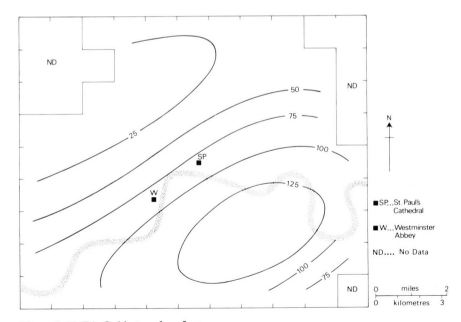

Figure 1.12 (D) Cubic trend surface

Sources and Further Reading

The sources for the maps of cholera data are as set out in Figure 1.3 of this Atlas.

Two standard accounts of trend-surface mapping are given in K.L. Millar and J.S. Kahn (1962), *Statistical Analysis in the Geological Sciences*, New York: John Wiley, pp.390–439 and in R.J. Chorley and P. Haggett (1965), 'Trend-surface mapping in geographical research', *Transactions of the Institute of British Geographers*, 37, pp.47–67. See also D.J. Unwin (1975), *An Introduction to Trend-Surface Analysis*, Concepts and Techniques in Modern Geography No. 5, Norwich: Geoabstracts, P. Haggett, A.D. Cliff and A.E. Frey (1977), *Locational Analysis in Human Geography*, second edition, London: Edward Arnold, pp.378–85, and B.D. Ripley (1981), *Spatial Statistics*, New York: John Wiley, pp.28–77.

Surfaces can be fitted using the standard regression programmes available on a microcomputer. See, for example, B.F. Ryan, B.L. Joiner and T.A. Ryan (1985), *Minitab Handbook*, second edition, Boston: Duxbury Press, pp.236–59.

Technical appendix

Using the notation established in equation (1.12.1), the polynomial trend surface model is formed by entering various power functions of the x_1 and x_2 cartesian coordinates as independent variables in a regression of the linear (in the parameters) form

$$Y = \sum_{i=0}^{p} \sum_{j=0}^{q} \beta_{ij} x_1^i x_2^j + \epsilon . \qquad (1.12.2)$$

Here the error terms, ϵ, are assumed to be independently normally distributed with mean zero and variance σ^2. The model is readily estimated by ordinary least squares, yielding all the standard tests of hypotheses.

Diagram (E) shows schematically the general shape of the surface produced by first, second and third order equations and, in addition, the equations and curves for the corresponding conventional polynomial regressions in two, rather than three, dimensions. It is apparent from these figures that the number of inflections which can be handled by any equation is one less than the order of the polynomial. The effects of combinatorial arithmetic imply that with a cubic surface, depending on which coefficients are non-zero, over 2,000 maps may be generated, each with its own distinctive surface form.

The results of fitting up to a third order surface to the London cholera data are summarized in Table 1.12.1. The origin (0,0) of the coordinate system was fixed at the southwest corner of each map. The cells in the last row of diagram (A) were given the coordinates (2, 2), (6, 2), (10, 2) and so on.

Table 1.12.1 *Trend surface analysis of London cholera data, 1849*

Terms in regression	Surface					
	Linear		Quadratic		Cubic	
	Coefficient	*t*-value	Coefficient	*t*-value	Coefficient	*t*-value
Constant	93.4300	8.99★★	79.2500	4.07★★	91.9700	3.29★★
x_1	1.4086	4.15★★	4.1010	2.90★★	−0.2690	−0.08
x_2	−3.0938	−7.75★★	−2.9880	−1.82★	0.4770	0.12
x_1^2			−0.0859	−2.84★★	0.1482	0.91
$x_1 x_2$			0.0720	1.92★	0.2686	1.61
x_2^2			−0.0557	−1.34	−0.5528	−2.42★★
x_1^3					−0.0052	−2.15★
$x_1^2 x_2$					0.0071	2.16★
$x_1 x_2^2$					0.0159	−4.54★★
x_2^3					0.0162	3.99★★
Degrees of freedom (df)	83.0		80.0		76.0	
R^2	0.47		0.53		0.68	

★ Significant at $\alpha = 0.05$ level (1-tailed test)   ★★ Significant at $\alpha = 0.01$ level (1-tailed test)

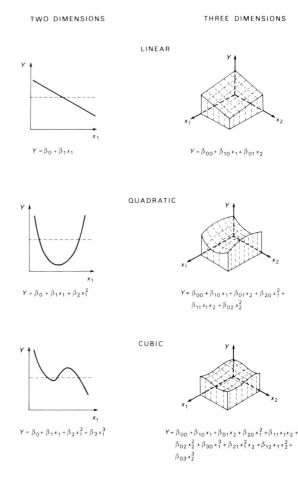

TWO DIMENSIONS   THREE DIMENSIONS

LINEAR

$Y = \beta_0 + \beta_1 x_1$

$Y = \beta_{00} + \beta_{10} x_1 + \beta_{01} x_2$

QUADRATIC

$Y = \beta_0 + \beta_1 x_1 + \beta_2 x_1^2$

$Y = \beta_{00} + \beta_{10} x_1 + \beta_{01} x_2 + \beta_{20} x_1^2 + \beta_{11} x_1 x_2 + \beta_{02} x_2^2$

CUBIC

$Y = \beta_0 + \beta_1 x_1 + \beta_2 x_1^2 + \beta_3 x_1^3$

$Y = \beta_{00} + \beta_{10} x_1 + \beta_{01} x_2 + \beta_{20} x_1^2 + \beta_{11} x_1 x_2 + \beta_{02} x_2^2 + \beta_{30} x_1^3 + \beta_{21} x_1^2 x_2 + \beta_{12} x_1 x_2^2 + \beta_{03} x_2^3$

Figure 1.12 (E) Polynomial equations in two and three dimensions

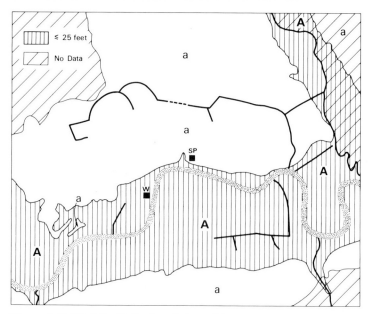

Figure 1.13 (A) The 'defective drainage' factor

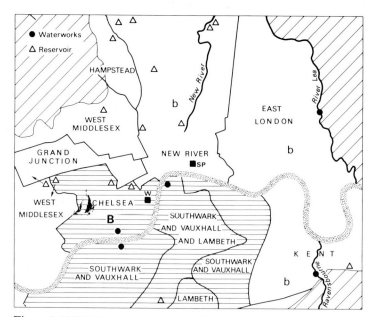

Figure 1.13 (B) The 'water company' factor

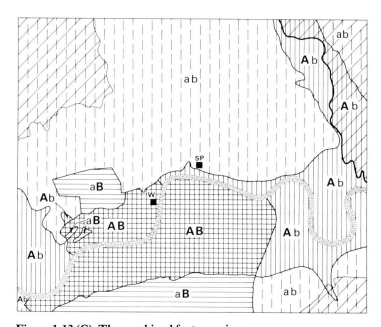

Figure 1.13 (C) The combined factor regions

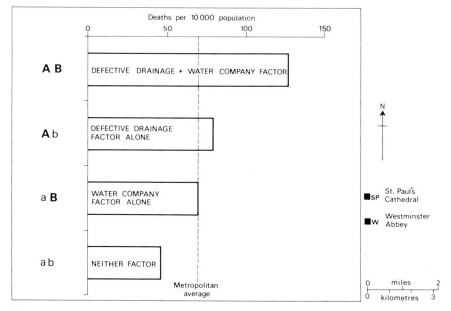

Figure 1.13 (D) Cholera death rates in the factor regions

1.13 MAPS AND HYPOTHESIS TESTING I: SIEVE MAPS

Hypotheses and factor regions

So far in this Atlas we have been concerned with problems of map production and design; that is, with the various cartographic techniques which may be employed to *display* data on maps to the best effect. However, maps are also devices for *analysis* and the use of sieve maps provides a powerful means of isolating the various factors which have shaped the geographical distributions of diseases. These factors may be both environmental and aetiological.

The basic idea behind the sieve map is straightforward. A series of factors are identified which it is believed will account, in part, for the spatial pattern of disease shown on a map. The map is then split into two categories on the basis of the first factor chosen. Category one comprises those areas in which the factor is present while category two comprises those areas in which the factor is absent. This process is repeated for each of the factors believed to influence the mapped distribution. Thus as many maps will be produced as there are factors, with each map split into the two categories of presence and absence of the factor mapped.

The factor maps are next superimposed like a stack of sieves in order to see which factor combinations are present in each of the map areas. The factor combinations which are most closely associated with areas of high and low disease incidence can then be isolated by overlaying the factor combination map on the disease distribution map.

The method is used here to relate (a) modern knowledge on the factors which contribute to the spread of Asiatic cholera to (b) the geographical distribution of deaths per 10,000 population from this disease in the 34 registration districts of London in 1849. Figure 1.8(A) records the number of deaths and the population of each district.

Cholera and water-related factors

Cholera is a water-borne disease and, as discussed in detail in Figure 1.1 of this chapter, its incidence is positively related both to poor drainage and to faecal contamination of water supplies. In Victorian London, its spread reflected the impoverished sanitary arrangements of the city. Raw sewerage was emptied into the River Thames at locations close to the waterworks of certain water companies and the river also formed the source from which these same companies drew their supplies for the pumps and taps of the metropolis. We might therefore expect to be able to relate the level of cholera deaths to proximity to the River Thames (a defective drainage factor, whereby sewerage was ineffectually discharged from the houses) and a water company factor (reflecting the differences in the sources of supply of the different water companies).

The defective drainage factor is illustrated in map (A). Those areas of the city less than twenty-five feet above the River Thames, which we have taken as our definition of 'defective drainage', are shown by vertical shading. These areas are all close to the River Thames and to its tributary, the River Lea. They are designated by the capital letter **A**. The areas of the city which are more than twenty-five feet above the Thames have been left blank and are designated by a lower case a. Areas for which no data on cholera deaths are available are diagonally shaded.

The water company factor is shown in map (B). Three water companies – the Chelsea, the Lambeth and the Southwark and Vauxhall – drew their water supplies from the Thames. The areas of the city served by these companies are shown by horizontal shading and are coded with a capital letter **B**. The areas of the city supplied by companies which drew their water from wells and reservoirs, rather than from the Thames, have been left white and are coded with a lower case b. As on diagram (A), areas for which no data are available have been diagonally shaded.

Factor combinations and cholera deaths

The interplay of the defective drainage and the water company factors is shown in (C) by superimposing the two maps, (A) and (B). Thus those areas of the city suffering from both defective drainage and contaminated water supplies appear as cross-hatched shading and are coded **AB**. Other combinations are **A**b, a**B**, and ab, each reflecting a particular combination of the two factors.

In diagram (D) the number of deaths per 10,000 population in the geographical areas covered by each of the factor combinations is shown on the horizontal axis as a bar chart. The average for the city as a whole is also plotted. The substantial excess of deaths in those areas covered by both factors **A** and **B** is evident. If the single-factor areas are considered, then it appears that defective drainage is more important than is the water company supplying the district. Areas in which neither factor operates have a substantial deficit of deaths.

Technical appendix

The statistical technique which provides an analytical equivalent of the sieve map is the *Model I Analysis of Variance* (ANOVA). The total variation in a set of observations (deaths from cholera per 10,000 population in the registration districts of London in 1849), as measured by the sums of squares of deviations from the mean of the observations, is separated into components associated with defined sources of variation (type of drainage and water supply) used as criteria of classification for the observations. For the example considered here, the analysis of variance table is given in Table 1.13.1.

The value of the death rate from cholera in each of the registration districts is assigned to one of the four categories defined by the two cross-classifying variables. The codings, **AB**, **A**b, a**B** and ab, link the sieve map approach to the ANOVA table. If equal numbers of observations appear in each category, the ANOVA table is said to be *balanced*. The total variation in death rates can be divided into four components as follows:

$$\text{Total } SS = \text{between-column } SS + \text{between-row } SS + \text{interaction } SS + \text{unexplained } SS. \quad (1.13.1)$$

In equation (1.13.1), SS is used to denote sum of squares. We are taking the total variation in death rates (total SS) and explaining all that is possible by means of the first nominal scale, namely defective drainage, to define a between-column SS. Of that which is left unexplained, a certain proportion can be accounted for by the second nominal scale (supplying water company), defining a between-rows SS. There will also be interaction effects between the two explanatory variables and, finally, an error term which represents the portion of the total variation which cannot be accounted for by the categorical variables. The sources of variation may be tested for significance using Snedecor's F-distribution.

The results of the ANOVA are given in Table 1.13.2. The design was unbalanced. To increase accuracy, the analysis was based upon data for the 124 parishes making up the 34 registration districts. Using this finer spatial mesh enabled a much closer degree of correspondence to be achieved between the factor regions shown in map (C) and the geographical distribution of death rates. Three hypotheses were tested. First, interaction was checked for, yielding an F-ratio of 1.7 which is not significant at

conventional levels. The interaction SS was then added back into the error term and this increased error component was used to test the two further hypotheses: (a) the population column means are equal, implying no defective drainage effect and (b) the population row means are equal (implying no water company effect). Both these hypotheses are rejected on the basis of the large F-ratios. We conclude that, as judged by the mean squares, the defective drainage effect is much more important than the water company effect, which is the same result as obtained in diagram (D) from the sieve map approach.

Sources and Further Reading

The sources for the maps of cholera data are as set out in Figure 1.3 in this Atlas.

The general issues raised in hypothesis testing are covered in standard statistical texts; see, for example, G.W. Snedecor and W.G. Cochran (1980), *Statistical Methods*, seventh edition, Ames, Iowa: Iowa State University Press, pp.64–82. An elementary introduction in a medical context is given in T.D.V. Swinscow (1983), *Statistics at Square One* (articles published in the British Medical Journal), eighth edition, London: British Medical Journal.

The specific problems of hypothesis testing in a spatial context are reviewed in W.C. Krumbein (1955), 'Experimental design in the earth sciences', *Transactions of the American Geophysical Union*, 36, pp.1–11, and in P. Haggett, A.D. Cliff and A.E. Frey (1977), 'Hypothesis testing', in *Locational Analysis in Human Geography*, second edition, London: Edward Arnold, pp.378–85. For computational methods see B.F. Ryan, B.L. Joiner and T.A. Ryan (1985), *Minitab Handbook*, second edition, Boston: Duxbury Press, p.193–217.

Table 1.13.1 *Two-way analysis of variance table for London cholera data, 1849*

Water company factor	Defective drainage factor	
	Low areas ($\leq$ 25 ft) **A**	High areas ($>$ 25 ft) a
Supplied from Thames[a] **B**	**AB**	a**B**
Not supplied from Thames[b] b	**A**b	ab

[a] Registration districts fed by Southwark and Vauxhall, Lambeth and Chelsea Companies.

[b] Registration districts fed by West Middlesex, Grand Junction, Hampstead, Kent, East London and New River Companies.

Table 1.13.2 *Results of analysis of variance for London cholera data, 1849*

Source of variation	Degrees of freedom	Sums of squares	Mean square	F-ratio
Defective drainage (between columns)	1	113091	113091	46.9*
Water company (between rows)	1	45977	45977	19.1*
Interaction	1	4003	4003	1.7
Error	120	288087	2401	

* Significant at $\alpha = 0.01$ level.

1.14 MAPS AND HYPOTHESIS TESTING II: REGRESSION ANALYSIS

Regression analysis

This technique provides a second method for establishing the relative importance of a series of factors which have been proposed to account for the observed features of a mapped distribution. The methodology is illustrated using the data of Figure 1.13. The death rates from cholera per 10,000 population in the 34 registration districts of London in the epidemic of 1849 constitute the dependent or effect variable whose distribution it is sought to explain, while the defective drainage and water supply factors are to be used as explanatory or independent variables. Given the aetiology of cholera outlined in Figure 1.1, it may be hypothesized that (a) death rates will increase with proximity to the poorly drained areas of the floodplain of the River Thames and (b) rates will also be higher in districts served by those water companies whose source of supply was the Thames, into which raw sewerage was discharged.

Elevation and cholera deaths

In diagram (A), the death rates from cholera in each of the 34 districts are plotted on the vertical axis of the two upper graphs against, on the horizontal axis, elevation (in feet) above the River Thames. One of the graphs is on an arithmetic scale and shows that death rates fall off rapidly in an exponential manner, with increasing height. The second of the graphs shows how such an exponential relationship may be readily transformed into a linear form by plotting the death rates on a logarithmic scale. The lower chart in (A) shows the relationship between death rates from cholera and elevation along a north to south cross-section (A–A′) across the study area. The location of the cross-section is marked on diagram (B).

Map (B) illustrates in two dimensions the relationship between elevation and death rates. Five different elevation classes have been delimited on the map by contours and the areas between each contour have been shaded. The course of the Thames is stippled. The highest region, in the northwest part of the map, is Hampstead Heath at an elevation of over 400 feet. The defective drainage area formed by the floodplains of the Rivers Thames and the Lea has been left white. Superimposed on the topographic base are a series of heavy 'contours' showing the death rates from cholera. Here the high death rate areas south of the Thames reach a peak of over two hundred.

Least squares regression

In order to construct map (C), the following regression relationship was first fitted using ordinary least squares. Let

y = the death rate per 10,000 population from cholera, by registration district;

x = the height in feet above Trinity Highwater mark as given in Great Britain Parliamentary Papers 1850 XXI, *Report of the General Board of Health on the Epidemic Cholera of 1848 and 1849*, by registration district.

Then

$$\log y = 2.376 - 0.469\log (1 + x), R^2 = 0.68.$$
$$(-8.42) \qquad\qquad (1.14.1)$$

The number in brackets is the t-statistic for the regression coefficient and implies that there is an extremely significant inverse relationship between death rates and height; that is, as height goes up, death rates go down so that 68 percent of the variability in death rates is accounted for by the height variable [cf. Diagram (A)]. The regression was based upon the logarithms of the variable values on the strength of diagram (A).

Residuals from regression

Map (C) shows the residuals from this regression. These residuals correspond with factor, a, in Figure 1.13 (that is, the component of death rates from cholera *not* accounted for by the defective drainage factor, as measured by height above Trinity HWM). The residuals have been mapped as (observed – regression) values. Thus positive residuals occur in registration districts in which death rates were underestimated by the regression relationship specified in equation (1.14.1). Negative residuals represent districts in which model (1.14.1) overestimated death rates. It is readily seen that the positive residuals are concentrated south of the River Thames. Comparison with Figure 1.13(B) shows that there is a substantial overlap of the positive-residual districts with the areas of London served by the Southwark and Vauxhall, Lambeth and Chelsea Companies. It will be recalled that these three companies, unlike the other metropolitan water companies, drew their water directly from the River Thames.

Water company and cholera deaths

Accordingly, to prepare map (D) the relationship between death rates and water supply was examined. With the variable y defined as before,

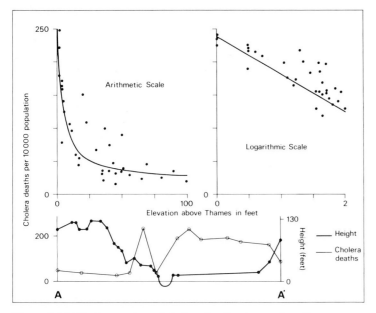

Figure 1.14 (A) Regression of cholera death rates on elevation

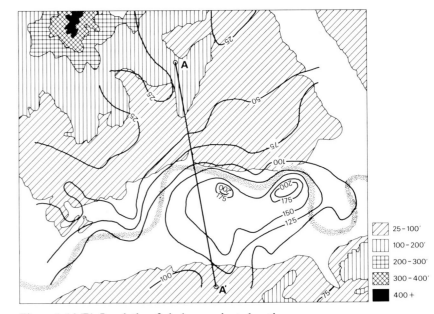

Figure 1.14 (B) Isopleths of cholera against elevation

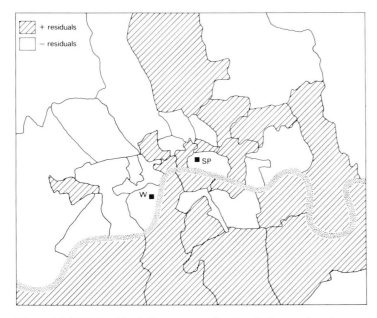

Figure 1.14 (C) Residuals from regression for cholera – elevation model

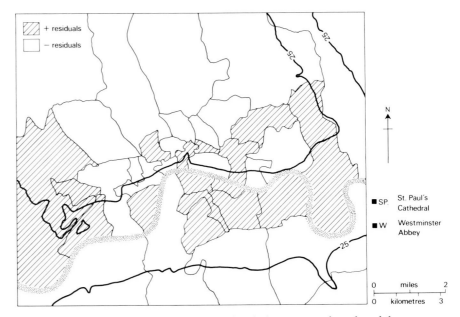

Figure 1.14 (D) Residuals from regression for cholera – water board model

the following explanatory variables were specified. Let

$x_1 = 1$ if the registration district was served by the Southwark and Vauxhall or Lambeth Companies,
  $= 0$ otherwise;
$x_2 =$ as x_1, but for the Kent Company;
$x_3 =$ as x_1, but for the East London Company;
$x_4 =$ as x_1, but for the Chelsea Company;
$x_5 =$ as x_1, but for the New River Company;
$x_6 =$ as x_1, but for the West Middlesex Company.

Then

$$\log y = 1.17 + \underset{(4.76)}{1.013x_1} + \underset{(4.19)}{1.030x_2} + \underset{(2.90)}{0.623x_3}$$
$$+ \underset{(2.35)}{0.528x_4} + \underset{(1.99)}{0.418x_5} + \underset{(0.88)}{0.217x_6}, R^2 = 0.71.$$
$$(1.14.2)$$

The values for t given in brackets and the signs of the coefficients imply, at the 99 percent significance level in a 1-tailed test, a positive relationship between death rates and districts supplied by the Southwark and Vauxhall, Lambeth, Kent and East London Companies. The water company variables account for 71 percent of the district to district variability in death rates. Although the results are not so unambiguous as those for equation (1.14.1), it is noteworthy that x_1, which represents the Southwark and Vauxhall and Lambeth Companies, is the most significant explanatory variable. These companies supplied most of the area south of the Thames which, as Figure 1.6 shows, experienced the highest rates of mortality.

Following exactly the procedure used to construct map (C), map (D) shows the residuals from (1.14.2). Positive residuals denote registration districts in which the death rate from cholera was underpredicted by the water company factor. It will be seen that these districts lie mainly in the floodplain of the River Thames within the 25 foot contour. We thus see the interplay of both factors – defective drainage and source of water supply – in accounting for the geographical distribution of cholera deaths. This suggests that a regression relationship using both factors might be fitted. If all the x variables defined in equations (1.14.1) and (1.14.2) are used in this fashion, an R^2 value of 0.80 is obtained. This is better than with either factor alone.

Sources and Further Reading

The sources for the maps of cholera data are as set out in Figure 1.3 of this Atlas.

The elements of regression modelling are described in standard statistical texts; see, for example, G.W. Snedecor and W.G. Cochran (1980), *Statistical Methods*, seventh edition, Ames, Iowa: Iowa State University Press, pp.149–74. An elementary introduction in a medical context is given in T.D.V. Swinscow (1983), *Statistics at Square One* (articles published in the British Medical Journal), eighth edition, London: British Medical Journal.

Advanced methods are covered in N.R. Draper and H. Smith (1981), *Applied Regression Analysis*, second edition, New York: John Wiley. For computational methods see B.F. Ryan, B.L. Joiner and T.A. Ryan (1985), *Minitab Handbook*, second edition, Boston: Duxbury Press, pp.218–59.

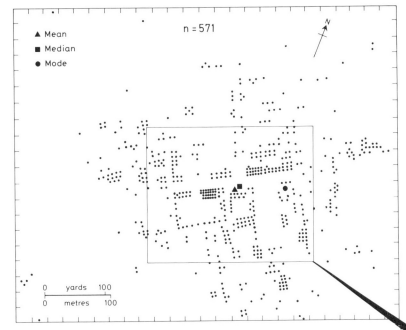

Figure 1.15 (A) Distribution of deaths on the map

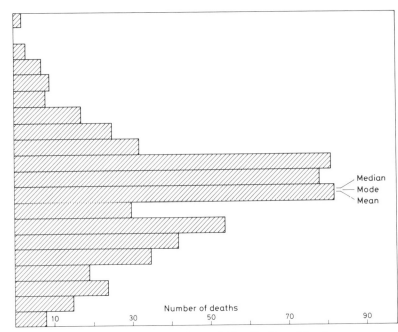

Figure 1.15 (B) Histogram of north-south distribution of deaths

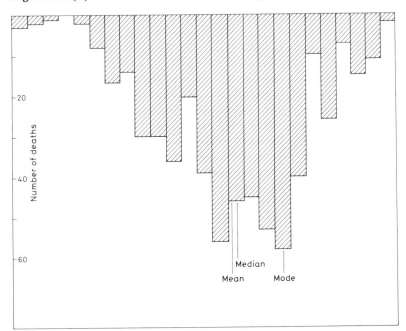

Figure 1.15 (C) Histogram of east-west distribution of deaths

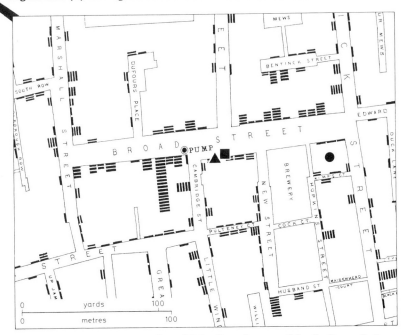

Figure 1.15 (D) Central section of John Snow's map of deaths from cholera in Soho, London, 1854

1.15 CENTRES OF MAP DISTRIBUTIONS

John Snow and the Soho cholera data

When examining the spatial distribution of some disease, it is frequently necessary to decide where the main centre of activity is located. To illustrate the way in which the *geographical centre* of an areal distribution can be calculated, we remain with the theme of deaths from cholera in Victorian London, but shift our focus from the epidemic of 1849 to that of 1854. This epidemic provided Snow with, as far as he was concerned, final proof of the water-borne nature of cholera although, as noted in Figure 1.1, he had established this as a working hypothesis in the latter part of 1848.

The geographical scale is reduced from that of the metropolis considered in earlier figures to a restricted area around the Broad Street pump in Soho. Of the conflagration, Snow himself wrote:

> The most terrible outbreak of cholera which ever occurred in this kingdom, is probably that which took place in Broad Street, Golden Square, and the adjoining streets, a few weeks ago. Within two hundred and fifty yards of the spot where Cambridge Street joins Broad Street, there were upwards of five hundred fatal attacks of cholera in ten days. The mortality in this limited area probably equals any that was ever caused in this country, even by the plague . . .   (Snow, 1854, p.38)

The outbreak began in the latter part of August 1854, with the real explosion of cases occurring on 31 August and 1 September. At the Middlesex Hospital, 128 cases were admitted in three days; 80 percent came from the Broad Street area, of whom two-thirds died. As soon as Snow "became acquainted with the situation and extent of this irruption of cholera, I suspected some contamination of the water of the much-frequented street-pump in Broad Street" (Snow, 1854, pp.38–9). In the terminology of this figure, Snow believed the geographical centre of the outbreak to be concentrated around one particular source of infection.

Measures of spatial centrality

Map (A) is taken from Snow's monograph and shows the locations of 571 deaths from cholera situated within a radius of about 250 metres of the Broad Street pump. The deaths are drawn as a point pattern with the underlying mesh of streets and dwellings omitted. Diagrams (B) and (C) are obtained directly from (A). In each, the numbers of deaths falling within a particular row or column of the lattice, as defined by the marginal ticks drawn round the perimeter of (A), are accumulated and plotted as histograms.

The concept of centrality in a spatial distribution can be described by three measures based on the elementary statistical parameters of the mean, the median and the mode. Computational formulae are given in the technical appendix to this figure. The position of each parameter is marked on the two histograms, (B) and (C). The location of the geographical centre, as defined by a particular parameter, is fixed at the intersection of the positions of the parameter in the row and column histograms. These are shown by the symbols on map (A). The mean and the median are relatively stable measures and are located within a few yards of each other; the mode is much more heavily affected by the shape of the histograms.

Spatial averages and the Broad Street pump

To emphasize this point, we have enlarged the central part of Snow's original map in (D). This shows that the locations of the spatial mean and median fall within a cricket pitch length of the offending pump. Although subsequent investigation revealed that the brickwork of the well sides was intact, the well drew its water from the base of gravel beds onto clay at a depth of 28–30 feet. 'The sewer, which passes [in the gravel] within a few yards of the well, is twenty-two feet below the surface' and contained 'the evacuations from the patients' (Snow, 1854, pp.52–3).

It is interesting to reflect that, had the measures of geographical centrality described here been available to Snow, they would have pointed unerringly to the probable source of the contaminated water.

Sources and Further Reading

The maps of cholera deaths are based on J. Snow (1854), *On the Mode of Communication of Cholera*, map with the second edition, London: Churchill Livingstone.

The various methods for establishing a centre for a geographic distribution are described in D.S. Neft (1966), *Statistical Analysis for Areal Distributions*, Monograph Series Number 2, Philadelphia: Regional Science Research Institute, University of Pennsylvania, and in R. Bachi (1963), 'Standard distance measures and related methods for spatial analysis', *Regional Science Association, Papers and Proceedings*, 10, pp.83–132. A further application of these methods is given in Figure 5.10 in this Atlas. These so-called 'centrographic methods' have been applied to a wide range of demographic phenomena; see for example the Russian examples in E.E. Sviatlovsky and W.C. Eels (1937), 'The centrographic method and regional analysis', *Geographical Review*, 27 pp. 240–54.

Technical Appendix

In the above analysis, the problem of determining the centre of an areal (two-dimensional) distribution has been tackled by fixing the centre at the intersection of the values of a particular parameter evaluated for two one-dimensional distributions. That is, the standard statistical formulae have been applied *separately* to the frequency distribution of deaths mapped first onto horizontal or x-axis of diagram (A) and then, second, to the frequency distribution of deaths mapped onto the vertical or y-axis of diagram (A). Let x_i denote the cartesian x-coordinate of the mid-point of class i of histogram (C), with a similar definition for y_i for histogram (B). Let f_i denote the number of deaths in class i. Then the locations of the means on the x- and y-axes, denoted by X and Y respectively are given by

$$X = \sum_i x_i f_i / \sum f_i$$
$$\text{and} \qquad (1.\,15.\,1)$$
$$Y = \sum_i y_i f_i / \sum f_i.$$

In computing the median for a histogram, we treat all deaths within a given class as though they are distributed at equal distances throughout the interval. Let the subscript i index the histogram class containing the median. Since the median is defined as the value which splits the number of deaths in the histogram in half, the median will be the $(N/2)$th observation, where N is the total number of deaths. Let (F_{i-1}) denote the cumulative frequency of deaths up to class $(i-1)$. Then, using M_x to denote the median of the x-axis histogram [diagram (C)], the computational formula is

$$M_x = l + [(N/2 - F_{i-1})/f_i] w_i \qquad (1.15.2)$$

with a similar definition for M_y, the median of the y-axis histogram [diagram (B)]. In equation (1.15.2), l denotes the lower limit of the class containing the median and w_i is the width of the interval containing the median.

The mode of a frequency distribution is simply defined as the class with the most number of deaths in it.

Matters become more complex if we treat an areal point pattern like that shown in diagram (A) two-dimensionally when locating the geographical centre,

rather than as two one-dimensional distributions. Let m_r represent the rth moment of an areal distribution evaluated with respect to any arbitrary location j on a map, where

$$m_r = \sum_k d_{jk}^r / N. \qquad (1.\,15.\,3)$$

In this equation, d_{jk} denotes the straight-line distance from j to each of the points k on the map, in addition to previously used notation. If there are f_k points located at k, then it will be necessary to weight the distances by the corresponding frequencies. The arithmetic mean centre of an areal distribution is the location of the minimum value of m_2 on the map. A suitable algorithm for finding this minimum-value location is given in Figure 5.10.

The median of an areal population is the location of the minimum value of m_1. This arises from the fact that, in a one-dimensional distribution, the median computed from equation (1.15.2) has the property that the sum of the absolute deviations of the values of the individuals in the frequency distribution from the median is at a minimum.

The mode is the high point of a surface constructed over the map.

Figure 1.15 (E) The John Snow public house at the corner of the present Broadwick and Lexington Streets, the site of the Broad Street pump.
(*Source*: Robinson, 1982, p.178)

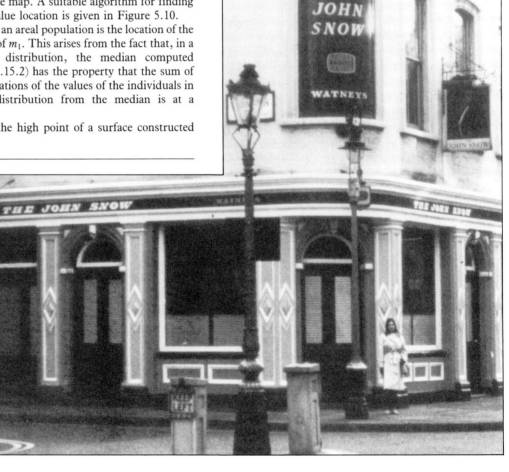

1.16 THIESSEN POLYGONS

Accessibility to a point source

It is often useful to be able to describe a population which is susceptible to a particular disease in terms of its access to a potential point source of that disease. Two such contemporary problems which have captured the popular imagination are the distribution of leukaemia deaths with respect to nuclear power stations (see Figure 3.8) and the possibility of a link between lung cancer and radon gas levels in dwellings (see Figure 3.9). Another, and very different example, in which the same general principle of access of a population to a point source is apparent, is the location of patients with respect to hospital facilities (see Figure 7.5).

The question of the degree of accessibility of any geographical area or population to a point source may be resolved using the method of *Thiessen polygons*. To illustrate the technique, we examine the geographical distribution of deaths from cholera in the Golden Square area of Soho, London, in August and September 1854 (see Figure 1.15). This outbreak, with its large and rapid mortality, was extensively studied by Dr John Snow as part of his classic work to demonstrate the water-borne nature of the disease. The basis of the method is outlined in diagram (A) which shows the distribution of water pumps in the area in relation to the street pattern as recorded by Snow on Map 1 of his monograph, *On the Mode of Communication of Cholera*. This map also gives the locations of the deaths from cholera in the area between 19 August and 30 September; an extract appears as Figure 1.15(D).

Snow believed the source of the outbreak was the pump located in Broad Street, whose water had become contaminated by excrement. The location of this pump is marked. His own words reveal that the question of access to this pump, as opposed to others in the area, was uppermost in his mind. The caption to Snow's map states: 'The situation of the Broad Street Pump is also indicated, as well as that of all the surrounding Pumps to which the public had access.'

If we assume that people generally visited the geographically nearest pump to obtain their drinking and cooking water then, under Snow's hypothesis, cholera deaths should be greater within the catchment area of the Broad Street pump than in the catchment areas of the other pumps. These *spheres of influence* of the pumps may be delimited by Thiessen polygons.

Procedure for constructing Thiessen polygons

The procedure for constructing the polygons is shown in diagram (B). Three steps are involved:

(a) lines are drawn joining a given pump to each adjacent pump;

(b) each of these inter-pump lines is bisected to give the midpoint of the line. The locations of these bisectors are shown by the ticks;

(c) from these midpoints, boundary lines are drawn at right angles to the original inter-pump lines to define a series of polygons.

The polygon around the Broad Street pump is shaded in diagram (B) and has been constructed in this way. Note that not all the midpoints on the inter-pump lines radiating from a particular pump are involved in this process.

The basic property of any Thiessen polygon is that it contains all the area of any map which is geometrically nearer to its point centre (here a particular pump) than it is to any other point centre on the map. The complete set of polygons around all of the pumps given on Snow's map is shown in diagram (C). The number of deaths within each is also recorded using Snow's data as mapped in Figure 1.15(A). The excess within the catchment area of the Broad street pump (348 as compared to the next largest of 64) is apparent.

Snow and the pump hypothesis

So far we have assumed that access to each pump was determined by 'crow-fly' distances. While the physical effort of carrying water meant that most people visited their nearest pump, recognition must be made of the complex street pattern in this area of London. Therefore in (D), the Thiessen polygons have been adjusted to take into account the patterns of access made possible by the street system shown in diagram (A). The modified polygons enclose areas which are closest to each pump in terms of street distance. The revised number of deaths within each has also been calculated. Again, the excess mortality in the catchment area of the Broad Street pump is evident.

Snow himself was sensitive to the influence of the street pattern upon accessibility. He wrote:

> With regard to the pump in Rupert Street [southeast of Broad Street], it will be noticed that some streets which are near to it on the map are in fact a good way removed, on account of the circuitous road to it. These circumstances being taken into account, it will be observed that the deaths either very much diminished, or ceased altogether, at every point where it becomes decidedly nearer to send to another pump than to the pump in Broad Street. It may also be noticed that the deaths are most numerous near to the pump where the

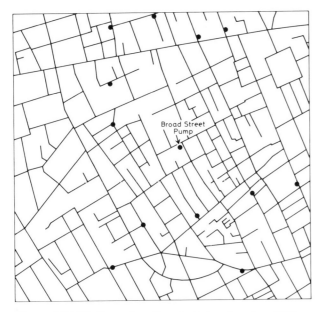

Figure 1.16 (A) Pump locations in Soho, London, 1854

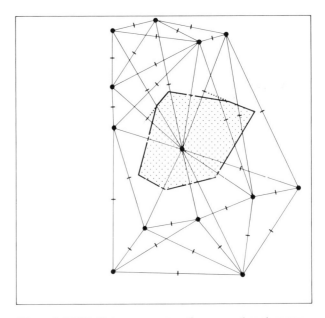

Figure 1.16 (B) Polygon construction around each pump

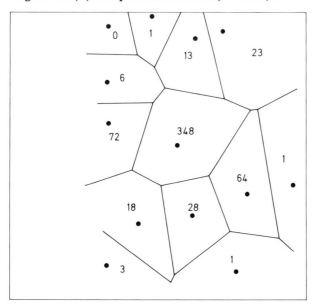

Figure 1.16 (C) Thiessen polygons (unadjusted)

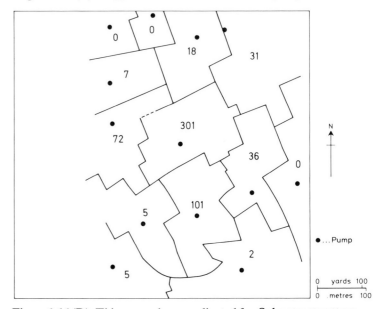

Figure 1.16 (D) Thiessen polygons adjusted for Soho street pattern

water could be more readily obtained. The wide open street in which the pump is situated suffered most, and next the streets branching from it, and especially those parts of them which are nearest to Broad Street.   (Snow, 1854, pp.46–7)

The proximity hypothesis occurred again in 1855 in a report by the Reverend Henry Whitehead, the curate of St Luke's, Berwick Street. Snow had presented Whitehead with his book on his investigations into the cause of cholera, but Whitehead was not convinced and wrote to Snow saying so. Whitehead then set out on his own enquiries and collected data which showed that, of those known to have drunk water from the Broad Street pump, 80 out of 137 contracted cholera while, among the non-drinkers, only 20 out of 299 succumbed. Whitehead also showed that the greatest contamination of the Broad Street pump water was on 31 August and that partial purification occurred by 3 September. This was followed by his most dramatic discovery. On 2 September, an infant whose attack of cholera began on 28 August died at 40 Broad Street. This house was nearest to the pump and the date of onset, allowing 24–36 hours incubation, matched the timing of the major outbreak (cf. Figure 1.15). The mother of the dead child had washed its napkins and emptied pails into the cesspool in front of the house, which was less than three feet from the pump well. Inspection of the brickwork of the cesspool showed decay and seepage with the well-known consequences. By this time, Whitehead had become a strong supporter of Snow. As a result of Snow's pressure on St James' Vestry, the Broad Street pump was disabled, contributing to the final extinction of an outbreak which was already past its peak.

Sources and Further Reading

The sources for the maps of cholera deaths are as in Figure 1.15 of this Atlas. See also the accounts in H. Whitehead (1856), *Report on the Outbreak of Cholera to St. James' Vestry, 1855*, and in M.R. Winterton (1980), 'The Soho cholera epidemic 1854', *History of Medicine*, 7, pp.11–20.

Methods of constructing Thiessen polygons are set out in D. Rhynsberger (1973), 'Analytic delineation of Thiessen polygons', *Geographical Analysis*, 5, pp.133–44; P. Haggett, A.D. Cliff and A.E. Frey (1977), *Locational Analysis in Human Geography*, second edition, London: Edward Arnold, pp.436–9; and R.J. Kopec (1963), 'An alternative method for the construction of Thiessen polygons', *Professional Geographer*, 15, pp.24–6. Ecological applications of Thiessen polygons are illustrated in E.C. Pielou (1969), *An Introduction to Mathematical Ecology*, New York: John Wiley/ Interscience, pp.140–56.

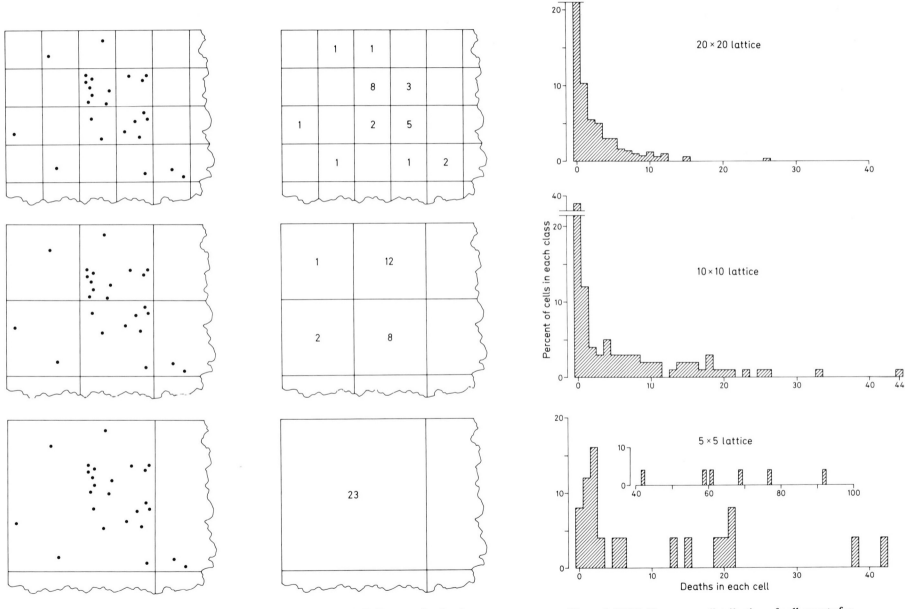

Figure 1.17 (A) Hypothetical distribution of deaths on map

Figure 1.17 (B) Cell counts for deaths mapped in (A)

Figure 1.17 (C) Frequency distribution of cell counts for John Snow's cholera map, 1854

1.17 REAL AND APPARENT CONTAGION

Real contagion

Many maps showing the geographical incidence of a disease as a point pattern appear to display 'clusters' when scanned by eye. The map of the distribution of deaths from cholera in the Broad Street area of London in 1854, depicted in Figure 1.15, provides an example. In the case of simple infectious diseases like measles, which are passed from person to person, these clusters are a real reflection of the transmission process involved. We may envisage some initial individual with the disease, called the parent, who passes the disease on to other susceptible individuals living nearby, called the offspring. Such a process will yield a cluster centre (the parent), surrounded by offspring whose geographical density will decline with increasing distance from the parent. The process described represents *real contagion* in the sense that the initial contact has been directly responsible for passing on the disease to others in subsequent generations.

Apparent contagion

If, however, we turn our attention to the distribution of cholera deaths in the Broad Street area of London as mapped by Snow, a different conceptualization is required. As shown in Figures 1.15 and 1.16, the point pattern of deaths is concentrated around the Broad Street pump. However, the contagion has not been produced by a straightforward person-to-person transmission process. Instead, as discussed in connection with Figures 1.15 and 1.16, spread occurred primarily through the intervention of contaminated water supply. In that the grouping is not primarily produced by person-to-person contact, but rather by spatial variation in some other factor, the pattern is described as bogus or *apparent contagion*. Geographically restricted areas of high and low levels of deaths will occur, reflecting spatial variations in the quality of the water supply. Areas with high death rates will appear visually as clusters embedded in areas with low death rates.

Process and point patterns

While the difference between real and apparent contagion can be appreciated for these examples because the underlying processes producing the patterns are well understood, for many geographical distributions of medical phenomena the generating processes are not properly identified. It is the task of the researcher to infer the process from the point pattern produced. That is, the researcher is attempting to reconstruct the causative mechanism from the end pattern displayed, rather than deciding the likely geographical result of a known disease process. In that many processes can produce the same end pattern (that is, they are *equifinal*), the difficulty of moving in the opposite direction, from pattern to process, can be appreciated and we need to recognize that errors may occur.

It was exactly this problem which faced investigators into the likely causes of cholera in the nineteenth century. Thus spurious correlations were found between cholera incidence and poverty-stricken parts of cities (and hence Divine retribution), foul air in low-lying areas, and so on. It so happened that the most decrepit areas of housing were associated with the poorest sanitation and drinking arrangements which were the root causes. Snow's theory was therefore regarded, at first, as yet another contender which partially fitted the observed patterns of deaths.

Cell-count observations

The series of diagrams which comprise this figure illustrate a related issue. The top part of diagram (A) shows part of a hypothetical point pattern of deaths, over which a regular lattice has been superimposed. The counts of the number of deaths in each cell or quadrat are given in the top part of diagram (B). The pattern displayed appears to be highly clustered. However, when cells are aggregated to form bigger quadrats, as in the second and third parts of diagrams (A) and (B), the apparently clustered point distribution disappears. Thus our ability to recognize clusters on a map in the first place is a function of the scale at which the process is studied.

This scale problem is illustrated further in (C). Snow's 1854 data, given in Figure 1.15(A), are used. The map was successively partitioned into 400, 100 and 25 rectangular cells using 20×20, 10×10 and 5×5 lattices. The frequency distribution of the number of cells with $0, 1, 2, \ldots$ deaths in them was constructed for each lattice and is shown in (C). The exponential decay in the cell frequencies for the 20×20 lattice is simple to interpret. Most cells have no deaths in them, while several have five or more; one has 26. Spatial clustering is implied but, without knowledge of the generating process, we could not be certain whether it is apparent or real. However, as cells are amalgamated to produce the 10×10 and 5×5 lattices, the frequency distributions lose their regularity and, by the time the 5×5 is reached, the spatial implications of the frequency distribution are difficult to determine.

Table 1.17.1   *Results of BW join count test on Snow's 1854 cholera map*

Statistical quantity	Lattice dimensions		
	20 × 20	10 × 10	5 × 5
BW	150.00	32.00	12.00
E(*BW*)	296.80	81.60	16.80
σ(*BW*)	10.84	6.01	2.49
Standard Normal score	−13.94	−8.25	−1.93

Clustering and contagion

This apparent yoking of our ability to distinguish 'clusters' to quadrat size is, however, paradoxically often our salvation in any attempt to distinguish real from apparent contagion. In general, true contagion implies small or tight clusters with point density falling off rapidly from cluster centres. As a result, the number of clusters overlapping quadrat boundaries is likely to be small. Conversely, apparent contagion usually implies that the mean point density will vary slowly over space in response to changes in the intervening factor. Then 'clusters' tend to cover much larger geographical areas and frequently cross quadrat boundaries. Thus the cell counts in neighbouring cells are likely to be highly correlated for a variety of cell sizes if the clustering is apparent rather than real. In the case of true contagion, high correlation will occur within, as opposed to between, clusters.

The *BW* join count procedure outlined in Figure 1.9 provides a suitable test of independence between neighbouring quadrats. This test was applied to Snow's map shown in Figure 1.15(A); 20 × 20, 10 × 10 and 5 × 5 lattices were used for comparability with diagram (C) of the present figure. A join was taken to exist between any pair of lattice cells if they shared a common

boundary, and the moments were evaluated under nonfree sampling. Cells were coded black, *B* if the number of deaths exceeded the average number per quadrat and white, *W* otherwise. The results of the analysis appear in Table 1.17.1. In all cases, a deficit of *BW* joins was detected at the 95 percent significance level in a 1-tailed test. The number of deaths in adjacent quadrats is not independent and so apparent contagion appears more plausible than true contagion on statistical grounds, which we know should be the case on aetiological grounds.

Sources and Further Reading

The distribution of cell values is based on John Snow's map described in Figure 1.15 of this Atlas.

The statistical questions of discriminating between real and apparent contagion are set out in A.D. Cliff and J.K. Ord (1981), 'The analysis of spatial point patterns', in *Spatial Processes: Models and Applications*, London: Pion, pp.86–117. See also A. Rogers (1974), *Statistical Analysis of Spatial Dispersion*, London: Pion, and the extensive bibliography in R.W. Thomas (1981), 'Point pattern analysis', in *Quantitative Geography*, edited by N. Wrigley and R.J. Bennett, London: Routledge and Kegan Paul, pp.164–76.

1.18 ISODEMOGRAPHIC BASE MAPS

Base maps

So far in this chapter we have been concerned with aspects of mapping on a geographical surface. A crucial property of such a surface is that a simple linear scale enables distances on the map to be equated with distances on the globe. Data have been plotted on base maps showing both administrative areas (such as the registration districts of London and the service areas of the metropolitan water companies in 1849) and subareas formed by partitioning a map with a regular lattice of cells. In all cases the spatial extent of the map and its subdivisions have formed a well-known, fixed matrix against which variability in disease incidence has been measured.

However, for some mapping problems it may be appropriate to use an alternative, non-geographical, metric to form the base map. One approach is through the use of isodemographic maps (from the Greek words *isos* meaning equal and *demos* meaning people). Here the areal extent of the districts or cells on the map is made proportional to the population size of the unit rather than to its geographical area. The procedure by which an isodemographic map is created is illustrated in the present figure using data on the number of deaths from cholera in the 34 registration districts of London in the epidemic of 1849. These data have already been plotted as a dot map on a conventional geographical base in Figure 1.3(B). The same data are replotted here on an isodemographic base.

Procedure for constructing isodemographic base maps

In diagram (A), the 34 registration districts shown in Figure 1.3(A) have been mapped as their nearest regular equivalents; district boundary lines have been replaced by straight-line segments and all bends are through 90 degrees. An identity number has been assigned to each district and the population, in thousands, of each is also given. For expository purposes, we focus upon the central area of map (A) which is delimited by the pecked line. This has been redrawn at a larger scale in diagram (B, I). The steps involved in the construction of the isodemographic base are:

(a) Select an appropriate size of cell to represent the units of population. Thus in diagram (B, II) we have chosen one cell to represent a population of 4000. This enables compact shapes to be drawn to represent larger population units.

(b) Using the compact shapes so defined and the population values of the registration districts given in diagram (A), a basic map of the central area shown in diagram (B, I) has been constructed as diagram (B, III). The compact shapes do not 'pack' properly so that, unlike a real map, holes are left at some locations where the demographic units meet. These areas have been shaded in (B, III). Note that the demographic units in (B, III) have been drawn in such a way that all the abutments of the registration districts on the original map, (B, IV), have been preserved.

(c) The map shown in diagram (B, III) is then adjusted so that all abutments are still preserved but the shapes of individual demographic units are changed to fill in all the gaps left in (B, III). The resulting configuration appears in diagram (B, IV).

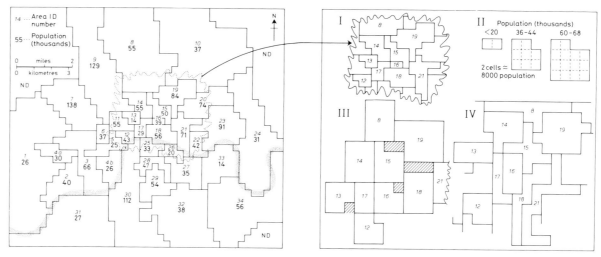

Figure 1.18 (A) District populations

Figure 1.18 (B) Stages in matching district area to district population

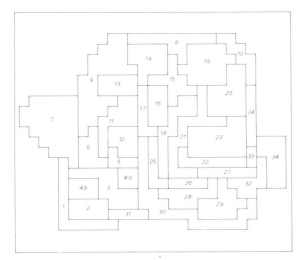

Figure 1.18 (C) Isodemographic base map

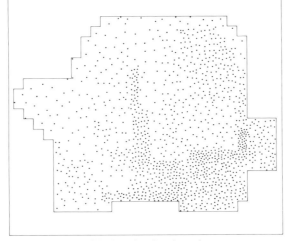

Figure 1.18 (D) Cholera deaths plotted on isodemographic base map

Isodemographic map of mid nineteenth-century London

The steps outlined above may be applied to the complete set of districts comprising the original base of diagram (A). The resulting isodemographic map appears in diagram (C). Comparison of maps (A) and (C) shows that area 10, for example, which is geographically very large on the conventional map (A) is relatively small in extent on the isodemographic map (C). Area 11 provides an example of the opposite case. One other striking feature of map (C) compared with map (A) is that many of the registration districts have become very long and thin. This is a common feature of isodemographic maps, especially near the margins, and arises from the need to pack the units properly while at the same time preserving the abuttments.

The number of deaths from cholera in the registration districts mapped as a point pattern in Figure 1.3(B) have been mapped onto the isodemographic base in diagram (D). The same scale of one dot to represent ten deaths has been used. Comparison of Figure 1.3(B) with diagram (D) shows that, while some concentration of deaths is still apparent in the southern part of the map, the density is not nearly so marked now that population extent has been allowed for.

A second example of an isodemographic map appears in diagram (E). This shows the counties of England and Wales in the early 1960s both as a conventional map and in their isodemographically equivalent form. As with the London example, the marked lineation of some of the demographic units, particularly on the west coast, is evident.

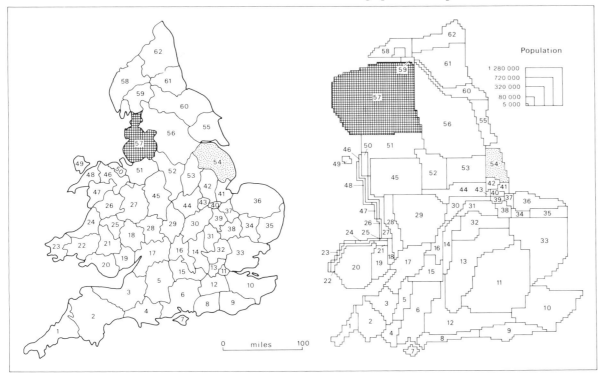

Figure 1.18 (E) Conventional and isodemographic county base maps for England and Wales

Sources and Further Reading

The sources for the maps of cholera data are as set out in Figure 1.3 of this Atlas.

An early example of a medical application of isodemographic maps is F. Forster (1966), 'Use of a demographic base map for the presentation of areal data in epidemiology', *British Journal of Preventive and Social Medicine*, 20, pp.156–71. Isodemographic maps are also used in a study of the spread of influenza in J.M. Hunter and J.C. Young (1971), 'Diffusion of influenza in England and Wales', *Annals of the Association of American Geographers*, 61, pp.637–53, from which diagram (E) is redrawn. See also a sub-continental application in L. Skoda and J. C. Robertson (1972), *Isodemographic Map of Canada*, Ottawa: Lands Directorate, Department of the Environment.

CHAPTER TWO

DATA SOURCES AND PROBLEMS

Figure over   Epidemiological sources

CENTERS FOR DISEASE CONTROL

MMWR

MORBIDITY AND MORTALITY WEEKLY REPORT

May 1, 1981 / Vol. 30 / No. 16

Epidemiologic Notes and Reports

Community-Acquired Methicillin-Resistant
Staphylococcus aureus Infections — Michigan

Ninety-eight patients have been hospitalized in medical center hospitals in Detroit, Michigan, since June 1980 in the first reported outbreak of community-acquired methicillin-resistant* *Staphyloccus aureus* (MRSA) infection. Nearly one-fourth of all *S. aureus* isolates from patients with invasive disease at 1 inner-city hospital have been methicillin resistant (Figure 1), and patients with MRSA infections continue to be admitted to Detroit area hospitals. Of the 98 patients discussed in this report, 96 had a history of intravenous heroin use.

*In this investigation, methicillin resistance was defined as either the failure of a 1-μg oxacillin disc to inhibit growth of *S. aureus* isolates in disc-diffusion tests *or* a broth-dilution minimal inhibitory concentration of >4 μg/ml.

FIGURE 1. Community-acquired *Staphylococcus aureus* at a Detroit receiving hospital, July-December 1980

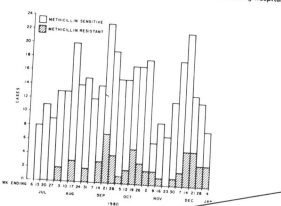

U.S. DEPARTMENT OF HEALTH AN...

ANNUAL SUMMA...
Issued September

CENTER FOR DISEASE CONTROL

MALARIA
SURVEILLANCE

TABLE OF CONTENTS

Heilbrigðisskýrslur
1978-79

Public Health in Iceland
With an English Summary

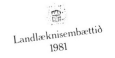

Landlæknisembættið
1981

Communicable
Diseases
Intelligence

ISSN 0725 - 314...

Bulletin number 88/1
Issue date: 18 January 1...

Contents:

TB and AIDS in New York (...
Japanese encephalitis — S...
Human salmonellosis surve...
Australia 4th quarter...
Notifiable diseases.

Editor Dr I.F. Cook
Asst. Editor L. Keo

...ng Scheme

...1 from Victoria, 4 from
...national exposure

EPIDEMIC OBSERVATION UNIT

OF THE

ROYAL COLLEGE OF GENER...

1975 - 1978

continuous morbidity obs...

Office of
Population
Censuses &
Surveys

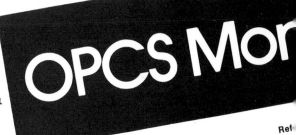

OPCS Mo...

Re...

Registrar General's Weekly Return for England and...

Week ended 26 DECEMBER 1986

CONTENTS

DATA SOURCES AND PROBLEMS

INTRODUCTION

One of the biggest single difficulties faced when trying to map disease data are their variable reliability over both space and time. There are several aspects to this problem.

First, there is the need to ensure that, when a particular disease is referenced in a statistical source, all the different countries in the international community are describing the same phenomenon. To this end, the International Classification of Diseases (ICD) has been developed, and Figure 2.1 examines the complex but common structure for disease reporting that it provides.

Second, despite the existence of this international list, enormous spatial variations in data quality still persist. Some of these variations can be attributed to country-by-country differences in the procedures employed to assemble disease data for international reporting. So we next examine the nature of disease statistics, the collecting methods (Figure 2.2), the variability from country to country in the resulting information (Figure 2.3), and the means by which the data can be cross-checked using multiple sources (Figure 2.4).

Third, even those data which have been meticulously gathered differ in ways which reflect the geographical location, year of collection and demographic characteristics of the population being described. Some diseases are found mainly in the tropics, some affect mainly younger populations, others are diseases of age, or relate to a particular occupation. Thus, when

interpreting data which have been amassed in different parts of the world, it is important to standardize the information to correct for these differences; aspects of the data standardization problem are considered in Figures 2.5–2.7.

Fourth, when disease data relating to a particular geographical location are examined over time, it commonly happens that the time-series is incomplete, with missing observations for some time periods. In the same way, when inter-area comparisons are made, observations may be absent or else complicated by changes in the boundaries of areas from one time period to another. Sometimes areas are split, sometimes amalgamated. If sensible inter-regional comparisons are to be made, we need to develop procedures both to interpolate the missing values and to correct for such boundary changes. Data 'cleaning' methods are a frequent prerequisite of the analytical techniques presented in Chapters 3–5, and we examine two of these, the missing data and boundary change problems, in Figures 2.8–2.11.

Fifth, changes in disease data need to be assessed in terms of a reference or an 'at risk' population. Such populations are constantly changing in both time and space and, in Figure 2.12, we illustrate these changes for the country which is used as an example in many of the plates of this Atlas, namely Iceland.

2.1 DISEASE CLASSIFICATION

Historical development of disease classification

The disease which formed the subject of the opening chapter of the Atlas was cholera. Cholera also happens to be the first disease in the International Classification of Diseases and it possesses the indicator, ICD 001. All diseases in the list carry a distinctive number; thus measles is ICD 055.

The ICD list was devised to promote international comparability in the categories under which information about disease mortality and morbidity is reported to the World Health Organization (WHO). The history of the ICD may be traced to classifications proposed by William Farr and Marc d'Espine. In 1855, a classification of 138 rubrics suggested by these two authors was adopted by the first International Statistical Congress (ISC). This initial attempt produced a grouping of diseases by anatomical site. Subsequently, Jacques Bertillon revised the classification, taking into account the similar classifications used in England, Germany and Switzerland.

The International Statistical Institute (ISI), the successor to the ISC, adopted the revised classification in 1893 and strongly encouraged its use by member countries in order to promote comparability in cause of death statistics. Under French guidance, the first International Conference for the Revision of the Bertillon or International Causes of Death was held in Paris in 1900. From then on, a revision Conference was held in each decade in order to update the Bertillon classification.

The early twentieth century work established that the International Classification of Diseases, as it has become known, refers to aetiology rather than just to site or manifestation. The major goals of the decennial review are to promote international comparability in cause of death statistics while maintaining a classification which uses current levels of medical knowledge as the criteria for including specific detailed codes or rubrics.

The Sixth Decennial Revision Conference was held in 1948 under the auspices of the World Health Organization which had been given responsibility for the revision of the classification. This meeting made a fundamental change in the gathering of international information on disease by defining the concept of underlying cause of death, by expanding the content of the classification to include both mortality and morbidity, and by initiating a programme of international cooperation in vital and health statistics. Although subsequent revisions have changed the ICD in a variety of ways, cause of death statistics since the sixth revision have been characterized by continuity.

Structure of the ICD table

The 1975 (ninth) revision is the current revision of the ICD and its broad form is illustrated in Figure 2.1. It consists of 17 main groups and each specific disease is given a three digit code identifying its aetiology. In the interests of greater specificity, however, more detail is pro-

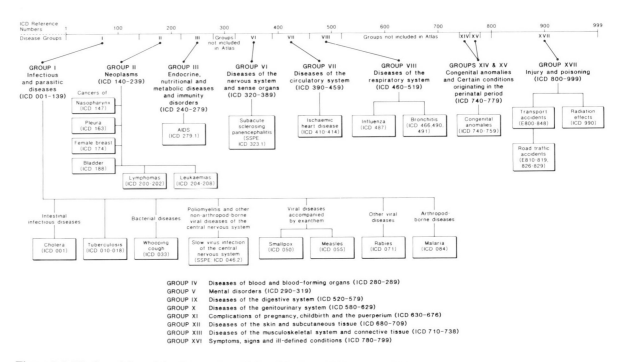

GROUP IV   Diseases of blood and blood-forming organs (ICD 280-289)
GROUP V   Mental disorders (ICD 290-319)
GROUP IX   Diseases of the digestive system (ICD 520-579)
GROUP X   Diseases of the genitourinary system (ICD 580-629)
GROUP XI   Complications of pregnancy, childbirth and the puerperium (ICD 630-676)
GROUP XII   Diseases of the skin and subcutaneous tissue (ICD 680-709)
GROUP XIII   Diseases of the musculoskeletal system and connective tissue (ICD 710-738)
GROUP XVI   Symptoms, signs and ill-defined conditions (ICD 780-799)

Figure 2.1 Ninth revision of the *International Classification of Diseases* (ICD) to show grouping of the diseases studied in this Atlas

vided in the ninth revision than in earlier versions by adding a fourth and sometimes a fifth digit to the code. For example, the emergence of AIDS since the 1975 revision has been handled, as shown in Figure 2.1, by coding the disease as 279.1; 279 denotes disorders involving the immune mechanism, which are located in the general group of endocrine, nutritional and metabolic diseases and immunity disorders (240–279). In addition, manifestation of disease may also be identified for the first time with the ninth revision, but it is not used to code cause of death.

Group I of the list covers all infectious and contagious diseases, Group II all neoplasms, Group III endocrine, nutritional and metabolic diseases and immunity disorders, and so on. Apart from Groups I (infectious and parasitic diseases), V (mental disorder), XI (complications of pregnancy, childbirth and the puerperium), XIV (congenital anomalies), XV (certain conditions originating in the perinatal period), XVI (symptoms, signs and ill-defined conditions), the groups generally classify disease according to anatomical site affected. The increasing urbanization and industrialization of society has produced very many more ways of being injured or dying – in accidents, from inadvertent poisoning and so on – so that group XVII (injury and poisoning) has been extended by the provision of a supplementary classification, prefixed by the letter E, of External causes of injury and poisoning.

Problems of comparability and complexity

Although every effort is made in the periodic revisions of the ICD list to maintain continuity of definitions, revisions required by increases in medical knowledge do result in lack of comparability. Thus inter-area comparisons (see Chapter 3) can be affected because different countries may adopt the new classification at different dates. Comparability over time may not be straightforward for some diseases that are studied as a time-series (see Chapter 4) if the time-series spans several revisions of the list. These difficulties affect our ability to analyse data. Changes in the list also produce time changes in the quality of the data collected. In principle, the data might be expected to become more refined and accurate the more recent they are. But the more refined the classification becomes, the greater is the need for expert clinical diagnosis of the cause of death. Throughout the developing world, few deaths occur in the presence of a doctor. Because the ICD contains many diagnoses that cannot readily be identified by a non-medical person, use of the level of detail implied by the full list can reduce inter-area comparability, particularly between countries where the level of medical services differs widely. Some of these problems are reviewed by Brockington (1975).

Adapted Mortality List

To go some way towards meeting these problems of comparability and complexity, a much coarser classification known as the Adapted Mortality List (AML), consisting of 55 mutually exclusive categories, was produced in conjunction with the ninth revision. The AML has substantial overlap by design with the 50-category abbreviated List B produced in conjunction with the eighth revision. Both are tied into the full ninth revision so that, with care, reasonably comparable data between countries for many diseases can be constructed going back over some 20 years. Exceptions can be found. Thus in List B, causes of death due to tuberculosis (B5 and B6) included late effects of tuberculosis, while in the AML (class AM4) these are excluded so that,

superficially, deaths due to tuberculosis will appear to be in decline in areas where they have been constant.

In the remainder of this book, the current ICD classification of every disease discussed is given. The range of diseases covered may be seen from Figure 2.1 where each disease considered at some point in the book has been listed and its relation to the subgroup and group within which it is classified shown.

Sources and Further Reading

The full ICD list containing detailed comments on comparability with earlier revisions is published by the World Health Organization as *Manual of the International Statistical Classification of Diseases, Injuries and Causes of Death*, ninth edition, Geneva. See also K. Kupka (1978), 'International classification of diseases, ninth revision', *WHO Chronicle*, 32, pp.219–25. The role of WHO in health statistics is evaluated in F. Brockington (1975), *World Health*, third edition, Edinburgh: Churchill Livingstone, pp.213–88. See also R.M. Acheson, editor (1965), *International Comparability in Epidemiology*, Washington, DC: Milbank Memorial Foundation. Sources of demographic and related statistics are reviewed in P. Wasserman and J. O'Brien (1983), *Statistics Sources: A Subject Guide*, eighth edition, Detroit, Mich.: Gale Research.

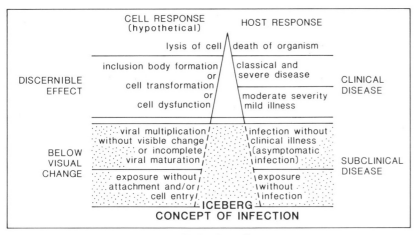

Figure 2.2 (A) 'Iceberg' concept of infectious diseases

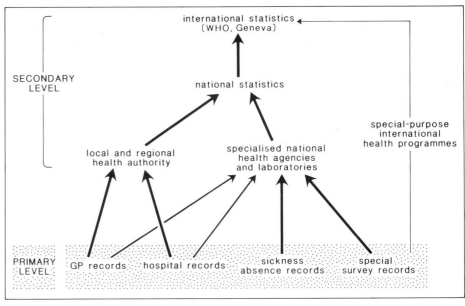

Figure 2.2 (C) Primary and secondary data collection networks

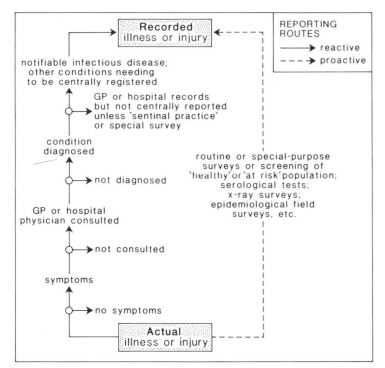

Figure 2.2 (B) Morbidity reporting at the primary level

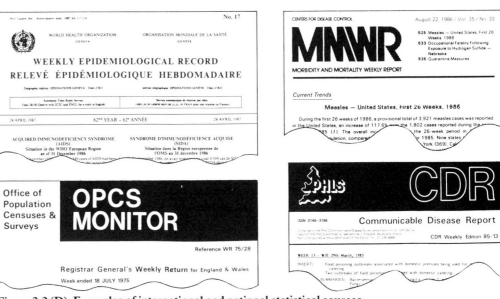

Figure 2.2 (D) Examples of international and national statistical sources

2.2 DISEASE STATISTICS I: COLLECTING NETWORKS

The maps which form the plates in this Atlas are all based on disease statistics – numerical values of the occurrence of illness, injury or death – which vary strikingly in their reliability over both time and space. Thus in the previous chapter we outlined a wide range of cartographic techniques for the display and analysis of cholera data relating to mid nineteenth-century London, but we did not address the issue of how these data were gathered nor their degree of reliability.

An understanding of the methods by disease data are compiled and the potential sources of error is a necessary prerequisite to their proper analysis. Each data set presents its own special problems, but we can appreciate their general nature by examining the way in which international disease statistics are assembled.

Disease and the individual

A wide gap and a complex reporting network separate the reality of a disease distribution from the statistics which appear at the international level. At the bottom of the reporting pyramid is the individual suffering illness or injury at a particular time and place; whether or not this event will ever appear as a number in international statistics depends on many factors.

As diagram (A) shows for infectious diseases, the human response to disease may be pictured as an 'iceberg'. At the tip is death of the cell or of the organism itself; below that clinically recognizable disease occurs, while below that again are subclinical attacks with no recognisable effects.

For viral diseases, Evans (1984, p.20) shows that the estimated subclinical:clinical ratio varies from 1000:1 (for example, poliomyelitis) through 2:1 (for example, rubella) to 0:100 (for example, rabies). Whether a patient with clinical symptoms seeks medical help depends on the severity of the disease and the culture of the individual; ability to seek help may depend on a complex of factors in which the availability or absence of doctors, their location with respect to the patient, and the economics of medical care all play some part.

Recording at the primary level

As chart (B) shows, a clear distinction must be drawn between the actual pattern of morbidity in a population and the recorded morbidity. The left-hand path describes a *reactive* process in which an individual may present himself to a physician (either in a general practice, a clinic or a hospital) and in which a particular condition may be diagnosed and reported. The critical link in the reporting chain is the individual physician or paramedic who diagnoses a clinical illness. While records will normally be kept as part of the confidential files of the practice, clinic, or hospital, only some of these observations will find their way into published statistical records. Some infectious diseases are *notifiable* and some non-infectious conditions must be *registered*. The quality of the data record for the various diseases will depend on many factors: the complexity of the disease, the diagnostic skill of the physician, the case load of other clinical work, and so on. Diagnosis may be uncertain (especially without expensive laboratory confirmation). Finally, lack of secretarial help or time may further reduce the reporting level even for required diseases. For example, Marier (1977) found that reporting rates for Washington DC hospitals varied from 50 percent (meningococcal meningitis) to 11 percent (tuberculosis).

The right-hand path in (B) shows a *proactive* path in which screening or survey of a 'healthy' or 'at risk' population may reveal diseases either unrecognized by the individual or for which medical advice was not sought. This part of the flow-chart represents a supplementary source to mainstream reporting (on the left). It includes serological surveys, routine X-rays, hospital and medical care statistics, absentee records (both from work and school), cancer registries, panels of cooperating physicians, screening programmes, and so on. The detailed monitoring carried out under schemes like the Virus Watch Programs established in New York City and Seattle (Cooney, Hall and Fox, 1970) indicates that considerably more disease activity occurs than actually finds its way into the 'mainstream' statistics network.

Secondary statistical networks

Above the primary recording level, in which morbidity or mortality is noted by a physician, is the secondary reporting network illustrated in diagram (C). Part of that network is geographically based, with local or regional medical offices forming an important intermediate tier in the data-collecting hierarchy. For example, in the United States, each of the fifty states has a State Epidemiological Service which collects and publishes periodic statistics; below that, the 3,000 counties have a responsible medical officer to whom certain morbidity and mortality statistics are reported. Alongside this geographically based system stand the specialist national agencies (for example, the cancer registries and national virological laboratories) through which certain records are chanelled.

At the top of the national hierarchy appear the specialist statistical bureaux. A typical example is the United States whose Centers for Disease

Control (CDC) in Atlanta, Georgia, publishes the *Morbidity and Mortality Weekly Report* (MMWR) shown in diagram (D). The weekly tables and reports in MMWR are supplemented both by *Annual Supplements* on notifiable diseases within the United States and by irregular *Surveillance Reports* on individual diseases (for example, measles, hepatitis, infectious mononucleosis). Further vital statistics are reported by other national agencies such as the National Center for Health Statistics at Hyattsville, Maryland.

In the United Kingdom, a parallel set of reports is published by the Office of Population Census and Surveys (OPCS), the Centre for Communicable Diseases [see diagram (D)] and the Department of Health and Social Security (DHSS). British health statistics are fully described by Alderson (1974).

International statistics

The main international source for world disease statistics is the World Health Organization (WHO) established by the United Nations in 1948. Its several objectives (the eradication of epidemic, endemic and other diseases; the improvement of nutrition, housing, sanitation and other aspects of environmental hygiene; the promotion of maternal and child health; and the promotion of research in the fields of private and public health) each generate a welter of statistical information.

Like the national agencies, WHO provides a wide range of information and data on disease incidence. A basic source is the WHO *Weekly Epidemiological Record*; see diagram (D). This publication is supplemented by the monthly *Epidemiological and Vital Statistics Report* and the multi-volumed *World Health Statistics Annual*.

Before World War II similar, though less complete records were published by its predecessor, the Health Office of the League of Nations. A parallel role to that of WHO is played by certain regional organizations for limited continental areas; the *Weekly Epidemiological Report* published by the Pan American Health Organisation (PAHO) is a case in point.

As diagram (C) has shown, the global surveillance of disease is articulated by WHO from its headquarters in Geneva and through its regional offices. Data and qualitative information from member countries are collected and then redistributed worldwide, both through its publications and through telex and computer links. The on-line and weekly WHO statistics are, to use a meteorological analogy, akin to daily weather reports which serve immediate roles in forecasting and control, while the monthly and annual volumes provide the equivalent of climatic statistics. Volume II of the WHO *World Health Statistics Annual* contains a summary of reportable diseases in terms of notified cases and deaths officially returned to WHO by individual countries. These figures are broken down by time into quarterly, monthly or four-weekly periods; their use is illustrated in Chapter 4.

As WHO stresses, these statistics are supplied by national members, and the international statistics are dependent for completeness and accuracy upon the quality and coverage of the national records. As Figure 2.3 will show for measles and influenza, that record may vary greatly from one country to another.

Thus what finally appears in the international statistics is an incomplete and fragmentary part of the reality of disease in the world population. At each stage in the data-collecting process, filters intervene to reduce the full flow of information upwards through the hierarchy.

Sources and Further Reading

Diagram (A) is from A.S. Evans, editor (1984), *Viral Infections of Humans*, second edition, New York: Plenum, Figure 2, p.20.

Critical reviews of the value of the WHO statistics as a data source are given periodically in the WHO's *World Health Statistics Report*. The pattern of health statistics reporting in the United Kingdom is described and critically assessed in M. Alderson (1974), *Central Government Routine Health Statistics*, London: Heinemann for Royal Statistical Society and Social Science Research Council (Vol. 2, no. 3, *Reviews of United Kingdom Statistical Sources*, edited by W.F. Maunder), and in M. Alderson and R. Dowie (1979), *Health Surveys and Related Studies*, Oxford: Pergamon for Royal Statistical Society and Social Science Research Council (Vol. 9, no. 16, *Reviews of United Kingdom Statistical Sources*, edited by W.F. Maunder.)

A wide range of epidemiological records is discussed in B. Benjamin, editor (1980), *Medical Records*, second edition, London: Heinemann. An example of special virological surveys is M.K. Cooney, C.E. Hall and J.P. Fox (1970), 'The Seattle Virus Watch Program', *American Journal of Public Health*, 60, pp.1456–65.

2.3 DISEASE STATISTICS II: GLOBAL VARIATIONS

Frequency of disease

Two measures of the frequency of disease in a specified population are normally calculated. *Incidence* is the number of instances of an event (for example, illness) *commencing* during a given time period. *Prevalence* is the number of instances of illness *without any distinction between new and old cases* (Brockington, 1975, p.246). Diagram (A) illustrates the application of these concepts to a hypothetical population, showing that prevalence may be defined either at a given point (such as at the beginning of a year) or over a given period (for example, during a year). The former is known as point prevalence and the latter as period prevalence.

Most of the data routinely published as time-series by the national and international collecting agencies relate to incidence and give, for example, the number of newly-occurring cases or deaths for different diseases in a given unit of time such as a month, and it is these data whose global variability we examine in this plate.

Attempts to measure incidence at the international level are undermined by geographical and time-based variations in the reporting of disease morbidity and mortality. While some countries (for example, Scandinavia) are remarkably thorough in their recording and have very high reporting rates of both disease morbidity and mortality, others have only fragmentary records. Although the deficiencies are particularly pronounced in the developing world, there are some surprising lacunae in the records of the developed nations. Since the pattern of reporting varies with each disease and from year to year, we illustrate these points here with reference to two infectious diseases, measles and influenza.

Spatial variability: measles morbidity

Measles (ICD 055) is discussed in a number of plates in the Atlas and its characteristics are described in Figure 3.3. It occurs throughout the world without any apparent relationship to the ethnic or genetic background of the population infected, or to the environment in which that population lives. It has been a notifiable disease in a few countries since the 1880s and in some places (for example, Denmark and Iceland) particularly complete historical records exist.

However, building up a picture of the worldwide incidence of the disease is made difficult because only a certain number make notification compulsory. This is evident from map (B) which shows by hatching the countries reporting the incidence of measles cases in 1970. There is an absence of records for much of Asia, while some countries with highly developed health services only note mortality from measles (for example, West Germany, Australia and New Zealand).

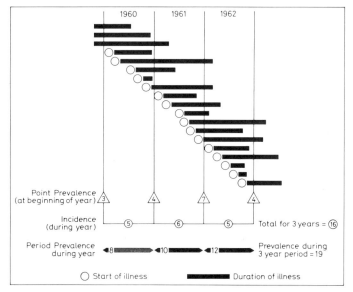

Figure 2.3 (A) Frequency of diseases in terms of incidence and prevalence

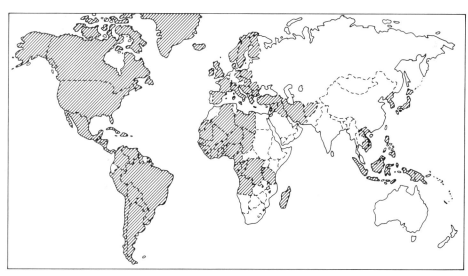

Figure 2.3 (B) Countries reporting measles morbidity to WHO in 1970

Such widespread geographical variation in the reporting pattern makes comparisons between countries very difficult. The problem is made more complex by the great differences, even among those countries collecting morbidity information, in the proportion of cases captured (see Figure 2.2). Thus in the United Kingdom, detailed clinical work by Stocks (1949) suggests that the reported cases are some 1½–2 times lower than the true figure. Similar work by Black (1966) on the relationship between number of reported cases and measles antibody levels as determined by titration in a sample of the resident population of 18 island communities led him to suggest that, at one extreme, in islands like Iceland and St Helena, the reporting rate was better than 40 percent of cases which actually occurred, while in islands like Guam and Bermuda it was less than 20 percent.

Temporal variability: influenza morbidity and mortality

Influenza (ICD 487) is discussed in section 6.4 of the Atlas and its characteristics are described there. Study of the international statistics for this disease reveals a picture as erratic in the time domain as that for measles in the spatial domain. The number of countries reported by WHO as recording influenza on a monthly basis from 1945 to 1977 averaged 95 a year for morbidity and 70 for mortality. As diagram (C) shows, the numbers have not been constant. For morbidity they range from a maximum of 124 countries in 1960 to a minimum of 48 in 1974. The number of countries reporting mortality data follows a generally similar time path to morbidity but at a lower level. Variations in the annual total of countries relate partly to the increase in the number of newly independent countries return-

ing information to WHO during the period and partly to gaps in the format and publishing programme of WHO's *World Health Statistics Annual* in the early 1970s.

The map in diagram (D) shows that there were only 16 countries around the world with more than thirty years of influenza morbidity reporting between 1945 and 1977; five in Europe, three each in the Pacific and Africa, two in Middle America, and one each in South America, West Asia and East Asia. For mortality, the coverage was poorer still; only four countries returned more than thirty years of data to WHO (Canada, England and Wales, Finland and France).

Thus, if we think of space as the weft and time as the warp of a space-time fabric, then it is evident that the threads are broken in many places. The many countries which have never made returns to WHO sever the weft and the missing observations in each country over time break the warp. Together, the resulting holes in the data matrix make the inter-regional and time-series comparison of morbidity and mortality data extremely complex.

Sources and Further Reading

See under Figure 2.4

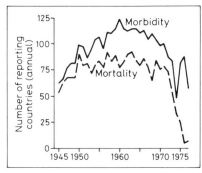

Figure 2.3 (C) Number of countries reporting influenza morbidity and mortality on a monthly basis to WHO

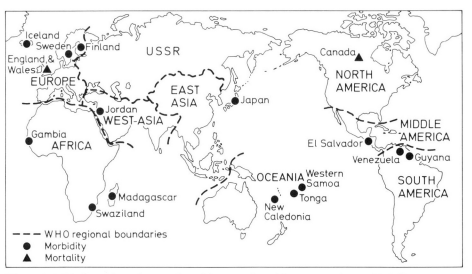

Figure 2.3 (D) Location of countries with more than thirty years of monthly influenza records

2.4 DISEASE STATISTICS III: MULTIPLE SOURCES

We have seen in Figures 2.2 and 2.3 some of the factors which contribute to the difficulties encountered when making comparisons of levels of disease morbidity and mortality between countries. These include places and times for which no data are recorded and, where information is available, marked under-recording of the prevalence of disease. A solution to the *missing data problem* is considered later in Figure 2.8. In the present plate, we show how multiple sources of data on a given disease may be used, when under-recording is suspected, to improve estimates of its prevalence.

The principles involved are illustrated by considering the measurement of influenza prevalence in the United Kingdom and the United States. This has proved much more difficult than for those infectious diseases such as measles with more clear-cut clinical signs. Influenza may lead to illnesses that are too slight to warrant medical attention and thus escape the medical record, or the illness may present symptoms which, though severe enough to call for medical attention, may be confused with those produced by other agents. At some times an influenza epidemic may so overwhelm medical personnel that recording becomes a minor priority. In addition many countries make no attempt to record the incidence of influenza morbidity.

Virus isolation in public health laboratories

Laboratory diagnosis of influenza depends on either (a) isolation and identification of the virus or (b) a rise in specific antibody titre between a serum specimen collected from the patient at the start of the disease and a specimen collected two or three weeks later. Virus isolation allows the antigenic character of particular influenza strains to be established, whereas serological tests provide a means of estimating the extent of virus infection in the community. The diagnostic procedures involved lie outside the scope of this Atlas but are discussed in full in the standard sources (Palmer *et al.*, 1975; Stuart-Harris *et al.*, 1985). Virus isolations are relatively expensive and are performed for only a minutely small fraction of the infected population. Isolations of influenza A and B viruses reported to the Epidemiological Research Laboratory, Colindale, England, over an eight-year period are shown in the top graph of (A). Note that, although the maximum number of isolates rarely exceeds 500 in any one week (about one for every 100,000 people in the resident population of Great Britain) the pattern of influenza outbreaks over time is very clearly shown.

Deaths

Influenza may be recorded on death certificates as a primary or as a secondary (associated) cause of death. The second graph of (A) shows the total number of deaths in England and Wales over an eight-year period; the association with peaks in virus isolations in 1969–70 and, to a lesser extent, in 1967–68 and 1972–73 is apparent.

Although influenza mortality must reflect in some way the prevalence of influenza in the community, the association is by no means a direct or simple one. Secondary complications of influenza can affect the cardiovascular and nervous systems as well as the lower respiratory tract. Increases in influenza may therefore show up in increased deaths from heart disease as well as in deaths from influenza and pneumonia. Thus, as long ago as 1847, Farr concluded that influenza attacks individuals with all sorts of diseases and terminates the life of many who are aged or chronically sick.

One approach to the problem of converting influenza mortality information into estimates of prevalence has been to try to identify severe epidemics of influenza through 'excess mortality'. Diagram (B) shows an application of this concept to weekly deaths attributed to pneumonia and influenza for 121 cities in the United States between 1976 and 1979. Two alternative models are illustrated. On the left graph, the curve for reported deaths is shown and, superimposed upon it, the expected curve and the epidemic threshold under a model proposed by Serfling (1963). From the graph, Serfling's model identifies excess deaths due to an influenza epidemic, and therefore above normal prevalence of influenza in the United States, in the first quarter of 1978. The right chart relates to a more sophisticated model developed by Choi and Thacker (1981). This plots the difference between the reported deaths from pneumonia and influenza and those which would be predicted on the basis of the model. Again a sharp peak indicates excess mortality (and so prevalence) from influenza in the first quarter of 1978.

The mathematical basis of these models is discussed in Cliff, *et al.* (1986, pp.20–22).

Morbidity records

In a few countries of the world, influenza is a notifiable disease and some information about prevalence can be gleaned from their published figures. A map of the countries with lengthy time-series of influenza morbidity appears earlier in Figure 2.3(D). But in the majority of countries, including the United Kingdom and the United States, where notification is not required, information of influenza morbidity has to be

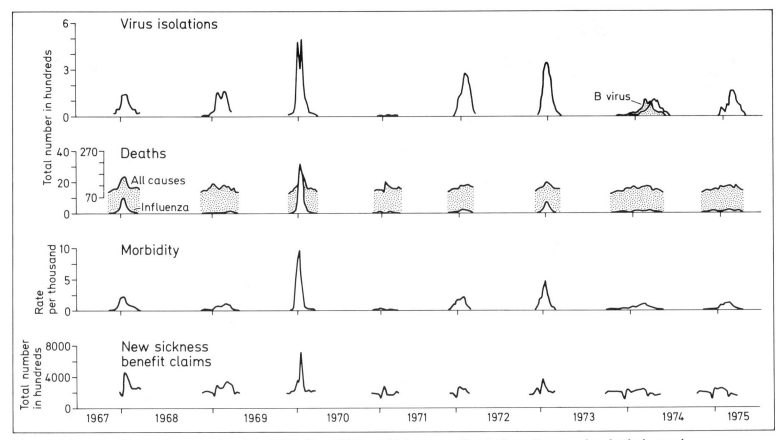

Figure 2.4 (A) Surveillance of influenza from July 1967 to June 1975 by multiple sources. Deaths from all causes given by the inset axis

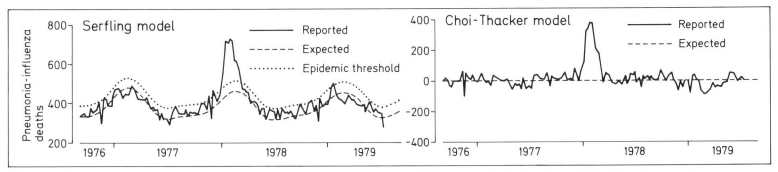

Figure 2.4 (B) Observed and expected weekly deaths attributed to pneumonia and influenza under the Serfling and Choi-Thacker models, United States, 1976–1979

derived from other sources.

In the United Kingdom an important indirect measure is obtained through 'sentinel practices'. A panel of general practitioners in different geographical regions of England and Wales notify the occurrence of cases of acute respiratory illness in their practice to the Epidemiological Research Unit of the Royal College of General Practitioners. The weekly totals of such returns are plotted for an eight-year period as the morbidity curve in (A). They give a sensitive index of influenza prevalence and can be further refined by tests on throat swabs from cases diagnosed as influenza. Similar sentinel practices exist in the United States.

Absentee records

A secondary measure of influenza morbidity shown on (A) is provided by the weekly data on new claims for sickness benefit in the working population as recorded in National Insurance returns. Although the sickness benefit claims are for all forms of illness, they also show a consistent seasonal increase in the winter half of the year. Large epidemics, such as that caused by the Hong Kong strain in 1969–70, stand out as major peaks in the sickness returns; small peaks coincide with the 1967–68 and 1972–73 epidemics.

Finally, we note that, in principle, useful local information could also be gained from school absence records but these are not preserved on a consistent national basis in the UK.

Informal records

In addition to the formal sources listed above, the progress of the disease may be caught by other non-medical sources. Newspaper accounts frequently highlight very severe peaks in an influenza epidemic with headlines such as 'Flu Sweeps West' or 'Local Schools Closed'. Individually, the value of such reports is limited, but collectively and particularly when subjected to quantitative analysis through such techniques as 'content analysis', they may yield useful results.

Conclusion

Each of the three main sources of information on influenza prevalence – virus isolations, excess mortality and morbidity – gives a partial and incomplete picture of the disease. Nevertheless, what is particularly striking about graph (A) is the consistency with which usually three of the four traces rise together in the years of major influenza epidemics such as 1969–70 and 1972–73. This enhances our confidence in recognizing these years as ones of large-scale influenza prevalence, even though any one source of information may be dubious as an indicator of excess prevalence when considered in isolation (for example, new sickness benefit claims in 1972–73). The success of the multiple source approach in identifying such years argues more generally for its use as a procedure for verifying levels of prevalence when single sources are deficient.

Sources and Further Reading

In Figure 2.3, diagram (A) is redrawn from F. Brockington (1975), *World Health*, third edition, Edinburgh: Churchill Livingstone, Figure 24.1, p.247. Geographical variations in patterns of reporting for measles are discussed in A.D. Cliff, P. Haggett, J.K. Ord and G.R. Versey (1981), *Spatial Diffusion: An Historical Geography of Epidemics in an Island Community*, Cambridge: Cambridge University Press, pp.40–6, from which Figure 2.3 (B) is taken. A parallel discussion for influenza appears in A.D. Cliff, P. Haggett and J.K. Ord (1986), *Spatial Aspects of Influenza Epidemics*, London: Pion, pp.88–96, from which Figures 2.3 (C) and (D) have been redrawn.

The degree of under-reporting in measles morbidity data in the United Kingdom is considered in P. Stocks (1949), *Sickness in the Population of England and Wales in 1944–47: Studies on Medical and Population Subjects, No. 2*, London: Her Majesty's Stationery Office. International variations are examined in F.L. Black (1966), 'Measles endemicity in insular populations: critical community size and its evolutionary implication', *Journal of Theoretical Biology*, 11, pp.207–11.

In Figure 2.4, diagram (A) is based on J.W.G. Smith (1976), *Surveillance of Influenza: Report of the Public Health Laboratory Service*, Epidemiological Research Laboratory, Colindale, London. Diagram (B) has been constructed from graphs in K. Choi and S.B. Thacker (1981), 'An evaluation of influenza mortality surveillance, 1962–79, 1: Time series forecasts of expected pneumonia and influenza deaths, 2: Percentage of pneumonia and influenza deaths as an indicator of influenza activity', *American Journal of Epidemiology*, 113, pp.215–26, 227–35.

The classic account of influenza is given in Sir Charles Stuart-Harris, G.C. Schild and J.S. Oxford (1985), *Influenza: The Viruses and the Disease*, third edition, London: Edward Arnold. See also the discussion in Section 6.4 of this Atlas.

2.5 STANDARDIZATION PROBLEMS I: GLOBAL VARIABILITY

One of the central problems in any Atlas which compares diseases on a world basis are the major contrasts in the overall pattern of morbidity and mortality between its major regions. We illustrate this by simply dividing the world's nations into two groups, the developed and the developing, based on standard United Nations definitions (see United Nations, 1980). Other and more complex divisions could, and should, be used but this binary split is sufficient to illustrate the general nature of a problem which is encountered in detail in many later parts of this Atlas.

Global variations by major cause of death

The bar charts in diagram (A) plot for the developed and for the developing nations the percentage of their total deaths recorded by WHO in 1980 in six general groups of diseases namely: (a) infectious and parasitic diseases, (b) degenerative diseases and diseases of the circulatory system, (c) neoplasms, (d) perinatal conditions, (e) injury and poisoning and (f) all other and unknown causes. The right-hand bar chart shows the global picture. The bar representing the biggest percentage of deaths has been coloured black on each chart.

Stark contrasts are evident. The widespread availability of antibiotics, high levels of nutrition and medical care mean that, in the developed nations, infectious and parasitic diseases and perinatal complications are relatively insignificant as causes of death compared with the

developing world. In the developed nations, these causes of death cover only 10 percent of all deaths, whereas in the developing nations, they contribute 48 percent. In contrast, degenerative diseases, diseases of the circulatory system and neoplasms produce almost 75 percent of the deaths in the developed world as against 25 percent in developing countries.

Diagram (B) uses pie-charts to show the distribution of deaths in the developed and the developing worlds by the broad age categories, 0–14 years, 15–44, 45–64 and 65+. The pie-charts have been constructed by drawing prop-

ortional circles (cf. Figure 1.3) in which the area of each circle is proportional to the total number of deaths; each circle has been divided into sectors whose areas represent the percentage of the total deaths falling in each age category.

Global variations by age of death

The population of the planet in 1987 was estimated at five billions by WHO. Of this total, 75 percent live in the developing nations. Just over 50 million deaths from all causes were

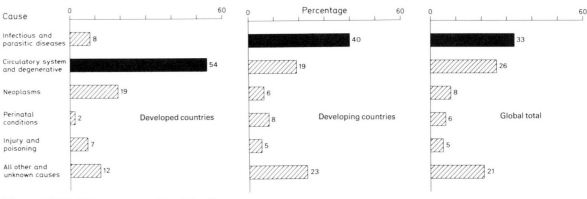

Figure 2.5 (A) Major causes of death by disease group

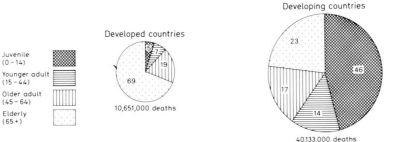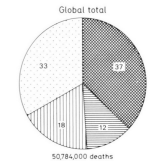

Figure 2.5 (B) Percentage deaths by age group

reported globally to WHO. Eighty percent occurred in the developing world, substantially in excess of the proportion expected on the basis of population totals. The reason is apparent from the pie-charts. Mortality among the young (0–14 years) accounts for nearly half of the total deaths in the developing world, in contrast to five percent in the developed countries. The corollary is that, in the developed countries, nearly 70 percent of deaths occurred in the 65+ age group.

The bar-chart and the pie-chart showing global mortality are, of course, weighted averages of those for the developed and the developing countries. The charts for the developing nations and the globe are broadly similar because, as we know, the bulk of the world's population lives in the developing nations.

The overall pattern which emerges from diagrams (A) and (B) is clear. In the developing countries, men (and even more so women) are likely to survive until old age and thus are most likely to die from the diseases of old age. In the developing nations, survival into adolescence is a matter of some chance, with infectious and parasitic diseases which are either naturally absent from, or else medically controlled in, the developed countries reaping a rich and early harvest. High birth rates run alongside the high mortality, whereas in the developed nations the population is scarcely replacing itself.

The implications of major global variations in the impact of disease for inter-area comparisons may be illustrated by supposing that we wished to compare the seasonal incidence of measles in the United States with that in an African country. From diagram (A) we would expect measles, as an infectious disease, to have a higher rate of incidence in Africa than the United States. Therefore, to detect seasonal variability in the United States, fluctuations must be looked for in the context of a much lower base level than in Africa, and we must recognize that what

constitutes a major seasonal upswing in the United States may very well be trivial alongside levels expected in Africa.

Years of potential life lost

Although global variations in disease intensity have been assessed in this plate by considering reported levels of mortality, alternative measures have been proposed which take into consideration the different ages at which deaths occur. A death in childhood might be considered to result in many more years of potential life lost than a death in old age. The idea was introduced by Dempsey (1947) in a study of tuberculosis, where the age of death was subtracted from life expectancy at birth. With the advent of computers more sophisticated calculations can be made in which the age of death can be taken from the remaining life expectancy based on a life table. For example, in the United States in 1984, a death at age 80 lost 8.2 years of potential life. In practice, the exact values will not only vary by sex but also with geographical location since, as we have seen in (A) and (B), life expectancy is itself regionally varying.

Chart (C) shows the ten leading causes of mortality in the United States in 1984 based on crude mortality and by years of potential life lost (YPLL) calculated from life-expectancy tables. Note that the YPLL method changes the relative rankings of seven of the main causes. Two, suicide/homicide and congenital anomalies, rise three places reflecting their concentration among the young as causes of death. Conversely, the three which fall two places (cerebrovascular disease, diabetes and pneumonia/influenza) do so because they generally appear as causes of death mainly in the elderly. Tables giving YPLL estimates of premature mortality are now regularly included in the Centers for Disease

Control's *Morbidity and Mortality Weekly Report.*

But in a global context, YPLL would need to be heavily modified. Since life expectancy varies greatly from one part of the world to another, the basis for its calculation also needs to change, and direct comparison from one reference population to another is not possible.

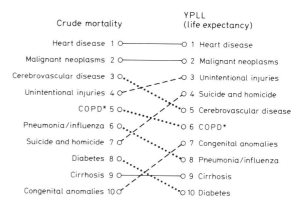

Figure 2.5 (C) Rankings of ten leading causes of death by crude mortality and years of potential life lost, United States, 1984

Sources and Further Reading

Charts (A) and (B) are based on demographic and mortality data in the United Nations *Demographic Yearbook* for 1980. Graph (C) is redrawn from Centers for Disease Control (1986), 'Premature mortality in the United States: public health in the use of potential life lost', *Morbidity and Mortality Weekly Report*, 35, Supplement 2, pp.1–11, Table 3. One of the earliest attempts to use loss of potential life statistics was M. Dempsey (1947), 'Decline in tuberculosis death rate fails to tell entire story', *American Review of Tuberculosis*, 56, pp.157–64.

2.6 STANDARDIZATION PROBLEMS II: AGE AND SEX

By comparing the developing and the developed nations, it was shown in Figure 2.5 that substantial differences in rates of mortality can arise on a given disease as a function of level of economic development and therefore geographical location. In the same way, we might expect there to be major differences within a country in mortality from different diseases which reflect the interplay of each disease with the demographic structure of the population being studied.

Age–sex distribution of a population

To illustrate this interplay, we examine patterns of mortality for six different diseases in relation to age and sex in Iceland since 1960. The reasons for using Iceland as an exemplar in this and many other plates in this Atlas is explained in the preface and in section 6.5.

The cartographic device used is the *age–sex pyramid*. In such a pyramid, age cohorts are plotted on the vertical axis, while the demographic variable of interest (here, percentage population and percentage deaths) is plotted on the horizontal axis. The score of each of the age cohorts on the demographic variable is plotted as a horizontal bar, with males to the left of the zero point and females to the right. On all the diagrams, the roman numbers give the total number of individuals involved for the single year, 1983, and the italicized numbers give the total in the decade 1961–70.

Diagram (A) shows the population pyramid of Iceland by five-year age groups for the year 1983.

The pyramid has been constructed by plotting the percentage of the total population of 238,416 in each age–sex category. The population aged 85 years and over is given as a single class. Unlike many developed countries, the demographic structure of Iceland displays a bias towards younger people, producing a bulge in the age–sex pyramid in the age groups up to 25. The natural increase in mortality with age ensures that the percentage population in each cohort generally falls as we move up the vertical axis, producing the characteristic pyramid-shaped survival diagram from which age–sex pyramids derive their name.

Age–sex distribution of all deaths

The age–sex distribution of deaths from all causes in Iceland is plotted in diagram (B) both for the single year, 1983, as a diagonally shaded pyramid and for the decade, 1961–70, by solid

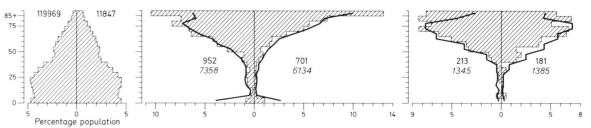

Figure 2.6 (A) Population, 1983   **Figure 2.6 (B) All deaths**

Figure 2.6 (C) Neoplasms (ICD Group II, 140–239)

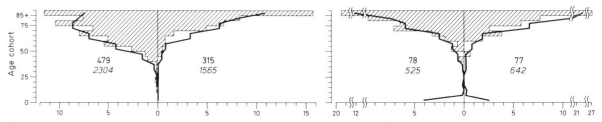

Figure 2.6 (D) Diseases of the circulatory system (ICD Group VII, 390–459)

Figure 2.6 (E) Diseases of the respiratory system (ICD Group VIII, 460–519)

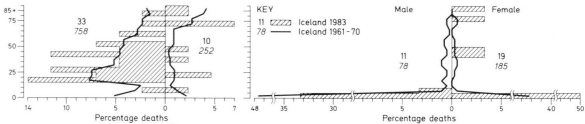

Figure 2.6 (F) Transport accidents (ICD Group XVII, E800–E848)

Figure 2.6 (G) Congenital anomalies and Certain conditions originating in the perinatal period (ICD Groups XIV and XV, 740–779)

lines. The two forms are used in order to contrast the variability in a single year with the more consistent pattern for a whole decade. The pyramid has a typical 'wineglass' shape. There is a relatively high proportion of the deaths in the youngest age class (0–4 years) which reflects the traumas of birth and the increased likelihood of death in the first year of life. Thereafter risk of mortality remains low until the end of the fourth decade, and the percentage of deaths then increases steadily. The well-known bias in western nations towards slightly earlier deaths for males is clearly seen, with a greater percentage of females surviving to die in extreme old age.

Neoplasms and circulatory diseases

Two major causes of death are shown in pyramids (C) and (D). The first plots deaths from all neoplasms (ICD classes 140–239) and the second deaths from diseases of the circulatory system (ICD classes 390–459). While an increase in percentage deaths with age is evident in both pyramids, mortality from diseases of the circulatory system only assumes significance from age 40 onwards; a substantial male bias between ages 45 and 70 is also apparent. In contrast, deaths from neoplasms are significant in the younger age groups because of population loss from childhood neoplasms such as leukaemia, and the disease strikes both male and female groups with similar severity from age 40 onwards. Since deaths from neoplasms and diseases of the circulatory system make up almost half of all deaths in Iceland, it is not surprising that their age–sex distribution is very similar to that of mortality from all causes shown in diagram (B).

Respiratory diseases

Pyramid (E) plots deaths from diseases of the respiratory system (ICD classes 460–519). The striking characteristic is the very high proportion of deaths occurring in the age group, 85 years and above. Note that the scale on the horizontal axis has been broken to permit deaths in this age cohort to be plotted on the same scale as the rest of the figure. This age category contains nearly one half of the deaths from these causes and reflects the loss each winter of the elderly from pneumonia in particular. A second feature of this pyramid is the contrast between the results for a single year and for a whole decade. In 1983, a relatively influenza-free year, there were no deaths recorded from respiratory diseases below the age of 40. In contrast the decennial curves show a significant peak in the youngest age category (0–4 years).

Accidents and anomalies

The last two pyramids illustrate deaths from relatively rare causes but which have interesting demographic characteristics. Pyramid (F) gives deaths from transport accidents (ICD classes E800–E848). These show the marked male bias found in all western nations, with particular peaks in the late teens and early twenties. Pyramid (G) plots the deaths from congenital anomalies and certain conditions originating in the perinatal period (ICD classes 740–779). Here the numbers are so small that regular patterns are difficult to establish. However, the very high incidence in the youngest age group is strongly marked and can only be plotted by breaking the horizontal axis of the graph.

It is evident from the examples given that diseases are age and sex specific in their impact. In assessing the importance of a particular disease in different geographical areas, it is therefore necessary to weight or to standardize the data by the demographic compositions of the populations of the areas being compared; otherwise our inferences may simply reflect these rather than geographical differences. Added to the need to allow for variations which are a function of level of economic development rather than intrinsic characteristics of the disease (Figure 2.5), as well as for country to country variations in reporting practices (Figures 2.2–2.4), the need for some method of standardizing data becomes overwhelming, and it is to this topic that we turn next.

Sources and Further Reading

The population pyramids for Iceland have been drawn from mortality data given in *Mannfjöldaskýrslur árin 1961–70* (Population and Vital Statistics), Reykjavík, 1975.

The cartographic device of population pyramids is discussed in F.J. Monkhouse and H.R. Wilkinson (1971), *Maps and Diagrams: Their Compilation and Construction*, third edition, London: Methuen, pp.365–9. While we have used the conventional method of plotting age–sex pyramids in this figure, we consider that more information might be gained about age and sex biases in mortality if the two halves of the pyramid were superimposed upon each other.

2.7 STANDARDIZED RATIOS AND SCORES

In the preceding plates it has been shown that comparison of diseases across different areas is handicapped by severe differences in recording levels (Figures 2.2 and 2.3), in geographical variability (Figure 2.5), and in age and sex demography (Figure 2.6). While such differences are at their most extreme in international comparisons (particularly between tropical and mid-latitude countries), they are also encountered at regional and local levels.

Benjamin (1968) has illustrated this by comparing the death rates in two English towns: Bournemouth and Corby. In 1954 the crude death rate in Bournemouth was 15.4 per 1,000 living and the corresponding rate for Corby was only 6.5. These two figures do not indicate the real difference in mortality risks in the two towns. Bournemouth is a coastal town attractive to retired people with 19 percent of its resident population aged 65 or more and a consequently high crude death rate. The reverse effect occurred in Corby which was, at that date, a new steel town with many young families which resulted in a deflated crude mortality rate.

The fact that mortality and morbidity are not independent of either the geographical environment or of the age–sex composition of the population restricts the comparisons which can be made of the impact of disease upon different areas, especially over time, unless the data are standardized in some way to remove their effect.

It is ways of standardizing which are considered in this figure.

Standardized mortality ratios

The usual way of standardizing data to allow for variations in the local age–sex composition of the population is to compute a *standardized mortality ratio* (SMR). The steps in the calculation are shown in diagrams (A) – (C) which are based upon data given in Benjamin (1968, pp.92–95). Diagram (A) gives the percentage of the total population falling in each of five age categories for two hypothetical districts A and B. The national picture is also given. For example, the total populations of the nation, district A and district B are 15.6, 3.12 and 3.06 millions respectively, while the corresponding percentages aged 4 and under are 9, 9 and 7 respectively. As the bar graphs show, the population balance in district A is 'young' compared with district B which is 'old'.

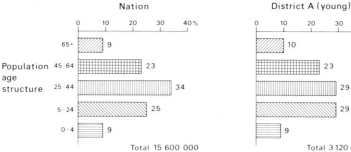

Figure 2.7 (A) Population age structure

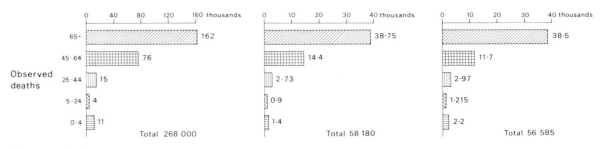

Figure 2.7 (B) Observed deaths by age groups

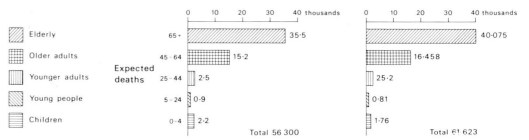

Figure 2.7 (C) Expected deaths, age adjusted

In the same way diagram (B) gives the total number of deaths in the nation and in districts A and B, as well as the distribution of deaths among the five age categories.

We have seen from the example of Bournemouth and Corby that the crude death rate suffers from the disadvantage that, as an average, the weights used in the denominator in its calculation are the local age group populations which vary from area to area. The basic idea behind the SMR is that some reference or standard population (which is to be the nation in the present figure) is used to generate expected death rates in districts A and B. This is done by multiplying the national death rate in a particular age (and/or sex) category by the population total in the districts in the same age (and/or sex) category. These expected deaths are then summed to give the total number of deaths expected in A and B on the basis of death rates in the standard population. The SMR for a given district is then formed as 100 (total observed deaths/total expected deaths).

Diagram (C) gives the expected deaths in districts A and B generated on this basis. For example, at the national level we know from diagram (A) that, out of a total population of 15600 thousands, 9 percent or $[15600 \times (9/100)]$ = 1404 thousands of individuals are aged 4 or under. From diagram (B), there were 11,000 deaths in the same age category so that the national age-specific death rate for the 0–4 age group is $(11000/1404)$ = 7.8 per thousand population. In district A, the total under-4 population is $[3120 \times (9/100)]$ = 280 thousands, so that the expected number of deaths is (280×7.8) = 2184 or, as shown in diagram (C), 2.2 thousands to one decimal place. Repetition of these calculations for all age categories in both districts A and B yields the expected deaths shown in diagram (C) which, when summed, produce the total

expected deaths of 56,300 in A and 61,623 in B. The SMR in district A is 100(58180/56300) = 103.3, while that in district B is 100(56585/61623) = 91.8. Thus, compared with the national picture, district A has substantially worse mortality than district B when differences in demographic structure are allowed for, whereas in terms of the crude deaths rates per thousand population of 18.6 and 18.5, there is apparently little to choose between them.

Standard scores for SMRs

A number of atlases which show the distribution of individual diseases varying across a population use SMR techniques to standardize either mortality or morbidity for age–sex differences. The *National Atlas of Disease Mortality in the United Kingdom* (Howe, 1970) is a good example.

Once the SMRs are calculated, they can be subjected to a wide range of analysis by applying the kind of techniques discussed in Figure 1.7. One common method is to reduce the SMRs to standard scores, in which values are expressed with reference to the average SMR for all areas (as reflected by a measure of central tendency) and to their variability (as reflected by a measure of range). The usual approach is to create the score, z_i, say, in area i by subtracting from the data values the mean and dividing through by the standard deviation. Thus, if x_i denotes the unstandardized value in area i, $\bar{x}$ is the mean of the x_i and s_x is the standard deviation, then the standard score is $z_i = (x_i - \bar{x})/s_x$. These scores have the important property that they are dimensionless; that is, independent of the units of the original data. In addition, the z_i have a mean of zero and a standard deviation of unity. As a result, it is possible to compare not only data for different areas but also for different

diseases because they will all have been mapped onto a new scale with the same mean and degree of variation.

The degree of standardization which is undertaken will depend upon the problem in hand. If variations within a single country on one disease are being studied, it will usually be sufficient to allow for demographic differences via SMRs. However, once comparisons between diseases and geographical areas are undertaken, computation of standard scores of a more complex kind (see Figure 2.10) may be necessary.

Sources and Further Reading

The properties of standard scores are discussed in any standard statistics texts; see, for example, G.W. Snedecor and W.G. Cochran (1980), *Statistical Methods*, seventh edition, Ames, Iowa: Iowa State University Press. An elementary introduction in a medical context is given in T.D.V. Swinscow (1983), *Statistics at Square One* (articles published in the British Medical Journal), eighth edition, London: British Medical Journal. A good account of the value of standardized mortality ratios is contained in Chapter 6 of B. Benjamin (1968), *Health and Vital Statistics*, London: Allen and Unwin. Examples of maps of SMRs are give in G.M. Howe, *National Atlas of Disease Mortality in the United Kingdom*, second edition, London: Royal Geographical Society.

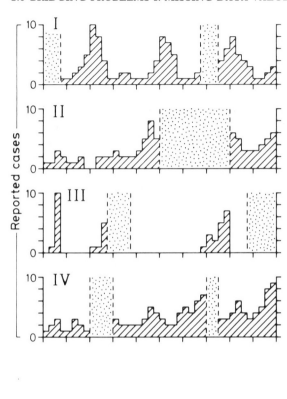

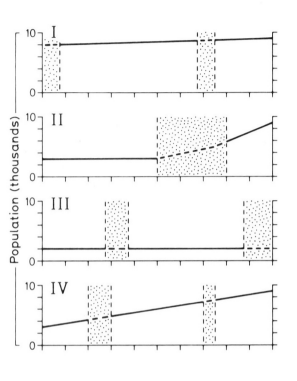

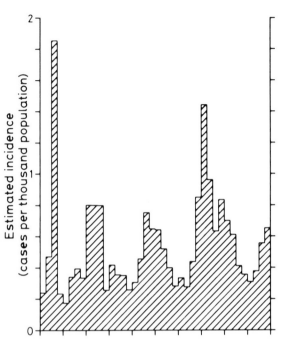

Figure 2.8 (C) Unbroken estimates of
incidence for all four areas combined

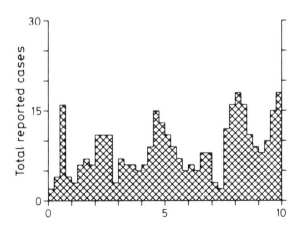

Figure 2.8 (A) Morbidity records
(incomplete) for four areas

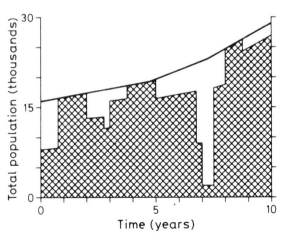

Figure 2.8 (B) Population records
(complete) for four areas

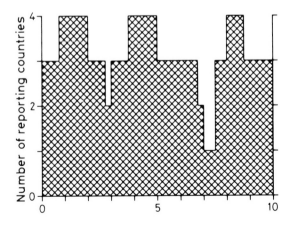

Figure 2.8 (D) Number of areas reporting in
each time period

2.8 BRIDGING PROBLEMS I: MISSING DATA VALUES

In an ideal world, when morbidity and mortality data relating to a set of areas are examined over time, the data matrix will be complete and there will be no missing observations. However, as we have seen in Figure 2.3, more usually this is not the case and we are frequently faced with broken time-series records for individual countries. The gaps may arise for any one of a number of reasons; changes in health reporting regulations and interruption by war are just two of the possible causes of lost observations.

The problems posed by missing observations are made more acute if inter-country comparisons of disease behaviour have to be made. It is common, when we take a set of time-series records relating to several areas, to find that the gaps in the data records of the countries do not coincide but vary from one country to another. In this plate we examine ways of constructing some sort of continuous record of the behaviour of a disease over time from fragmentary data. Here we provide a hypothetical example, while in Figure 2.10 a specific illustration is given using data from the South Pacific.

Missing observations

The morbidity records for four hypothetical areas over a period of ten years are shown in graphs I–IV of diagram (A). Diagonally shaded histograms have been used on each graph to plot the total number of reported cases of some disease. The years in the data record for which cases were not reported (missing observations) are delimited by stippled bands. The bottom graph in diagram (A) gives the total number of reported cases as a cross-hatched histogram; this has been obtained by summing the corresponding values in graphs I–IV. It is evident that this running total is misleading since no allowance has been made either for the presence of gaps in the data records of the individual areas or for the population sizes of the areas.

The question of population size is addressed in the graphs plotted in diagram (B). This shows, for the same four areas and for the same time period, changes in the total population of each area as a line trace (graphs I–IV). The years in which there were missing observations in the disease record of each of the four areas, as given in diagram (A), have been transferred to the population graphs of diagram (B); they are marked, as before, by stippled bands. The bottom graph of diagram (B) shows two population curves. First, the total population of the four areas, obtained by summing the four curves for the separate areas, is shown as a solid line trace. This takes no account of the stippled bands of missing observations. Second, the cross-hatched histogram gives the total population of only those areas which were reporting cases of the disease in each year. As a consequence, it has a very ragged outline.

One way of estimating the incidence of the disease in terms of cases per thousand population is shown in diagram (C). This has been con- structed by dividing the total reported cases plotted in the cross-hatched histogram of diagram (A), by the total population of areas reporting as plotted in the cross-hatched histogram of diagram (B). For example, in year 1 the observation for area I is missing, while the total number of cases reported by areas II–IV is 2 (1 + 0 + 1, respectively). The total population (in thousands) of these reporting areas is 8 (that is, 3 + 2 + 3, respectively), so that the estimated incidence (cases per thousand population) plotted in year 1 of diagram (C) is (2/8) = 0.25. Diagram (D) gives the number of countries reporting in each year of the time-series. Note the contrast between estimated disease incidence as plotted in diagram (C), where it has been corrected both for population size and missing observations, and the raw totals given in diagram (A). For example, the crude totals suggest that, over and above the oscillations, there is an increase over time in the general severity of the disease. However, the adjusted totals show a series of oscillations about an essentially constant mean. The maximum value in the crude series comes in years 8 and 10, while in the adjusted series the maximum occurs in year 1.

In interpreting the adjusted series, we have to recall that it has been patched together from the separate records relating to a number of areas, each of which is incomplete. The reason for plotting the number of areas reporting in diagram (D) is that it provides a measure of reliability for the adjusted series. We may place more confidence in an adjusted value calculated when all four areas have reported than when the value is based on the data for just one area.

2.9 BRIDGING PROBLEMS II: BOUNDARY SHIFTS

When analysing time-series of medical data which have been collected for a set of geographical areas, a recurring problem is that the boundaries of the recording units may differ from one time period to the next. These boundary movements may simply reflect administrative convenience or they may be related to more significant events such as marked changes in the population size of an area. Failure to adjust for boundary movements will invalidate inter-area comparisons.

This figure shows some of the possibilities which may occur and the strategies that can be adopted to overcome them. Diagram (A) illustrates the simplest case. Here no boundary changes occur in area A between time periods t_1 and t_2 and a continuous record of disease intensity can be readily plotted. Diagram (B), however, shows one common kind of boundary change which affects area B between times t_1 and t_2. Area B is divided into potentially several parts, taken for illustrative purposes as two in the diagram, namely B_1 and B_2. The separate time-series for B_1 and B_2 must then be added together to recover as a complete time-series the continuous record relating to the old area B. Figure (C) shows the reverse situation. Two areas, C and D which were separate at time t_1 have been combined by time t_2 to form a single geographical unit. Just as in diagram (B) where the problem was solved by adding together the time-series for the two small units to create a time-series for the large unit, B, so we must proceed in the same way here and be content with the time-series for the combined unit of C plus D over the entire study period.

In reality, very few boundary changes are as simple as those illustrated in diagrams (B) and (C). They are usually a complex mixture of subdivision and amalgamation. This is shown in diagram (D). At time t_1, three separate areas, E, F and G are assumed to exist. First, however, areas E and F are amalgamated but G remains separate. By time t_2, the situation has been made even more complex by the adding of part of E and F into G. The stipple demarcates the original area F of time period t_1 which has completely disappeared as a result of these boundary movements. The dendrogram in diagram (D) plots the changes. Again, the best we can do is to form a common time-series by taking the largest or coarsest geographical unit, that is, E + F + G to form our time-series of disease intensity for analysis. In fact this rule turns out to be general; boundary changes are always resolved by going to the coarsest geographical mesh to generate consistent time-series for study.

In Figure 2.11, we examine a practical example of boundary changes over time by studying the medical districts of Iceland for a 100-year period; see also Figure 3.8 where boundary changes of local authorities in England and Wales cause statistical complications.

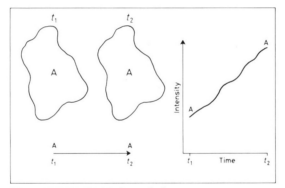

Figure 2.9 (A) Stable boundaries

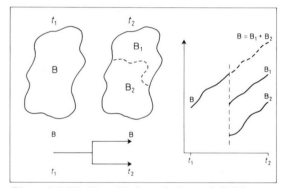

Figure 2.9 (B) Unstable boundaries: subdivision

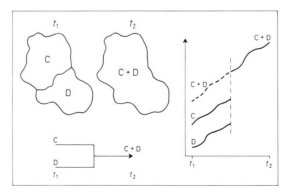

Figure 2.9 (C) Unstable boundaries: Aggregation

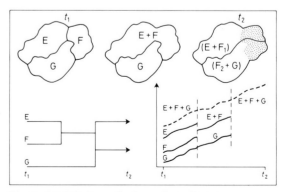

Figure 2.9 (D) Complex boundary changes

2.10 MISSING DATA VALUES: A REGIONAL EXAMPLE

In Figure 2.8, we looked at the general problem of patching together a continuous time-series of disease incidence from a set of geographical areas, each of which had an incomplete time-series record of its own. In the present figure, a specific regional application of the methodology is given using data on the incidence of measles in some island systems of the southern Pacific Basin between 1946 and 1981.

Measles in the Pacific Basin

Study of the incidence of measles in the Pacific Basin depends on a number of sources. We have used here the papers available from the World Health Organization, from the South Pacific Commission, and archival material in the Australian National Library. Using these sources, it is possible to build up a sequence of monthly records of measles morbidity for twenty Pacific countries; the geographical locations of the countries are plotted later in Figure 7.2.

The resulting matrix is shown in diagram (A) for the period from January 1946 to December 1981 (432 months). In diagram (A), each month in which a particular country made a report of measles morbidity has been shaded black, so that the black bars show the completeness of the data record for each territory. It is apparent from this bar chart that the availability of measles data is intensely variable. The countries have been arranged in a sequence from that with the fullest record down to that which is most fragmentary. They range from Fiji, with a complete time series, to Norfolk Island where published data are available for only nine percent of the time

period. Two countries with records, but with no recorded measles cases, Pitcairn and Tokelau, were eliminated from further consideration.

The implications of the broken time-series are shown in the shaded histograms. That in diagram (B) gives the number of months with recorded cases for each individual territory. The histogram in diagram (C) shows the number of countries with recorded cases for each of the 432 months of the time-series. Only in two time periods in the late 1970s was the record complete, spanning all 18 territories. In contrast, the 1940s and the early 1970s were times in which

fewer than half of the territories were publishing information on measles morbidity. We stress 'publishing' since data may exist in archives which did not find their way into WHO records.

It is clear from the discussion of the way in which morbidity records are compiled (see Figure 2.2) that the number of measles cases recorded in a particular Pacific country cannot be accepted at face value. The numbers will reflect the quality of the local reporting network (for example, the number and location of medical practitioners) at a given moment, as well as the cases occurring. The time-series plotted in

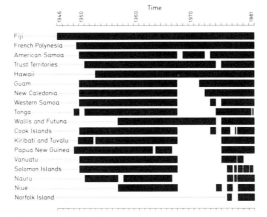

Figure 2.10 (A) Space–time data matrix

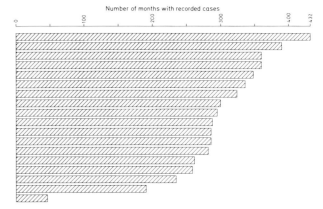

Figure 2.10 (B) Sequence of countries by length of record

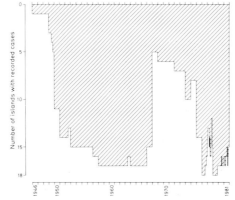

Figure 2.10 (C) Number of countries reporting in each time period

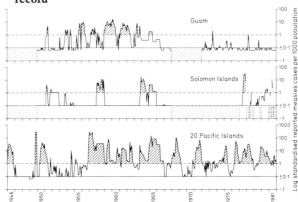

Figure 2.10 (D) Individual measles records (Guam and Solomons) and regional record (20 Pacific islands)

diagram (D) are therefore based upon data which have been expressed as standard scores (cf. Figure 2.7); the precise form of the standardization is given in the technical appendix to this figure. The series therefore represent a transformed index of measles incidence. This has the advantage that each separate series is adjusted by its own internal average level of reporting and variability.

Individual and composite series

Two examples of individual countries are shown, namely Guam and the Solomon Islands, followed by a composite series based upon the combined records of twenty Pacific island countries. The months of missing observations in the time-series of the individual countries have been stippled. The diagonally shaded areas of the line traces are more than one standard unit away from the average level of measles incidence in each series and represent the main epidemics.

It is evident that, while the individual series have serious gaps in them which make interpretation difficult, it is possible to build a relatively complete series for the Pacific as a whole. Clearly its accuracy is not consistent over time but it represents a best approximation given the fragmentary data available. There is some evidence of a change in the style of recording in that there is a discontinuity 1956; thereafter the series becomes much more regular showing the repeating cycles of measles waves so commonly recorded in the developed nations (cf. Figure 4.7).

Sources and Further Reading

The diagrams have been prepared from work described in A.D. Cliff and P. Haggett (1985), *The Spread of Measles in Fiji and the Pacific: Spatial Components in the Transmission of Epidemic Waves through Island Communities*, Publication HG18, Canberra: Australian National University, Research School of Pacific Studies, Department of Human Geography, Figure 13, p.69.

The background epidemiology for this region is described in N. McArthur (1967), *Island Populations in the Pacific*, Canberra: Australian National University Press. The statistical theory behind the methods used is discussed in B. Abraham (1981), 'Missing observations in time series', *Communications in Statistics A*, 10, pp.1643–53, and S.Y. Barham and F.D.J. Dunstan (1983), 'Missing values in time series', in *Time Series Analysis: Theory and Practice*, vol. 2, edited by O.D. Anderson, Amsterdam: North Holland.

Technical appendix

One approach to the standardization of morbidity data is the following. The inputs to the procedure, x_{it}, are the recorded number of cases for each time period, t (usually a calendar month but for some countries a four-week period) in the ith country. The steps are then:

(1) The number of recorded cases is converted into a monthly incidence rate per thousand population by dividing through by the population in thousands of the recording country. Since population estimates are usually available only for mid-year or census points, linear interpolation to give a monthly population is also required.

(2) Prevalence rates will reflect both genuine variations in virus activity and artifical variations in the collecting practices of a particular country. To reduce the role of the latter, the monthly incidence rate can be converted to an incidence index by subtracting some measure of average value (the mean or the median, say) and by dividing through by some measure of range (standard deviation or interquartile range). This standardization implies that the time-series values of a particular country are re-expressed in terms of the average level of reporting and the variability established within that country by its own recording practices. If the data are positively skewed, as with the Pacific measles records, the values may be normalized by taking logarithms prior to standardizing.

(3) A composite series like that for measles in the Pacific Basin shown in diagram (D) can be constructed by adding together all the individual standardized series and then taking in each month the arithmetic average of the values combined to give that monthly total. Alternatively, the contribution of individual series to the average can be weighted, prior to adding the individual series together, by multiplying each by, for example, the respective population totals or the number of months in the time-series with published morbidity records. This gives greater weight to series from larger countries, which might be expected to be more reliable, and to more complete series. In diagram (D), the individual series were weighted by the square root of the population size of the island territory concerned, which gives a positive weight to larger islands but in a reduced form compared with multiplying by population totals alone.

2.11 BOUNDARY SHIFTS: A REGIONAL EXAMPLE

In Figure 2.9 we looked at some simple examples of the ways in which the geographical boundaries of medical reporting districts can change from one time period to the next, and the consequent problem of patching together a consistent time-series of observations for each unit. In this figure, we give a specific example of the difficulties created by these shifts and the patching which proved necessary.

Iceland has the most complete epidemiological record both in time and space of any country in the world. Data are available for about 35 common infectious diseases, as well as for other non-communicable diseases on the ICD list, on a monthly basis for some fifty geographical areas back to 1896, and more irregularly for over 100 years before that. The basic reporting unit for these data is the medical district (*læknishérað*). In the period since 1896 there have been many changes both in their number and in boundary locations. In order to bring these districts to a common geographical mesh, it is necessary to work with the smallest administrative spatial unit in Iceland, the *hreppur*, which is roughly equivalent to the English parish and to the American township, and to build up the medical districts from these.

Medical districts are composed of *hreppar* and major boundary revisions were undertaken in 1875, 1899, 1907, 1932 and 1955. With the exception of 1875, legal documents exist defining which *hreppar* make up which medical districts. Using these legal documents and a base map of the *hreppar* it is possible to prepare the branching diagram shown in Figure 2.11(A). This shows all the known changes in the medical district boundaries and their date of occurrence. Thus

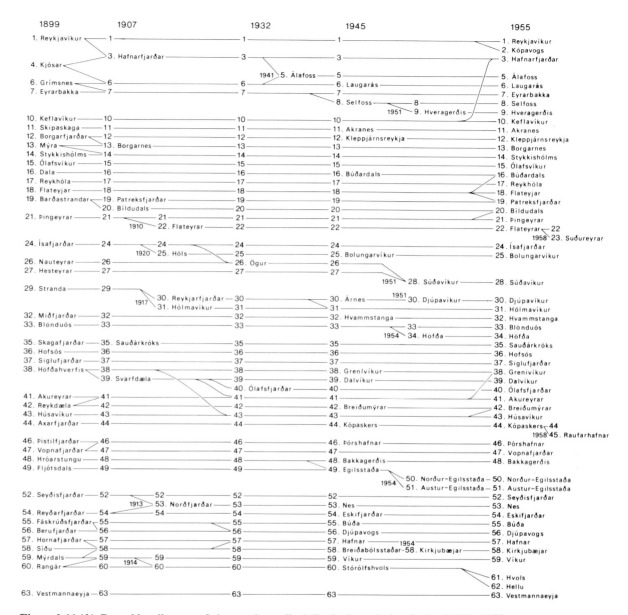

Figure 2.11 (A) Branching diagram of changes in medical district boundaries, Iceland 1899–1955

we can see that medical district 1, Reykjavíkur, existed throughout the study period but that district 3, Hafnarfjarðar was first created in 1907 by an amalgamation of Kjósar (district 4) with part of Reykjavíkur. The branching diagram may be converted into a geographical format to produce maps of the boundaries of the medical districts from base-maps of the *hreppar* at each of the major boundary-revision dates; these are shown in Figure 2.11(B). The identity numbers in each of the districts correspond with the branching diagram and the stipple indicates areas affected by boundary changes.

The map for 1945 plots the set of medical districts used for all the Icelandic examples discussed elsewhere in this book. Minor boundary changes were sometimes made between the major revisions and these are recorded in either *Heilbrigðisskýrslur* (Public Health in Iceland) or *Mannfjöldaskýrslur* (Population and Vital Statistics).

As Figure 2.9 emphasized, spatial continuity and temporal continuity represent irreconcilable goals. If we are to preserve a consistent time series, then we need to sacrifice (through amalgamation) a great deal of spatial detail. Conversely, if we wish to retain the maximum amount of spatial detail then we can only have very short and broken time series.

Sources and Further Reading

Diagrams (A) to (G) are based upon work undertaken by the authors in Iceland summarized in A.D. Cliff, P. Haggett, J.K. Ord and G.R. Versey (1981), *Spatial Diffusion: an Historical Geography of Epidemics in an Island Community*, Cambridge: Cambridge University Press; see figures 4.1 and 4.2, pp.55–61. Another example of the shifting boundary problem is the revision of Local Authority Area boundaries in 1974 in England and Wales; see Figure 3.9 of this Atlas.

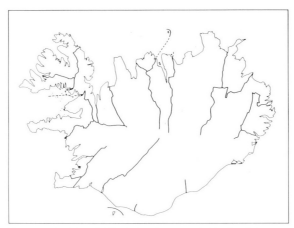

Figure 2.11 (B) Medical district boundaries in 1875

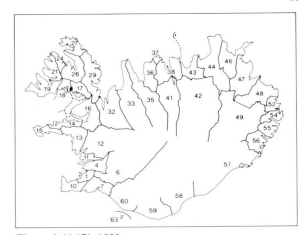

Figure 2.11 (C) 1899

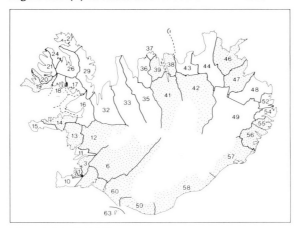

Figure 2.11 (D) 1907

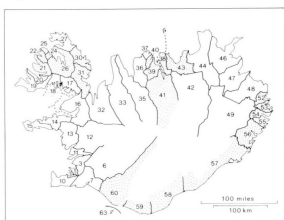

Figure 2.11 (E) 1932

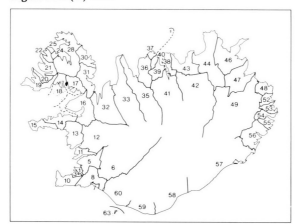

Figure 2.11 (F) 1945

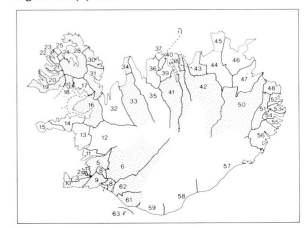

Figure 2.11 (G) 1955

2.12 POPULATION SHIFTS: ICELAND

So far in this chapter, it has been tacitly assumed that the analysis of disease statistics has taken place in populations which are fixed in size and geographical location. The comparison of disease statistics from area to area and from one time period to the next is particularly hazardous when time-based changes occur in either or both of the population totals and the age–sex composition of the populations concerned. Fixed incidence in a growing population will yield declining rates (and vice versa) and the same is also true as the population totals of geographical regions rise and fall. In the same way, if the population age–sex structure changes over time, a variable influence will be exerted upon incidence rates (see Figures 2.6 and 2.7). These changes must be taken into account if a proper assessment is to be made of statistical information.

To illustrate the profound changes which may occur in both the demographic structure and geographical distribution of a population, we examine the population dynamics of Iceland between 1751 and 1971.

Changes in totals

Diagram (A) shows the population totals and migration history of Iceland over the last two centuries. It is evident that the total population was stable at around 40–60,000 between 1751 and 1900 when a remarkable growth set in; the population approximately trebled between 1900 and 1970 to about 200,000. Up to 1950, this growth was concentrated mainly in the capital, Reykjavík. Since then Reykjavík and the rest of

Iceland have grown at about the same rate. The excess of immigrants over emigrants during this century has accounted for part of this growth but, as will be seen later in Figure 6.5(C), the decline in infant mortality linked to the higher birth rates (especially since 1940) shown in (A) are the main reasons.

Changes in geographical distribution

Diagrams (B) and (C) use the method of proportional circles (see Figure 1.3) to show the distribution of population by medical districts in 1911 and 1971. Population change is also given. Map (B) illustrates vividly the coastal location of the population in a country whose central area is occupied by tundra and a permanent icecap. The second striking feature of the map for 1911 is the relatively small degree of variability in the sizes of the circles from one medical district to another; the geographical distribution of the population was then relatively homogeneous.

By 1971 [map (C)], the pattern was very different. To define percentage change, the percentage of the total population of Iceland found in a given medical district was calculated for 1911 and 1971. Denote these percentages by P_{1911} and P_{1971} respectively. Percentage change was then defined as $(P_{1971} - P_{1911})$. Map (C) shows enormous growth in two areas of the country both in absolute and relative terms. These are located in the southwest of the country around the capital, Reykjavík, and on the north coast near the city of Akureyri. Only these two locations display a net population increase over the 60 years (stippled circles); all other districts have suffered a net loss (black circles).

Map (D) shows this population loss through rural depopulation in a fishing and farming region of northwest Iceland (see also Figure 5.5).

The pattern has been one of total abandonment of settlement except in two of the broader, more southerly, lowland embayments. Over time, the retreat has been broadly from northwest to southeast, with the earliest abandonments (denoted by triangles) occurring in the most isolated parts of the northwest peninsula.

Changes in age–sex structure

Diagrams (E) – (H) illustrate the changing age–sex structure of the Icelandic population in the present century. Using the method of age–sex pyramids (cf. Figure 2.6), charts (E) and (F) give the percentage of the population in 18 age categories in 1901 and 1981. Comparison of the two shows the classic 'ageing' of the Icelandic population over the course of the century which is characteristic of all developed countries. The percentage of the population aged 15 and under has fallen while the number surviving past 50 has increased.

Diagram (G) shows these trends in a different way by plotting, from 1921–74, the percentage of the total population under the age of 1 and the percentage over the age of 65. The very high birth rates of the period from 1940–65 [see also Figure 6.5(C)] have not been sustained, while the percentage over age 65 has grown steadily. The large number born between 1940 and 1965 have moved through the population to account for the bulge in the age–sex pyramid (F) in the age cohorts, 15 to 40.

For comparison, the cumulative percentage of the total population of all the Nordic countries (Iceland, Norway, Sweden, Denmark and Finland) in six age categories appears in chart (H) for the years between 1921 and 1983. Like (G) it shows the same features of decline in the younger age groups and an increase in the percentage

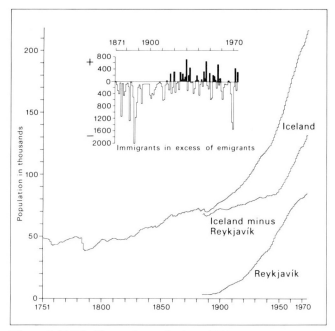

Figure 2.12 (A) Change in totals since 1751

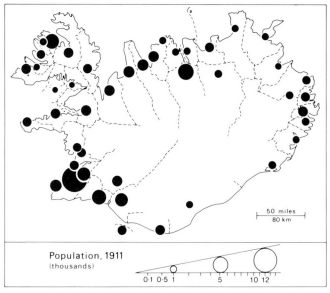

Figure 2.12 (B) Geographical distribution, 1911

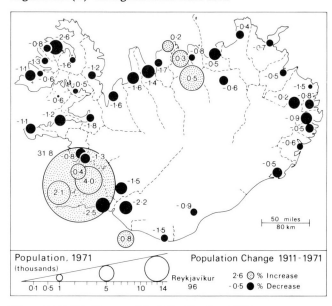

Figure 2.12 (C) Geographical distribution, 1971

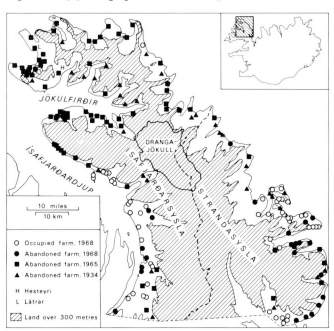

Figure 2.12 (D) Local changes through rural depopulation, 1934–1968

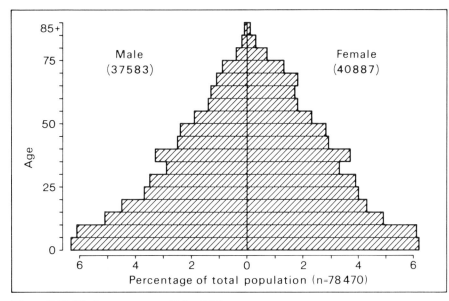

Figure 2.12 (E) Age–sex pyramid for 1901

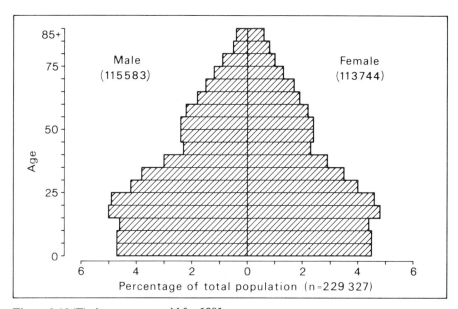

Figure 2.12 (F) Age–sex pyramid for 1981

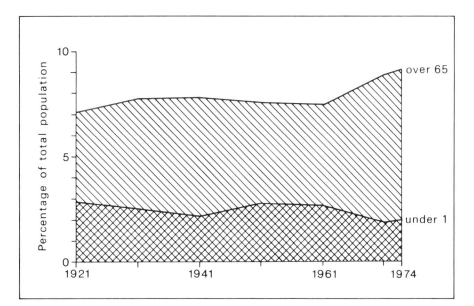

Figure 2.12 (G) Changes, 1921–1974 in the percentage of the Icelandic population aged under 1 and over 65

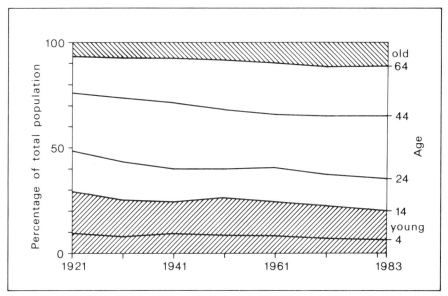

Figure 2.12 (H) Percentage of the total population of all Nordic countries under certain ages

aged 65 and over. However the dramatic changes in these categories shown in (G) for Iceland are not nearly so evident in the Nordic countries as a whole.

Sources and Further Reading

The source of demographic data for Iceland is *Manntal á Íslandi* (Population Census of Iceland), covering the period from 1703, and *Mannfjöldaskýrslur* (Population and Vital Statistics) which covers the period since 1911 in greater detail. Both series are published by the Statistical Bureau of Iceland in Reykjavík. A general review of Iceland's population growth is given in A.D. Cliff, P. Haggett, J.K. Ord and G.R. Versey (1981), *Spatial Diffusion: An Historical Geography of Epidemics in an Island Community*, Cambridge: Cambridge University Press, pp.46–53, upon which diagrams (A) – (D) are based. Comparable data for the Nordic countries (see diagrams (E) – (H)) are available in the *Yearbook of Nordic Statistics 1984*, 23, edited by the Nordic Statistical Secretariat, Stockholm: Nordic Council, 1985. The Icelandic pattern of change from 1920 to 1962 is set in a global context in N. Keyfitz and W. Flieger (1968), *World Population: An Analysis of Vital Data*, Chicago: University of Chicago Press, pp.374–9.

CHAPTER THREE
SPATIAL CROSS-SECTIONS

Figure over   Scanning electron micrograph showing (at left and right) two cancer (tumour) cells in the final stage of division, linked by fine cytoplasmic strands. Two lymphocytes, types of white blood cells, are seen above and below the cancer cells.
Source   Nina Lampen/Science Photo Library.

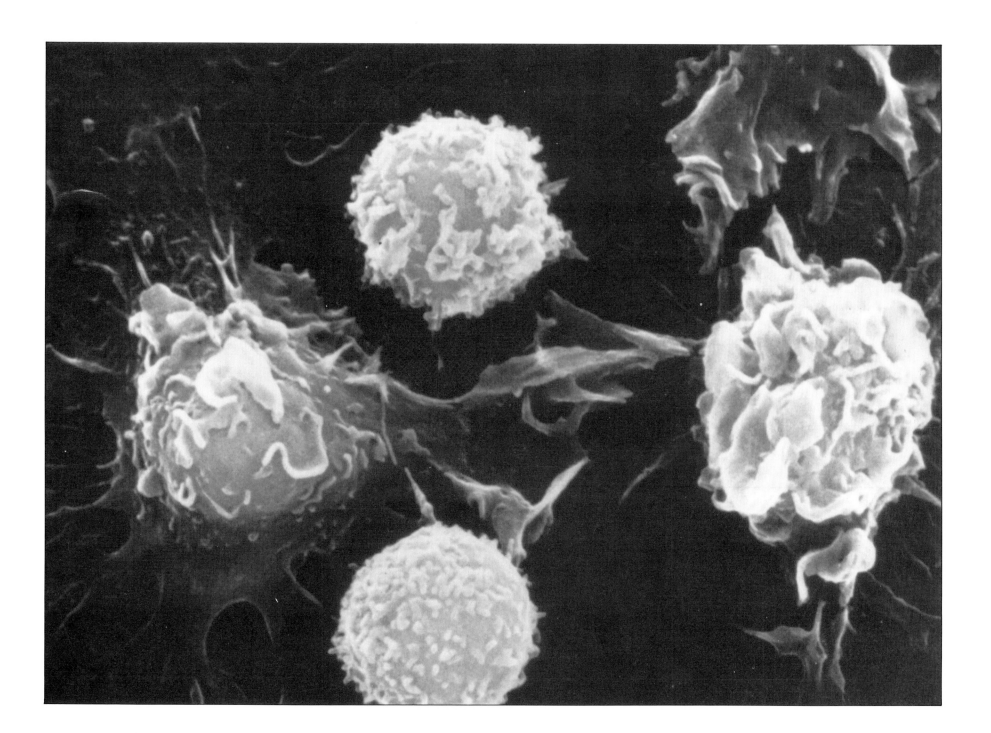

CHAPTER THREE

SPATIAL CROSS-SECTIONS

INTRODUCTION

The conventional way of collecting disease data is to record for an *observation unit* (such as a patient or a country) information on a set of *variables* (such as age, sex and disease symptoms). The recorded data are gathered at specific geographical locations (such as the hospital to which the patient has been referred) and at particular points in time. At any given spatial location, the progress of a disease, whether in a particular patient or in a geographical area, is monitored by repeated recording of information on the same variables in successive time periods. In this way, a temporal or dynamic element is added to the data record. The same pattern of observation and recording is, of course, repeated from hospital to hospital and from country to country so that, at any point in time, we will have a picture of the particular disease across a set of geographical locations. In general, then, we may regard each piece of disease data as having associated with it *spatial* and *temporal dimensions* which tell us where and when it was collected. We may thus display disease data in the form of a cubic data matrix with the dimensions (u, v, z) in which information is stored in terms of its spatial coordinates (u, v), its temporal coordinate z and the variable of interest. It is the purpose of this chapter to provide methods of analysis for the spatial dimension and examples of their use.

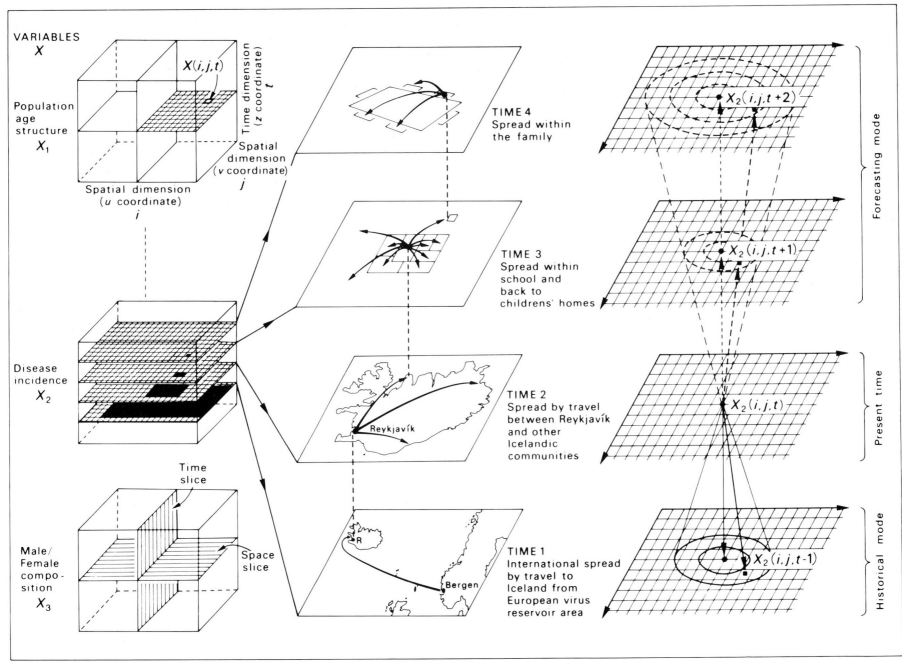

Figure 3.1 (A) Data matrices with spatial (*u*, *v*) and temporal (*z*) dimensions

Figure 3.1 (B) Example of spatial cross-sections at four time periods and four geographical scales

Figure 3.1 (C) Space, time, and forecasting modes in disease mapping

3.1 GEOGRAPHICAL DATA MATRICES

Matrix structure

In diagram (A), each variable is denoted symbolically by the letter X with the subscript 1, 2 . . . to identify the particular variable referenced. Thus X_1 refers to population age structure, X_2 to disease incidence and X_3 to the male/female composition of the population. Values of the variable are measured at various geographical locations whose representative positions on a cartesian grid we may fix symbolically as (i, j) corresponding to the u and v coordinates respectively. The variables are recorded at different time periods, denoted symbolically by t on the vertical axis, z. Where there are several variables, we therefore obtain, as in diagram (A), a series of space-time matrix cubes, one for each variable, stacked on top of each other. Horizontal cross-sections through any of the cubes (space slices) give the values of a variable across the map at a given point in time. Vertical or longitudinal sections (time slices) give the values in selected locations through time.

Analysis of the data matrices can proceed in a variety of ways. Purely spatial or cross-sectional analysis focuses upon the geographical variability in disease incidence at a given point in time and requires interpretation of horizontal slices through the data matrices. A second approach is to study the time-series behaviour of different observation units by examining the longitudinal slices. The most sophisticated analysis involves simultaneous study of both the time-series and spatial behaviour of observation units. This recognizes that observation units are generally not independent of each other. Disease may pass from individual to individual, area to area and country to country with time lags separating the observed events.

Spatial cross-sections and geographical scale

The binding together of time and space with the process by which disease is produced in an observation unit is illustrated by the simple example given in diagram (B). In a study by the authors (Cliff, Haggett, Ord and Versey, 1981) of measles epidemics in Iceland in the twentieth century, it was shown that the Icelandic population is not large enough to maintain a permanent reservoir of the measles virus. Instead, the virus is introduced into the population at regular intervals by international travel to cause periodic epidemics separated by quiescent periods when the island is free of the virus. If the observation unit is the patient attended by the local doctor on an Icelandic farm [time 4 in diagram (B)], then the patient will have been bound into a particular time-space location in the data matrix by several preceding steps.

At the earliest time period [time 1 in diagram (B)] and in a different spatial location, a measles epidemic will have been in progress and the virus brought by international travel to Iceland (cf. section 6.5, later). The usual reservoir for Iceland is Scandinavia. This step in the chain of events is represented in diagram (B) by virus movement from Bergen in Norway to the capital city of Iceland, Reykjavík, R. The next step in the chain sees time advance to time 2 in diagram (B) and the virus diffused to more spatial locations in the data matrix by travel between Reykjavík and other Icelandic communities. At time 3, spread occurs within a particular settlement to a school and finally, at time 4, a child comes home from school to spread the disease to brothers and sisters at the dining table and produce the observation units recorded by the doctor.

This example also shows how the *geographical scale* at which spatial cross-sections are examined may change from time period to time period; these scale changes are indicated by the successively smaller solid black rectangles marked on the spatial cross-sections in diagram (A) linked to the spatial slices in diagram (B).

Space, time and forecasting

The interrelationships between temporal and spatial locations in the data matrices implied by diagram (B) are formalized in diagram (C). Here we go inside the data matrix for any one variable of diagram (A). An event at a spatial location on the present time cross-section through the data matrix is related to events on past time planes (an historical mode) and will, in its turn, affect events at other locations on future time planes. These relationships create 'cones' of influence projecting back through time and forwards into the future. If we can understand the structure of the time-space matrix in sufficient detail, then diagram (C) shows that we may be able to forecast future events (a forecasting mode) and so address the issue of disease control more effectively.

Space, time and the Atlas structure

The ideas discussed form the structure around which the remainder of this Atlas is built. As noted in the chapter introduction, methods for the analysis of spatial cross-sections through matrices of disease data are considered here. In Chapter 4, the analysis of longitudinal slices is examined and a series of approaches to the study of the time-series behaviour of single observation units are outlined. Techniques which permit time and space slices to be handled simultaneously are presented in Chapter 5, so that the complex interactions between time periods and spatial locations may be disentangled.

In all these chapters, the cartographic and statistical techniques described are illustrated by brief examples. In Chapter 6, detailed substantive case studies of the space-time matrix produced by four different diseases, namely AIDS, smallpox, influenza and measles, are described in a variety of geographical settings. In terms of diagram (C), the account of AIDS emphasizes the forecasting part of the space-time matrix. As a contrast, the discussions of smallpox and influenza focus upon the historical element. Our treatment of measles examines both the historical and forecasting components of the matrix. An account of past patterns of epidemics in the island community of Iceland is provided and used as a framework within which future prospects for virus elimination are examined. It leads on naturally to Chapter 7 where the forecasting issue is taken up in more detail and some mathematical models for forecasting future maps are outlined and exemplified.

Structure of the chapter

In the present chapter we have tried to illustrate some of the main disease groups found within the *International Classification of Diseases* discussed in Figure 2.1. Six of the 17 groups are represented. The diseases examined are presented in the order imposed by the ICD list. Although obviously not designed for the present purpose, the sequence followed by the ICD list is also helpful from a geographical point of view.

We begin our study of spatial cross-sections by considering diseases like measles and malaria from Group I (infectious and parasitic diseases) which have a clear geographical structure and ready explanations. We then move on to study diseases from Groups II (neoplasms), VII (diseases of the circulatory system) and XIV (congenital anomalies). Some have marked geographical patterns for which there is a known explanation while others display spatial patterns for which the generating processes producing the geographical concentration are not properly understood. These include, for example, some neoplasms. Finally we examine, as an example of events which have a significant impact upon medical services, but which are not disease-related, the striking spatial patterns produced by road-traffic and other accidents (ICD Group XVII) at different geographical scales.

Sources and Further Reading

The general concepts of space, time and space-time cross sections are discussed in P. Haggett, A.D. Cliff and A.E. Frey (1977), *Locational Analysis in Human Geography*, second edition, London: Edward Arnold. For an Icelandic application, see A.D. Cliff, P. Haggett, J.K. Ord, G.R. Versey (1981), *Spatial Diffusion: An Historical Geography of Epidemics in an Island Community*, Cambridge: Cambridge University Press.

Some of the general concepts behind the spatial and environmental study of disease are set out in R. Doll (1959), *Methods of Geographical Pathology*, Oxford: Oxford University Press, in J.S. Simmons, T.F. Whayne, G.W. Anderson and H.W. Horack (1944–54), *Global Epidemiology: A Geography of Disease and Sanitation*, Vols 1–3, Philadelphia: Lippincott, and in R. Doll, editor, *The Geography of Diseases*, London: Churchill Livingstone. For a set of maps of disease distribution at the world scale see American Geographical Society (1950–5), sheets of the 'Atlas of diseases', *Geographical Review*, 40, pp.648–9; 41, pp.272–3, 638–9; 42, pp.98–101, 282–3, 628–30; 43, pp.89–90, 253–5, 404; 44, pp.133–6, 408–10, 583–4; 45, p.416, 572. A commentary on some of the maps is included in J.M. May (1959), *Ecology of Human Disease*, New York: MD Publications.

3.2 RESPIRATORY TUBERCULOSIS IN WALES

TUBERCULOSIS (ICD 010–018; see Figure 2.1) is an infectious disease of man and animals caused by the tubercule bacilli *Mycobacterium tuberculosis* and *M. bovis*. The principal form of the disease in man is pulmonary (ICD 011). The disease is world-wide in its distribution. It has declined steadily in importance in the twentieth century in the developed nations largely as a result of vaccination and general improvements in hygiene. In addition, the large-scale elimination of bovine tuberculosis, along with the pasteurization of milk, has removed a common source of infection for man. At the present time, the death rate is highest in densely populated countries in the developing world where poor hygiene is common. In general, tuberculosis rates are higher in urban than in rural communities because of crowding and greater opportunity for infection. Public health practice and education are important in control. Higher rates are generally found in males than in females, and among the economically disadvantaged as opposed to the advantaged. Tuberculosis is almost always transmitted by inhalation of the bacilli from the sputum of persons with active pulmonary tuberculosis. Infection of the gastrointestinal tract following ingestion of contaminated foodstuffs is now rare.

County map patterns

In this figure, the cartographic technique of *choropleth mapping* (see Figures 1.5 and 1.6) and the statistical method of *probability mapping* (see Figure 1.7) are used to study county-by-county variations in Wales in the average annual female mortality from tuberculosis of the respiratory system between 1959 and 1963. Diagram (A) shows the average annual number of deaths, 1959–63, while, to allow for variations in the population size of the different counties, the crude death rate per 10^7 females living has been mapped in diagram (B). The names of the counties are associated with the data values in Table 3.2.1. Those counties whose crude death rate exceeded the average for Wales as a whole have been shaded to produce a choropleth map in diagram (C), and those in which the crude death rate exceeded the average for the United Kingdom have been shaded in diagram (D); the significance of the cross-hatching is discussed below. In diagrams (E) and (F), counties have been stippled if they fell below the average for Wales and the United Kingdom respectively.

The information contained in the six diagrams is to some extent conflicting. The average annual number of deaths mapped in (A) focuses attention upon the 'high' of 26 in county Glamorgan, a value far greater than that in any other county. However, once the data are scaled by populations and mapped as crude death rates, the beacon shifts from county Glamorgan to county Cardigan (1085 per 10^7 females living) on the west coast. Comparison of the county values with the averages for both Wales as a whole and the United Kingdom [diagrams (C) – (F)] highlights a split between the eastern and western halves of the country. The above average rates are found around the coast and the below average values are found mainly inland in the border region with England.

The position of Glamorgan

The diagrams illustrate the difficulty of working back from spatial patterns to generating processes. Centred on the Welsh coalfield, county Glamorgan is the most heavily urbanized part of Wales, and the excess mortality recorded there is consistent with the epidemiology of the disease outlined above. Most of the main towns in the principality are scattered around the coast and this may go some way towards accounting for the west–east split in tuberculosis intensity. It is, however, dangerous to proceed further without first asking whether the county values displayed are greater than or less than those we would expect by chance alone; that is, we need to know whether the patterns are 'significant', and therefore worth interpreting at all.

Poisson interpretations

As we have seen in Figure 1.7, one approach to the problem of determining which geographical areas in a spatial cross-section display either 'surprisingly high' or 'surprisingly low' incidence of a disease is to compare the observed values with those expected under a random (Poisson) distribution. From Table 3.2.1, the death rate per thousand population in Wales as a whole was 0.037 (that is, 50/1352.26). We may therefore compute the expected number of deaths in each county by multiplying the population value of each county (in thousands) by 0.037 to obtain data column three in the table. The actual deaths in column two can then be compared with these expected deaths using the Poisson formula discussed in the technical appendix to Figure 1.7. The expected deaths in each county are used to estimate the Poisson parameter, λ. The method is thus being used to determine which of the Welsh counties have significantly high and low levels of deaths from tuberculosis, as judged by their departure from Poissonian expectation. The probabilities appear in data column five of Table 3.2.1, and county Cardigan (main town, Aberystwyth) is identified as a significant tuberculosis black spot compared with the rest of Wales.

If we broaden the basis of comparison and examine the spatial pattern with reference to the death rate per thousand females of 0.032 for the

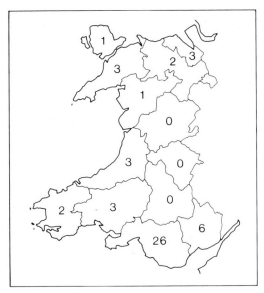

Figure 3.2 (A) Average annual number of female deaths 1959–1963

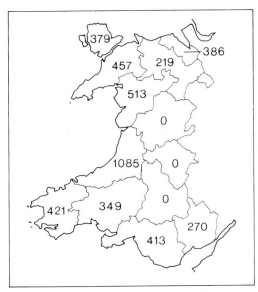

Figure 3.2 (B) Crude death rate per 10^7 females living

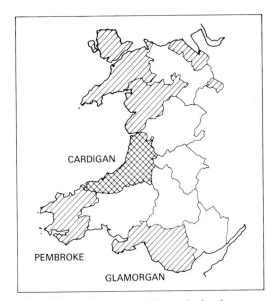

Figure 3.2 (C) Counties with crude death rates exceeding the average for Wales

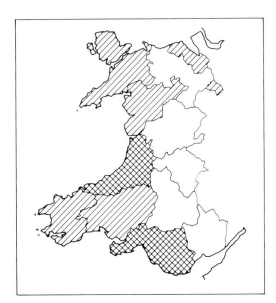

Figure 3.2 (D) Counties with crude death rates exceeding the average for the United Kingdom

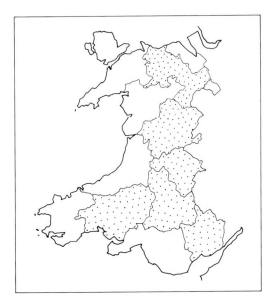

Figure 3.2 (E) Counties with crude death rates below the average for Wales

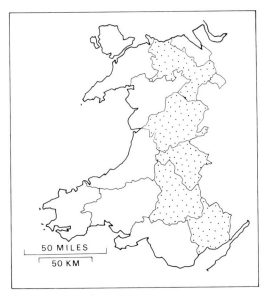

Figure 3.2 (F) Counties with crude death rates below the average for the United Kingdom

United Kingdom as a whole, then the probabilities in data column six of Table 3.2.1 are obtained. These confirm the high risk in Cardigan and suggest that Glamorgan is also substantially worse off than the United Kingdom as a whole. These high-risk areas have been cross-hatched in diagrams (C) and (D). They imply that only in two counties is it worth seeking an aetiological or environmental explanation for concentration of the disease, despite the seeming patterns thrown up by the cartographic techniques.

Table 3.2.1 also brings out the difference between frequencies of occurrence and probabilities. Pembroke has a mortality rate of 0.0421 per thousand, slightly higher than that in Glamorgan. However, the former is based on only two deaths observed as against 26 in Glamorgan. The Poisson probabilities place Glamorgan ahead of Pembroke in terms of risk compared with Wales as a whole and even worse off compared with the United Kingdom as a whole.

Finally we note from Table 3.2.1, again confirming the known epidemiology of the disease, the greater death rate in urban rather than rural areas.

Table 3.2.1 *Average annual female deaths from tuberculosis, 1959–1963, in the Welsh counties and Poisson probabilities compared with Welsh and UK averages.*

County	Popn. (000)	Observed deaths (rates in brackets)	Expected deaths using (a)	(b)	Probability based on (a)	(b)
Anglesey	26.38	1(0.0379)	0.976	0.844	0.255	0.207
Brecknock	27.29	0(0.0000)	1.010	0.873	0.364	0.418
Caernarvon	65.59	3(0.0457)	2.427	2.099	0.227	0.161
Cardigan	27.64	3(0.1085)	1.023	0.884	0.021★	0.013★
Carmarthen	86.06	3(0.0349)	3.184	2.754	0.606	0.298
Denbigh	91.16	2(0.0219)	3.373	2.917	0.345	0.442
Flint	77.82	3(0.0386)	2.879	2.490	0.326	0.240
Glamorgan	629.28	26(0.0413)	23.283	20.137	0.247	0.083★
Merioneth	19.51	1(0.0513)	0.722	0.624	0.164	0.130
Monmouth	222.62	6(0.0270)	8.237	7.124	0.285	0.431
Montgomery	22.09	0(0.0000)	0.817	0.707	0.442	0.493
Pembroke	47.52	2(0.0421)	1.758	1.521	0.258	0.197
Radnor	9.30	0(0.0000)	0.344	0.298	0.709	0.742
Totals						
Urban	947.47	35	35.056	30.319	0.395	0.132
Rural	404.79	15	14.977	12.953	0.469	0.319
Wales	1352.26	50				

(a) Welsh death rate; (b) UK death rate
Probabilities give the chance of obtaining, under the null hypothesis, observed deaths as big or bigger than those recorded for counties exceeding expectation, and as small or smaller for counties below expectation. Asterisked values are significant at the 10 percent level (1-tailed test).

Sources and Further Reading

Maps are redrawn from data in G.M. Howe, editor (1970), *National Atlas of Disease Mortality in the United Kingdom*, second edition, London: Royal Geographical Society, pp.56–7, 66–9. Further analysis of the data appears in A.D. Cliff and P. Haggett (1981), 'Mapping respiratory disease', in *Scientific Foundations of Respiratory Medicine*, edited by J.G. Scadding, G. Cumming and W.M. Thurlbeck, London: Heinemann, pp.30–43. Other maps of tuberculosis distribution are in M.J. Gardner, P.D. Winter and D.J.P. Barker (1984), *Atlas of Mortality from Selected Diseases in England and Wales, 1968–1978*, Chichester: John Wiley, pp.12–13, 42.

The epidemiology of tuberculosis is discussed in M.W. McNicol (1982), 'Tuberculosis', in *Epidemiology of Diseases*, edited by D.L. Miller and R.D.T. Farmer, Oxford: Blackwell Scientific, pp.31–9. A classic paper illustrating the application of probability concepts to a disease distribution in Poland is M. Choynowski (1959), 'Maps based upon probabilities', *Journal of the American Statistical Association*, 54, pp.385–8. See also the discussion of the Normal and Poisson distributions in Figure 1.7 of this Atlas.

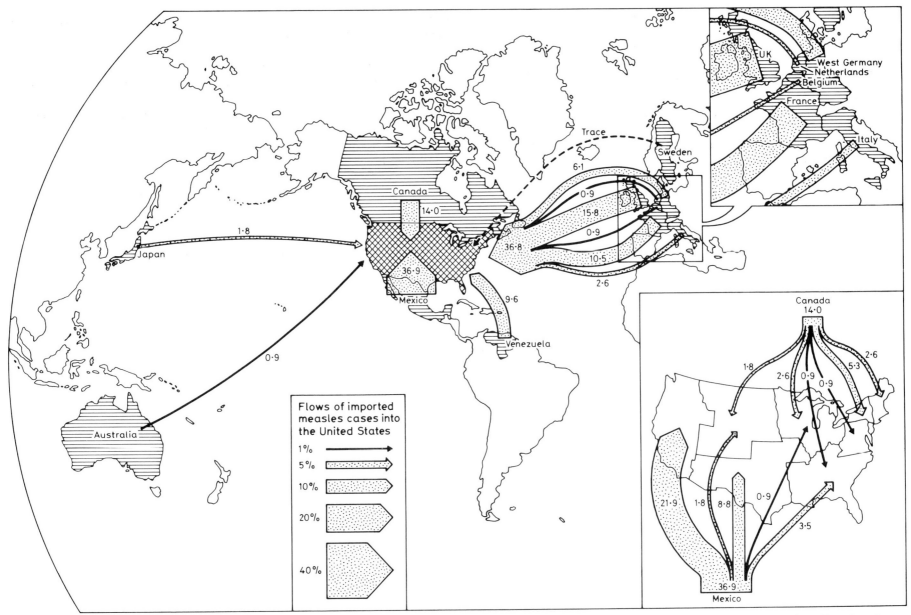

Figure 3.3 (A) International flows into the United States

Figure 3.3 (B) Regional flows from Canada and Mexico

3.3 MEASLES IMPORTS INTO THE UNITED STATES I: FLOW MAPS

MEASLES (*morbilli*, ICD 055; see Figure 2.1) is an epidemic disease of world-wide distribution. In each outbreak almost all persons who have never previously had the disease or been vaccinated against it are attacked. The causative virus was isolated by J.F. Enders and T.C. Peebles in 1954 and is one of the paramyxoviruses. The sequence of measles virus infection in an individual host normally involves three stages. First, a latent period of 7–14 days occurs during which the virus establishes itself and multiplies rapidly within the host; this period extends from initial exposure to the virus to the first appearance of cold-like symptoms. These symptoms herald the prodromal period of 2–4 days in which the patient shows upper respiratory catarrhal disorder and fever. It culminates in the third stage or external rash period. Here a distinctive raised red rash occurs, appearing initially behind the ears, spreading to the face and thereafter to the body and limbs. This stage may last from 4–10 days. The disease is highly infectious from the prodromal period onwards and, in the absence of control measures, spreads rapidly from susceptible contact to susceptible contact and from geographical area to geographical area.

Measles in the United States

Although measles is a highly infectious disease with a world-wide distribution, its presence in certain countries has been greatly reduced by vaccination. In the United States, the first licensing of attenuated-live and killed-virus vaccines against measles in 1963 saw the evolution from the mid-1960s onwards of a systematic programme of measles eradication from that country (see Figure 4.9).

By the mid-1980s, annual case levels in the United States had been so reduced by vaccination that attention was turned in the measles elimination programme from internal sources of measles outbreaks to external sources of infection. Studies of measles outbreaks by the Immunization Division of the Centers for Disease Control indicated that future importation of measles into the United States will be related, obviously, both to the level of measles incidence in the foreign country and to the level of exchange in terms of travel flow between that country and the United States. The specific risk in a particular part of the United States is further linked to the concentration of flow from a foreign country into particular 'gateway' cities and states where, for example, major international airports are located.

Mapping measles imports

The movements of infected cases into the United States may be represented using *flow maps*. There are two main types: those which simply symbolize the direction of flow by means of a line, usually with an arrowhead, and those which also portray the amount of flow by the width of the line. In this figure, the latter are used to examine the sources of measles importation into the United States. Notice also in the map the use of 'tributary' flows from various European countries which join to cross the Atlantic. Such tributaries should always be drawn entering the main flow smoothly to enhance the visual impression of movement.

Diagram (A) shows the known external sources of measles cases brought into the United States in the years 1980 and 1981. The width of the flow line from any country is proportional to its percentage share of the total number of measles cases in the United States which were

attributed to external sources. The immediate neighbours of the United States, Mexico and Canada, provided just over half of the externally generated cases, while the United Kingdom and France dominated the flows emanating from Europe.

When the gateways into the United States are examined in map (B) in the larger of the inset maps, then the association of the Canadian flow with the heavily populated and traditional industrial areas of the northeastern United States and the Midwest is apparent. In the same way, the dominance of southern California as a collecting area for cases originating in Mexico is marked. This flow is made up of both illegal immigrants and seasonal agricultural and hotel workers employed in large numbers in California. It is evident that the regions within the United States which act as the chief 'sink' areas for cases arriving from both Canada and Mexico all have close physical proximity to the originating countries; flows collapse rapidly with increasing distance from the source areas. The main European gateway is New York, focused upon J.F.K. international airport.

Modelling spatial flows

A wide variety of *spatial interaction* models have been developed in geography which can be fitted to data on flows between areas. In general terms, these models recognize that flows are likely to be directly proportional to the size (for example, in population) of the origin and destination areas of any flow, and inversely proportional to the distance between them. We have already seen this distance-decay effect in the way in which measles importations from Mexico and Canada rapidly diminish with distance from their international frontiers with the United States. In the same way, the larger population areas of Europe

(France, United Kingdom) generate bigger measles flows to the United States than do the smaller areas (Netherlands, Belgium), even though their distance from the United States is roughly the same.

The structure of these spatial interaction models is examined in detail in the next figure and one version is applied to the data considered here. These models are important because, once fitted to current data, they can then be used either to predict future flow levels or else to estimate flows between areas where data are missing.

Sources and Further Reading

The maps are based on unpublished data on imported measles cases provided by the Centers for Disease Control, Atlanta, through the courtesy of Dr A.R. Hinman. The cartographic methods used in the flow maps are described in A.H. Robinson, R.D. Sale, J.L. Morrison and P.C. Muehrcke (1984), 'Mapping with line symbols', in *Elements of Cartography*, fifth edition, New York: John Wiley, pp.307–36.

Measles is described at length in K.B. Fraser and S.J. Martin (1978), *Measles Virus and its Biology*, London: Academic Press, and by F.L. Black (1984), 'Measles', in *Viral Infections of Humans: Epidemiology and Control*, second edition, edited by A.S. Evans, New York: Plenum, pp.397–418. Variations in measles mortality in relation to crowding and malnutrition are reviewed in P. Aaby (1988), 'Measles mortality', *Review of Infectious Diseases*, 10, pp.451–91. The eradication programme in the United States is described by A.R. Hinman, A.D. Brandling-Bennett and P.I. Nieburg (1979), 'The opportunity and obligation to eliminate measles from the United States', *Journal of the American Medical Association*, 242, pp.1157–62. See also Figures 3.4 and 4.9, and Section 6.5.

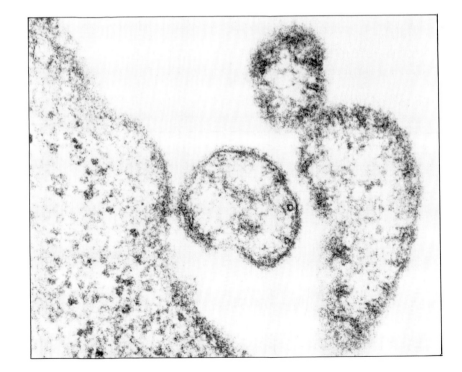

Figure 3.3 (C) Complete measles virion at a magnification of × 120,000
(Source: Electron micrograph by courtesy of Dr K.B. Fraser and Dr S.J. Martin, of the Department of Microbiology and Immunology and the Department of Biochemistry, at The Queen's University, Belfast.)

3.4 MEASLES IMPORTS INTO THE UNITED STATES II: MODELLING FLOWS

In the previous figure, we saw how the flows of measles cases (for disease description see box in Figure 3.3) between a set of originating areas or zones (countries in this instance) and a set of destination areas (US regions) could be represented pictorially by a flow map. Such maps contain a limited amount of quantitative information and we must turn to *spatial interaction* models if we are to provide a more general quantitative description of the flows shown.

Gravity models of flows

In studying flows, a simple gravity formulation suggests that interaction is directly proportion to the 'masses' of the origin and destination zones generating and receiving the flows and inversely proportional to some function of distance between them. In the context of disease incidence and the movement of disease from one area to another, we might use the population sizes of the origin and destination zones as measures of 'mass'; naively, larger populations might be expected to generate greater incidence of disease, although more subtle measures of mass might be used which allow for, say, vaccinations, demographic structure and so on. In the same way we would expect, *ceteris paribus*, zones which are closer together to have larger flows between them than zones which are further apart.

Mathematically, these ideas may be represented in the following way. Let T_{ij} denote the flow (of measles) between some origin area i and a destination area j. O_i is used to represent the total outflow from area i to all other areas, and D_j indicates the total inflow into area j from all other areas. Finally, L_{ij} gives the geographical distance, travel time, travel cost, or some other measure of deterrence between i and j. Then a generalized flows model (Wilson, 1970), is written as

$$T_{ij} = (A_i O_i)(B_j D_j)[\exp(cL_{ij})], \qquad (3.4.1)$$

subject to

$$\sum_j T_{ij} = O_i, \quad i = 1,2, \ldots ,n, \qquad (3.4.2)$$

$$\sum_i T_{ij} = D_j, \quad j = 1,2, \ldots ,n, \qquad (3.4.3)$$

and $\quad \sum_i \sum_j T_{ij} L_{ij} = C. \qquad (3.4.4)$

Here, C is a global cost constraint and n is the number of areas in the spatial cross-section. This model may be estimated using *entropy maximising* techniques. Then the quantities, A, B and c are functions of Lagrangean multipliers which describe flows in a general way in terms of the contribution of mass and distance to the process of interaction. The masses are positively related while interaction is assumed to decline as a negative exponential function of distance; this implies A, $B>0$ and $c<0$.

Observed and predicted flows

In equations (3.4.1) – (3.4.4) we have taken as the $\{O_i\}$ the proportion of the total number of measles cases attributed to foreign sources which originated in each of the 12 countries (see Figure 3.3) and, as the $\{D_j\}$, the proportion finishing in each of the eight US regions. Since we might expect the proportion of cases originating in country i and finishing in region j to be directly related to passenger traffic flows between the two, a simple measure of deterrance is provided by setting

$$L_{ij} = P_{ij} d_{ij} \qquad (3.4.5)$$

Here P_{ij}, given in Table 3.4.1, is the proportion of foreign arrivals in the US which left country i and arrived in region j. The quantity, d_{ij}, denotes the geographical distance (in statute miles) between i and j and, although more complex measures can be suggested, was used as a surrogate for cost of movement because of ease of measurement. Equation (3.4.5) implies that large passenger flows moving over long distances generate a high 'cost' of connection between i and j, and vice versa. The average cost of movement over all flows was 2610 units and this was used to estimate C in equation (3.4.4).

From the matrix of flows between all origins and destinations produced by the model, we have mapped in diagram (A) those originating in Mexico and Canada; solid black arrows are employed to represent the observed flows of measles cases between the two countries and US regions, with horizontally line-shaded arrows superimposed to denote the flows predicted by the model. As in Figure 3.3, flows are proportional to the width of the arrows. There is reasonable agreement between observed and predicted flows but, as is commonly found with such models, there is some degree of spatial smoothing in the predicted values. The largest flow (for example, Mexico to Far West) is underestimated, while positive flows are predicted for some links where none was observed (for example, Mexico to Eastern Gateway).

Interpreting Lagrangean multipliers

Diagram (B) uses columns to show the Lagrangean multipliers associated with the origin

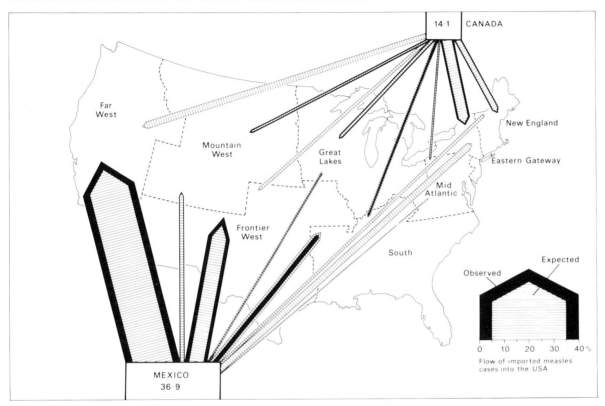

Figure 3.4 (A) Observed and predicted flows of measles into the US from Canada and Mexico

countries [A_i in equation (3.4.1)] and with the destination regions (B_j); the former have been stippled and the latter have been horizontally line-shaded. The $\{A_i\}$ discriminate broadly between countries close to the United States (small A_i) and those peripherally located (large A_i). The multipliers associated with the destination regions fall from west to east across the United States, with the largest D_j found in the western regions and the smallest on the Atlantic seaboard.

The exponent of distance in equation (3.4.1) was estimated by the model as $c = -0.97$, consistent with a fairly rapid fall-off of flows with distance.

Table 3.4.1 *Percentage of total foreign arrivals in eight United States travel regions from twelve principal countries.*

Country	New England	Far West	Eastern Gateway	The South	Great Lakes	Frontier West	Mid Atlantic	Mountain West
Canada	25.8	10.8	6.2	7.6	6.0	1.4	1.7	2.8
Mexico	0.3	4.9	1.1	1.4	0.7	4.3	0.4	0.3
UK	0.6	1.1	1.6	0.6	0.6	0.4	0.9	0.2
W. Germany	0.2	0.9	1.2	0.5	0.4	0.5	0.4	0.3
Japan	0.1	1.7	0.7	0.2	0.3	0.3	0.2	0.1
France	0.2	0.5	0.8	0.4	0.2	0.3	0.3	0.1
Australia	0.1	0.2	0.4	0.2	0.2	0.3	0.3	0.2
Italy	0.1	0.3	0.6	0.1	0.1	0.2	0.3	0.1
Netherlands	0.1	0.3	0.2	0.1	0.2	0.1	0.1	0.1
Venezuela	0.0	0.1	0.3	0.5	0.0	0.1	0.1	0.0
Sweden	0.1	0.2	0.3	0.1	0.2	0.1	0.1	0.0
Belgium	0.0	0.1	0.2	0.1	0.1	0.1	0.1	0.0

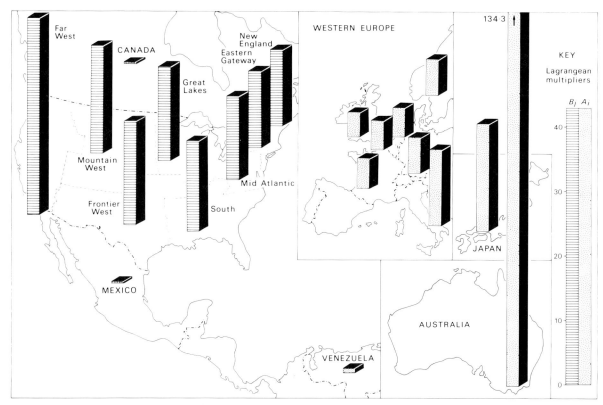

Figure 3.4 (B) Langrangean multipliers associated with origins (*A*ᵢ) and destinations (*B*ⱼ)

Sources and Further Reading

The measles data are described in Figure 3.4 of this Atlas. Additional demographic data on migration movements are based on US Department of Commerce (1975), *Arrivals and Departures by Selected Ports, Calendar Year 1975*, Washington, DC: Government Printing Office; US Department of Commerce (1979), *Analysis of International Travel to the United States*, Washington, DC: Government Printing Office; US Department of Transportation (1980), *International Travel Statistics, Calendar Year 1980*, Cambridge, Mass.: Transport Information Division.

The models used are described in A.G. Wilson (1970), *Entropy in Urban and Regional Modelling*, London: Pion. See also the review in P. Haggett, A.D. Cliff and A.E. Frey (1977), *Locational Analysis in Human Geography*, second edition, London: Edward Arnold, pp.25–63. There are relatively few cases where spatial interaction models have been applied in an epidemiological context but see R. Earickson (1970), *The Spatial Behaviour of Hospital Patients: A Behavioural Approach to Spatial Interaction in Metropolitan Chicago*, Chicago, Ill.: University of Chicago Press, Department of Geography Research Papers No. 124, Chicago: University of Chicago Press.

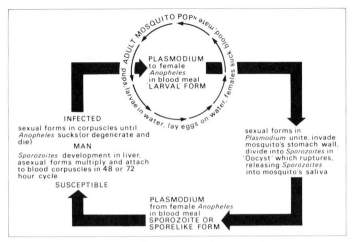

Figure 3.5 (A) Life cycle of the *plasmodium* parasite

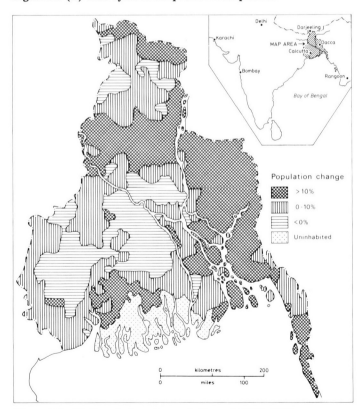

Figure 3.5 (C) Population change in Bengal, 1901–1911

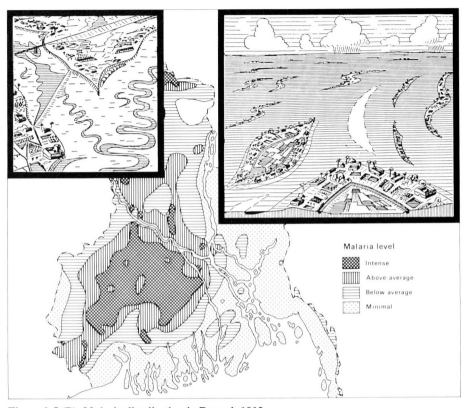

Figure 3.5 (B) Malaria distribution in Bengal, 1913

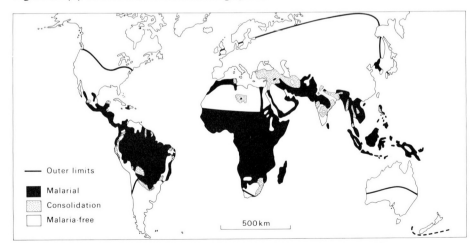

Figure 3.5 (D) World distribution of malaria in relation to WHO eradication programmes

3.5 MALARIA IN BENGAL

MALARIA (ICD 084; see Figure 2.1) is an infection produced in man by several species of protozoan parasites which are members of a single genus, *Plasmodium*. The parasites are transmitted naturally by the bite of an infected female anopheline mosquito. These mosquitoes are the only known vectors of human malaria and some 60 different species perform this function in various parts of the world. The mosquitoes undergo an aquatic larval stage, pupate and hatch into flying adults in about ten days, depending upon the temperature of the water. While the males feed on plant juices, the females require blood meals to produce fertile eggs. Usually their flight range is one mile or less from the source of human blood and infection. After the mosquito has ingested a blood meal containing the infectious forms of the parasite, the parasite penetrates and creates cysts on the outer wall of the mosquito's stomach. These cysts rupture and the organisms make their way through the body cavity to the salivary glands where they lie in wait until the female bites a susceptible human being. There are four recognised species of the parasite that produce malaria in man and each has an asexual part of its life-cycle in the tissue and blood of man, while the sexual stage can complete development only in a mosquito. Thus the parasite must be returned from man to a female mosquito via another bite and blood meal to complete its development. As shown in diagram (A), the cycle then repeats itself.

The symptoms produced include alternate bouts of chill, followed by high fever, sweating and prostration. The time intervals between these episodes are a function of the precise species of the parasite involved. Death often results, especially if complications like blackwater fever ensue.

Epidemiology of malaria

Malaria is one of the most ancient infections known to man and was noted in the records of Hippocrates in the fifth century BC. It is a world-wide disease and there are probably more cases of it than of any other infection. It is most common in the tropics, where climatic conditions are favourable for the mosquito throughout the year ($70°$–$80°$F and 70–80 percent relative humidity).

Our initial account highlights the critical interaction of man and insect in the propagation of the disease. The *plasmodium* parasite requires residence at certain stages in its life cycle in both man and mosquito, and the female mosquito requires human blood meals for the maturation of her eggs. Hence the geographical intensity of the disease is highest where dense human populations live within flying distance (as already noted, up to one mile) of the breeding grounds; these grounds depend upon the species of mosquito involved. The Ganges delta region of northeast India and Bangladesh (formerly Bengal) illustrated in diagrams (B) and (C) provides an ideal area in which to examine the interplay of these factors. Here the main vector is *Anopheles philippinensis* whose preferred water for breeding includes tanks, pools, borrow-pits, ditches and clear, uncontaminated water with marginal vegetation and dense growth of sub-aqueous bushes.

The maps given in diagrams (B) and (C) are historical and show the level of malaria in the Ganges delta region in 1913 and the changing distribution of population between 1901 and 1911. They are based upon maps in C. A. Bentley's 1916 *Report on Malaria in Bengal*. Choropleth techniques have been used (see Figure 1.6). Apart from the mouth where the river enters the Bay of Bengal, the maps are almost mirror images of each other. Greatest population growth has occurred in the least malarial areas of the 'active' eastern delta. Here, the purging action by spread flooding of water channels and water bodies flushes most breeding places free of the larvae of *A. philippinensis* at the very time when temperature, rainfall and humidity would be most favourable (in the autumn). In the 'dying' delta of the west, a multiplicity of breeding places exist, together with a lower water table which also appears to encourage breeding of this vector. In the pen sketches of diagram (B), water areas are drawn in horizontal line shading. The sketch in the east delta shows the flushing of water channels in (then) East Bengal at the height of the flood season, while that in the west delta illustrates breeding places around settlements in (then) West Bengal.

WHO eradication campaign

The community health problem posed by malaria is so extensive that, at the end of the Second World War, it was estimated by the New York Academy of Medicine that upwards of 3 million malarial deaths and at least 300 million cases of malarial fever were occurring annually throughout the world. The World Health Organization responded at its Eighth Assembly in 1955, which had as its goal 'the world-wide eradication of malaria' (WHO, 1955, p.31). For the next fifteen years the programme was as follows in each targeted country: (a) a preparatory phase characterized primarily by geographical reconnaissance and staff training; (b) an attack phase with total coverage spraying; (c) a consolidation phase, during which total coverage spraying ceased and surveillance was carried out; and (d) a maintenance phase from the time malaria was eradicated.

The attack phase in each country was dominated by the use of residual insecticides, especially DDT, against the adult mosquito. Anti-larval measures like draining were also employed against the water-bodies used as breeding grounds, and improved therapeutic and prophylactic drugs have also played a part. As a result, the white areas on diagram (D) between the 'past limits' line and the shaded areas formerly occupied by mainly seasonal but locally severe malaria were cleared by the mid 1970s either incidentally by improved agricultural technology or else by specific campaigns. The lightly shaded areas of diagram (D) have been virtually freed of malaria as a result of eradication programmes and are in the consolidation phase. The darkly shaded areas represent regions where the malarial cycle has not been interrupted. These coincide with the great tropical forest belts where control with residual insecticides is difficult and jungle, rather than house, haunting species of *Anopheles* exist.

shown in graph (E). The figures exclude China up to 1976 and Africa since 1981. The resurgence was reinforced by lack of resources in the countries affected and by the emergence of drug-resistant forms of *plasmodium*, handicapping treatment of human hosts. Although some decline has occurred in the 1980s, the latest preliminary data still show recorded malaria cases well above their early 1970s level. The Eighteenth Report of the WHO Expert Committee on Malaria (WHO, 1986) recognized this problem and has called for a redoubling of effort. The hope for a world without malaria is a long way off.

Sources and Further Reading

Diagrams (B) and (C) and the pen-sketches have been redrawn from A.T.A. Learmonth (1957), 'Some regional contrasts in the regional geography of malaria in India and Pakistan', *Transactions of the Institute of British Geographers*, 23, pp.37–59. The world distribution map is based upon a diagram in WHO (1974), *ICAS Report on Malaria*, Geneva.

A general account of the world geography of malaria is given in A.T.A. Learmonth (1977), 'Malaria', in *A World Geography of Human Diseases*, edited by G.M. Howe, London: Academic Press, pp.61–108. The continuing fight against malaria is recorded in the reports of the WHO Expert Committee on Malaria; see World Health Organization (1986), 'WHO Expert Committee on Malaria: Eighteenth Report', *WHO Technical Report Series*, 735. One detailed African case study is R.M. Prothero (1965), *Migrants and Malaria*, London: Longmans Green.

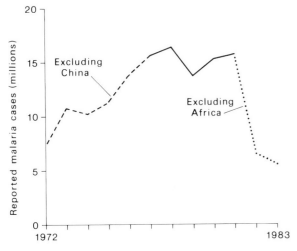

Figure 3.5 (E) Global malaria cases reported to WHO annually, 1972–1983

Although the use of DDT revolutionized the campaigns, the emergence of resistant forms of mosquito and the later widespread abandonment of DDT as an insecticide because of its persistence in food chains meant that, while the incidence of malaria at first declined, it began to increase again from the mid 1970s. This trend is

3.6 CANCER IN ENGLAND AND WALES: PLEURAL AND BLADDER

A **MALIGNANT NEOPLASM** (ICD 140–208 and 230–239; see Figure 2.1) is an autonomous new growth of tissue. It possesses an atypical structure of the body tissues or organs in which it originates, serves no useful purpose in the economy of the individual and exhibits unlimited and uncontrolled power of growth. It has the ability and tendency to spread locally by contiguous growth and to metastasize to distant locations where it may lodge and assume a renewal of growth. It is composed of cells or of cells and intercellular substances which tend to differentiate as cells do normally from the tissues in which the malignant neoplasm arose.

Role of cancer atlases

Although it may seem unpromising to look for causal factors which produce regional variations in cancer incidence, Doll (1983) has pointed out that, prior to 1914, knowledge of the causes of cancer grew almost entirely as a result of recognizing that different types of cancer occurred characteristically in men and women who lived in a particular part of the world or who were engaged in a particular occupation; we examine two such occupational cancers in this plate.

There is a growing belief from the world-wide differences observed in the incidence of different types of cancer that all the common types may be avoidable, and that they may be caused by some mixture of dietary, cultural, social and environmental factors. In this Atlas, both the extreme geographical concentration of nasopharyngeal carcinoma among the southern Chinese (Figure 3.7) and of Burkitt's lymphoma in parts of Africa and New Guinea (Figure 5.16) provide examples of malignancies which, because of their peculiar spatial patterns, have provoked intensive searches for environmental causes or environment triggers for biological processes.

The recognition that regional variations do exist in the incidence of different cancers has brought new interest to the medical tradition of mapping cancer incidence both on a global scale and at a local level within individual countries. Several recent atlases of cancer mortality have resulted. The standard work in the United Kingdom is M.J. Gardner, P.D. Winter, C.P. Taylor and E.D. Acheson (1983), *Atlas of Cancer Mortality in England and Wales, 1968–1978* (Chichester: John Wiley) which summarizes some of the research of the internationally known Medical Research Council Environmental Epidemiology Unit at the University of Southampton and Southampton General Hospital. The equivalent United States publication is by T.J. Mason, F.W. McKay, R. Hoover, W.J. Blot and J.F. Fraumeni (1975), *Atlas of Cancer Mortality for United States Counties: 1950–1969* (Washington, DC: Government Printing Office).

Cancer in England and Wales

As an illustration of the work being undertaken, we have selected in the present figure two cancers considered in Gardner *et al*. These are, in diagram (A), male and female mortality from mesothelioma of the pleura (ICD 163) and, in diagram (B), male and female mortality from cancer of the bladder (ICD 188). The data cover the period from 1968–78, and relate to 1,366 local authority areas in England and Wales. In both diagrams, the category, 'significantly high', includes those local authorities with standardized mortality ratios [SMRs (cf. Figure 2.7)] in the top tenth (that is, in the top 137) of local authorities in England and Wales and those with SMRs significantly greater than 100 at the 99 percent level when judged against a Poisson distribution (cf. Figure 1.7). The category, 'significantly low', consists of the corresponding local authorities in the lower tail of the distribution.

Pleural mesothelioma

MESOTHELIOMA OF THE PLEURA (ICD 163; see Figure 2.1) is a cancer of the pleura, which is the delicate serous membrane lining each half of the thoracic cavity and folded back over the surface of the lung of the same side.

In diagram (A), the pattern of excess mortality in males reflects the location of (a) the main naval dockyards and ports (Plymouth, Portsmouth, Southampton, London, Liverpool, Barrow-in-Furness, Teesside and Tyneside; (b) railway and carriage works (Crewe and Watford) and (c) textile towns in northern England (Rochdale, Leeds).

Pleural mesothelioma is specifically linked to exposure to asbestos dust, especially crocidolite (blue asbestos). So specific is it as a disease that of the 1,366 local authority areas, 916 for men and 1,133 for women had no deaths from this cause during 1968–78. Before the carcinogenic nature of asbestos was established, it was widely used in the shipbuilding and railway industries for fire resistance and for heat and soundproofing purposes. Asbestos yarns, impregnated with graphite and suitable greases were used for steam pipe and pump packings; as yarn, it also appeared in brake linings and other friction materials. Woven into cloth it was employed to form fireproof wall linings. The map of female

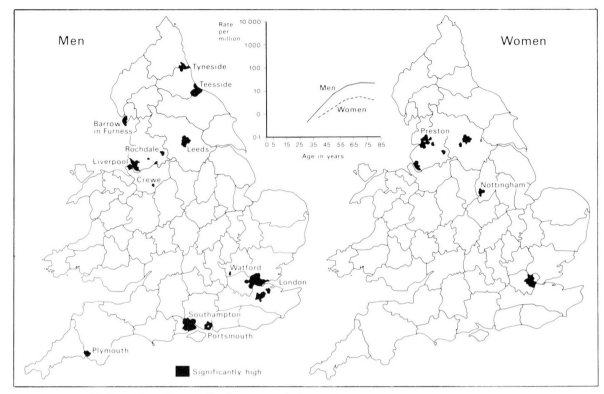

Figure 3.6 (A) Male and female mortality from mesothelioma of the pleura

mortality shows the same features to a lesser degree.

Cancer of the bladder

CANCER OF THE BLADDER (ICD 188; see Figure 2.1) is almost always the warty form of cancer known as epithelioma. It usually springs as a sessile growth from the mucous membrane of the floor near the opening of one of the ureters, or at the base and trigone of the bladder. It is one of the severest forms of cancer owing to the local changes it produces and its tendency to cause a fistulous opening between bladder and rectum in the male or vagina in the female. The most common type is primary carcinoma of the bladder. Secondary cancer is usually due to an extension of growth from the rectum or uterus. It often produces an initial symptom of haematuria or blood in the urine which may be associated with frequent urination and pain. In extreme cases the entire bladder may be removed surgically for the preservation of life.

Bladder cancer has a higher incidence than pleural mesothelioma. Many of the areas with raised SMRs are located in parts of north-central England where there have been concentrations of the dyestuff and rubber industries which used known carcinogens as part of the manufacturing process. In the dye industry aniline, benzidine and betanaphthylamine have been particularly implicated. Several high incidence areas occur in southeast England where this explanation is not relevant and a search for causes is being initiated by workers at the Southampton Environmental Epidemiology Unit. The example is important because it illustrates how unexplained features arising in mapped distributions can stimulate investigative research.

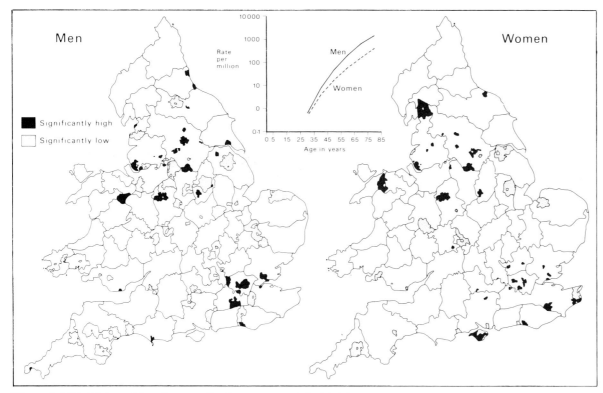

Figure 3.6 (B) Male and female mortality from cancer of the bladder

Sources and Further Reading

Diagram (A) has been compiled from M.J. Gardner, P.D. Winter, C.P. Taylor and E.D. Acheson (1983), *Atlas of Cancer Mortality in England and Wales, 1968–1978*, Chichester: John Wiley, pp.28–9 and p.46, while diagram (B) was prepared from pp.32–3 and p.48.

One of the standard references on the possible role played by various factors in the causation of cancer is R. Doll and R. Peto (1981), *The Causes of Cancer*, Oxford: Oxford University Press. A relevant paper is M.J. Gardner, P.D. Winter, E.D. Acheson (1982), 'Variations in cancer mortality among local authority areas in England and Wales: relations with environmental factors and search for causes', *British Medical Journal*, 284, pp.784–87. See also G.M. Howe (1979), 'Mortality from selected malignant neoplasms in the British Isles: the spatial perspective', *Geographical Journal*, 145, pp.401–15; R.J. Berry (1982), 'Carcinoma of the bladder', in *Epidemiology of Diseases*, edited by D.L. Miller and R.D.T. Farmer, Oxford: Blackwell Scientific, pp.266–72, and G.M. Matanoski and E.A. Elliott (1981), 'Bladder cancer epidemiology', *Epidemiologic Reviews*, 3, pp.203–29.

Geographical aspects of the distribution of malignant neoplasms are reviewed by C.R. Gillis (1977), 'Malignant neoplasms', in *World Geography of Human Diseases*, edited by G.M. Howe, London: Academic Press, pp.507–34. A major world atlas of cancer distributions is G.M. Howe, editor (1986), *Global Geocancerology: A World Geography of Human Cancers*, Edinburgh: Churchill Livingstone. See also R. Doll, C. Muir and J. Waterhouse (1970), *Cancer Incidence on Five Continents*, vol. 2, Geneva: World Health Organization, and B.J. Glick (1982), 'The spatial organization of cancer mortality', *Annals of the Association of American Geographers*, 82, pp.471–81.

Cancers have frequently been mapped at the national level. See for example T.J. Mason, F.W. McKay Jr, R. Hoover, W.J. Blot and J.F. Fraumeni Jr (1975), *Atlas of Cancer Mortality for United States Counties, 1950–69*, National Institute of Health Publication 75–780, Washington, DC: Government Printing Office and W.J. Blot and J.F. Fraumeni (1978), 'Geographic patterns of bladder cancer in the United States', *Journal of the National Cancer Institute*, 61, pp.1017–23. A number of other cancer atlases are listed in Part 2 of the References at the end of the Atlas.

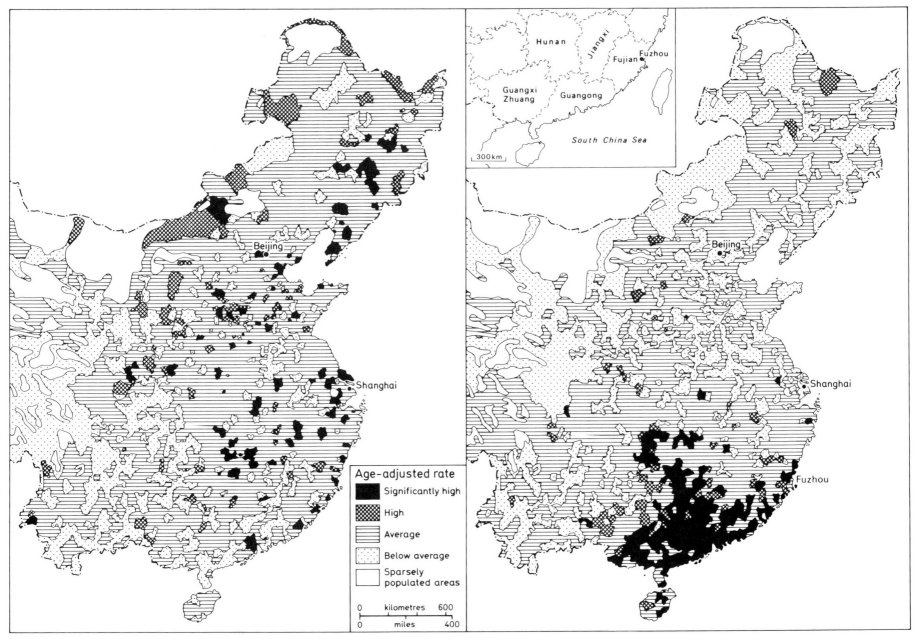

Age-adjusted rate

■ Significantly high

▨ High

☰ Average

⋰ Below average

□ Sparsely populated areas

0   kilometres   600

0   miles   400

Hunan   Jiangxi

Fujian Fuzhou

Guangxi   Guangong
Zhuang

South China Sea

300km

Beijing

Shanghai

Fuzhou

Figure 3.7 (A) Distribution of control cancer (female breast cancer)   **Figure 3.7 (B) Distribution of nasopharyngeal carcinoma in females**

3.7 NASOPHARYNGEAL CARCINOMA IN CHINA

NASOPHARYNGEAL CARCINOMA is disease 147 in the ICD list. See Figure 2.1. The tumorous process often infiltrates underneath an apparently normal mucosa. The vast majority of nasopharyngeal carcinomas (NPCs) arise from the nasopharyngeal epithelium and should be considered as variants of squamous cell carcinomas, irrespective of their appearance on light microscopy. The biological behaviour of the tumour may be metastatic, invasive, or both.

Cancer maps of China

For the vast majority of population groups, the incidence rates for NPC are below one per 100,000 per annum. In persons of Chinese descent, however, much higher rates have been found and distinctive regional patterns exist. The present figure shows the age-adjusted mortality rate per 100,000 population from female breast cancer [diagram (A)] and from female NPC [diagram (B)], in relation to the national rates in the main settled regions of the People's Republic of China. The data cover the period from 1973–75 and have been mapped at a county by county level using choropleth techniques (see Figure 1.6). The map for female breast cancer (ICD 174) has been included as a control since strong regional variations are not generally claimed for this disease. The patterns displayed serve to emphasize the enormous geographical concentration of NPC in the southern part of China in the provinces of Guangdong, Hunan, Fujian and Jiangxi, and in the autonomous region of Guangxi Zhuang. Mortality rates from NPC generally decline northwards.

Epidemiology of NPC

Such a distinctive regional pattern has resulted in a large number of studies which have attempted to discover the cause. The concentration appears epidemiological in nature and, as with Burkitt's lymphoma (BL) discussed in Figure 5.16, led to the suggestion of intervention by biological and/or environmental factors. It was discovered that, like BL, there exists the same serological and virological association between the tumour and the Epstein-Barr virus (EBV), with the strong implication of a causal relationship. The EBV is a member of the herpes group of viruses. It is the cause of heterophil-positive infectious mononucleosis, of some heterophil-negative cases, and of occasional cases of tonsillitis and pharyngitis in childhood. However, EBV is globally ubiquitous. Antibody to EBV has been demonstrated in every population tested, including very isolated tribes in Brazil, Alaska and other remote areas where even measles and influenza antibody are often lacking. Given the world-wide distribution of EBV, any triggering mechanism to release the oncogenic properties of the virus remains to be discovered for both BL and NPC.

There is little doubt that the concentration of NPC in individuals of Chinese descent reflects to some degree immunogenetic susceptibility; female incidence rates per annum of between 3

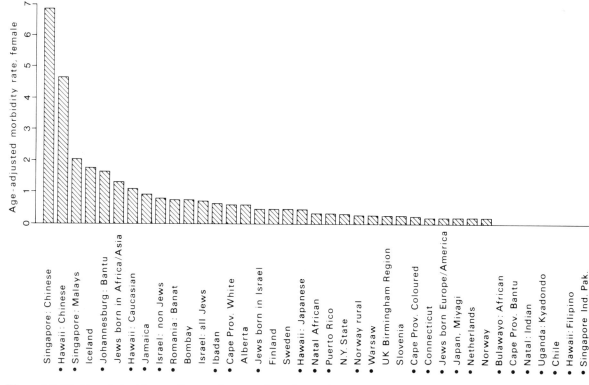

Figure 3.7 (C) Female incidence of narsopharyngeal carcinoma by ethnic groups

and 11 per 100,000 population may be contrasted with the general world rate of about 1 given earlier. Available morbidity data plotted in diagram (C) show that, for the vast majority of cancer registries, not only are the age-adjusted rates below 1 per 100,000 per annum, but also many rates are based on fewer than 10 cases [spotted in diagram (C)]. Moreover, within the general Chinese susceptibility, descriptive epidemiology has established that persons of southern Chinese descent, no matter where they live, or southeast Asian populations who have genetic similarities to southern Chinese such as Malays, are at high risk from this cancer. As diagram (B) shows, the disease is less common in north China and rare in the Japanese who are also of north Mongoloid origin.

Cultural factors in south China

Inevitably, a geographical concentration of disease on a scale like that shown in diagram (B) has led a large number of workers to seek an environmental explanation. Dietary, atmospheric (air pollution, smoking) and occupational factors have been tested against control groups, largely without success. The only real suspicion attaches to the use of salted fish in southern China which has been found to contain traces of dimethylnitrosamine (nitrosodimethylamine). This comestible is a traditional food in southern but not northern or central Chinaa and is eaten from early childhood on. While this may be difficult to investigate, it is known from animal experiments that a single dose of N-nitroso-dimethylamine is capable of inducing tumours in more than 70 percent of rats.

As might have been anticipated, there are unlikely to be any easy answers. The control of NPC is a major public health problem in southern China and in some parts of southeast Asia. Almost certainly, the aetiology will be multifactor, and the sieve-map approach described in Figure 1.13 may prove to be useful in that context.

Sources and Further Reading

The maps have been simplified and redrawn from large-scale versions in the Chinese Academy of Medical Sciences (1981), *Atlas of Cancer Mortality in the People's Republic of China*, Shanghai: China Map Press, pp.77–8, 85–6.

In addition to the general sources on malignant neoplasms described in Figure 3.6, see G. de-Thé, J.H.C. Ho and C. Muir (1984), 'Nasopharyngeal carcinoma', in *Viral Infections of Humans: Epidemiology and Control*, second edition, edited by A.S. Evans, New York: Plenum, pp.621–52. The Epstein-Barr virus is discussed in the same volume of essays; see A.S. Evans and J.C. Niederman, 'Epstein-Barr virus', pp.253–82. The standard works are G. de Thé and X. Yto, editors (1978), *Nasopharyngeal Carcinoma: Etiology and Control*, Lyons: IARC, and E. Gzundman, G. Kzueger, E. Gzundman, G.R.F. Kzueger and D. Ablashi, editors (1981), *Nasopharyngeal Carcinoma*, Stuttgart: Fischer Verlag. One geographical study of local variations is R.W. Armstrong, K. Kannan Kutty and S.K. Dharmalingham (1974), 'Incidence of nasopharyngeal carcinoma in Malaysia, with special reference to the state of Selangor', *British Journal of Cancer*, 30, pp.86–94. A general account of cancer variation in China is given in B. Armstrong (1980), 'The epidemiology of cancer in the People's Republic of China', *International Journal of Epidemiology*, 4, pp.305–15.

3.8 RADIATION AS A CANCER RISK I: MAN-MADE SOURCES

LEUKAEMIA is a term embracing a group of malignant diseases (ICD 204–208) in which the bone marrow and other blood-forming organs produce increased numbers of certain types of white cells (leucocytes). This overproduction of abnormal forms suppresses the production of normal white cells, red cells and platelets. Leukaemias are classified into *acute* and *chronic* depending on the rate of progression of the disease, and into *lymphoblast* and *myeloblast* forms depending on the type of white cell that is proliferating abnormally. Symptoms include increased susceptibility to infection, anaemia, bleeding, and enlargement of the spleen, liver and lymph nodes. Leukaemias are treated with radiotherapy or cytotoxic drugs aimed to suppress the production of abnormal white cells or, in appropriate cases, by bone marrow transplantation.

Cancers and radiation hazards

Ever since the Chernobyl accident of 1986 (see Figure 5.3), there has been growing concern about the possibility of elevated risks to the population living near nuclear installations. As the Black Report emphasizes, in its study of the possibility of increased incidence of cancer in West Cumbria (Black, 1984), a clear difference needs to be drawn between three levels of risk: (a) *actual risk* during normal operation of a plant, (b) *potential risk* should something go wrong, and (c) *perceived risk* which may be loosely equated with concern.

The scientific evidence for (a) is sometimes greatly at odds with the public perception for (c). Risks are perceived as very much higher than objective figures suggest and such groups as SCREAM (South Coast Radiation Elimination Movement) keep the levels of risk before the public in an exaggerated way. One might argue that the best antidote to panic are comparative statistics but, even where these are agreed and available, public reaction varies greatly. Thus newspaper headlines following the Black Report varied from 'Sellafield leukaemia allegations supported' to 'Cancer link not proven'.

Leukaemia is one of the cancers that the Hiroshima-Nagasaki evidence suggests is especially sensitive to radiation effects (Ichimaru, *et al.*, 1978) and leukaemia, particularly amongst children, has become a special focus of concern. Several studies have appeared to show a concentration of young leukaemia patients into spatial 'clusters' and the location of such clusters in the vicinity of nuclear installations; McHarry's (1985) report of a cluster of childhood cancers in Lydney across the river from the Berkeley and Oldbury stations in southwest England is a case in point. A large literature has grown up on leukaemia clusters in which many locations, age-groups, distance zones and time periods have been encompassed. In an extensive review, Smith (1982) concludes that the large number of statistical tests undertaken would have been expected, merely by chance, to show some significant results and that, when taken together, they provide little support for the notion of space-time clustering.

Choice of test areas

Given the degree of public concern, governments have set up several studies to try and resolve the problems which are inevitably involved when numbers of cases are small and when results are open to a very wide range of interpretations. In the Cook-Mozaffari study (Cook-Mozaffari, *et al.*, 1987), the incidence of, and mortality from, different types of cancer amongst people living near to nuclear installations in England and Wales [see map (A)] was compared with the average rates for the regions in which the installations are located and with the levels observed in control areas. To illustrate the method, the Severnside area has been chosen [see map (B)].

The spatial units used in the study are the local authority areas (LAAs) as they existed before the major boundary reorganization of 1974; they are recorded in the Registrar General's *Annual Report* for 1971. In order to decide which LAAs were 'close' to a nuclear installation, the installations were first located on large scale maps. Concentric circles of 10 miles radius were then drawn around each installation and, using parish data within each LAA, the population was accurately located with respect to the nuclear installation. As a result all LAAs were included which had at least one third of their population living within ten miles of an installation. More detailed studies at closer distances within the ten-mile ring were also carried out to see if a spatial trend in leukaemia incidence with distance from the installation could be detected.

Choice of control areas

Controls outside the 10-mile rings to match against each of the test areas were selected by searching for an area of (a) approximately similar population size, (b) located within either the same county or a contiguous county, and (c) of matching rural/urban status; that is, rural district (RD) with RD, and metropolitan borough (MB) or urban district (UD) with MB or UD. In map (B), different shading types have been used to discriminate between test and control areas, while the matched pairs have been linked by vectors.

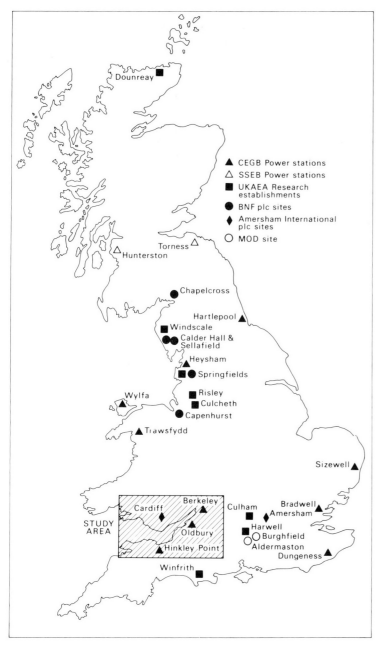

Figure 3.8 (A) Nuclear establishments in the United Kingdom

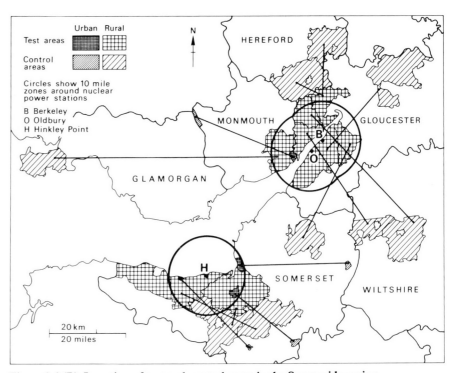

Figure 3.8 (B) Location of test and control areas in the Severnside region

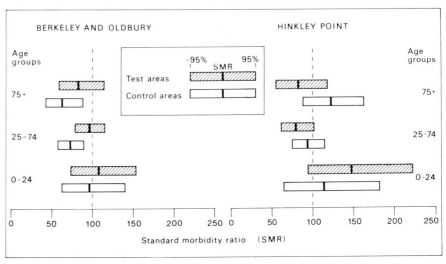

Figure 3.8 (C) Standardized morbidity ratios for test and control areas for Berkeley/Oldbury and Hinkley Point

Initially it was planned to use a fourth criterion (d), similarity of social class structure within the populations, but this was dropped (except for county boroughs, CBs) when it was found that, once requirements (a) through (c) had been met, there was rarely a choice.

Controls were, as far as possible, chosen from (e) within the same cancer registration region. This was important since standards of completeness of registration differ between regions and, before 1971, there was no system for identifying duplicate registrations which might contaminate results. Finally, controls were chosen wherever possible (f) from within the same standard region, and the standardized morbidity ratios used below (SMRs; see Figure 2.7) were calculated on a regional basis. In the case of the Berkeley–Oldbury study, some matching districts lie in Wales but the South West Standard Region has been used as a reference in view of the lack of adequate incidence data for the Welsh Region.

The study was complicated by the boundary shift problem described in Figures 2.9 and 2.11, in that in 1974 the old district boundaries were redrawn to give a new local authority system. Special tabulations had to be provided by going down to the parish and ward level and disaggregating data for the new units onto the pre-1974 grid.

Comparison of test and control areas

Over the twenty-year period of the study, the number of leukaemia cases registered in the Berkeley–Oldbury test area was 185 and in the Hinkley test area 117. The comparative figures for the two control areas were 149 and 138. This overall total of 589 cases in a mid-period population of just under one million (974

thousand in the 1971 census) has little meaning until it is converted into SMRs.

Diagram (C) shows the SMRs for the test and control areas for both Berkeley-Oldbury (left) and Hinkley (right). Note that the population is divided into three age strata at 0–24, 25–74, and 75+ years. Tabulations are by persons rather than for the two sexes separately.

As a guide to the significance of the geographical variations between the six SMRs, 95 percent confidence limits have been derived assuming that the observed value is a Poisson variate (Hill and Pike, 1976); for observed values in excess of 400 cases, a Normal approximation was used. The differences between the two distributions are discussed in the technical appendix to Figure 1.7. Only the Berkeley/Oldbury control, age 27–74, departs significantly from the expected SMR of 100.

Significance of differences

Routine tests cannot usefully be made of the differences between the SMRs in the test areas and those in the matching control areas; the numbers of observations are so small that they are subject to large sampling variability. Analysis of national figures for leukaemia and for all malignancies (involving therefore much larger numbers) shows no consistent pattern of raised incidence adjacent to nuclear installations. Nonetheless public concern remains so high that it would be surprising if detailed study were not to continue and that analytic field studies will be conducted wherever there is a risk of a positive association being detected.

Sources and Further Reading

Diagrams (A), (B) and (C) have been drawn from data in P.J. Cook-Mozaffari, F.L. Ashwood, T. Vincent, D. Forman and M. Alderson (1987), *Cancer Incidence and Mortality in the Vicinity of Nuclear Installations, England and Wales 1959–80*, Office of Population Censuses and Surveys, Studies on Medical and Population Subjects, Publication No. 51. London: Her Majesty's Stationery Office.

The general question of leukaemia epidemiology is discussed in R.J. Berry (1982), 'The leukaemias', in *Epidemiology of Diseases*, edited by D.L. Miller and R.D.T. Farmer, Oxford: Blackwell Scientific, pp.146–51. The question of leukaemia clusters is discussed in E.G. Knox (1964), 'Epidemiology of childhood leukaemia in Northumberland and Durham', *British Journal of Preventative and Social Medicine*, 18, pp.17–24. The space-time pattern of leukaemia is also described in R.R. White (1972), 'Probability maps of leukaemia mortalities in England and Wales', in *Medical Geography: Techniques and Field Studies*, edited by N.D. McGlashan, London: Methuen, pp.173–86, and in A.W. Craft, S. Openshaw and J.M. Birch (1985), 'Childhood cancer in the northern region, 1968–80: incidence in small geographical areas', *Journal of Epidemiology and Community Health*, 39, pp.53–7. On the relation of leukaemia to radiation hazards see also W.M. Court-Brown, F.W. Spiers, R. Doll, B.J. Duffy and M.J. McHugh (1960), 'Geographical variations in leukaemia mortality in relation to background radiation and other factors', *British Medical Journal*, 1, pp.1753–9. Compare with Figure 3.9 of this Atlas on natural radiation sources and with Figure 5.3.

Another approach to the detection of leukaemia clusters based upon comparing observed patterns with those simulated under a geographical Poisson process is described in S. Openshaw, A.W. Craft, M.Charlton and J.M. Birch (1988), 'Investigation of leukaemia clusters by use of a geographical analysis machine', *Lancet*, 1, pp. 272–3.

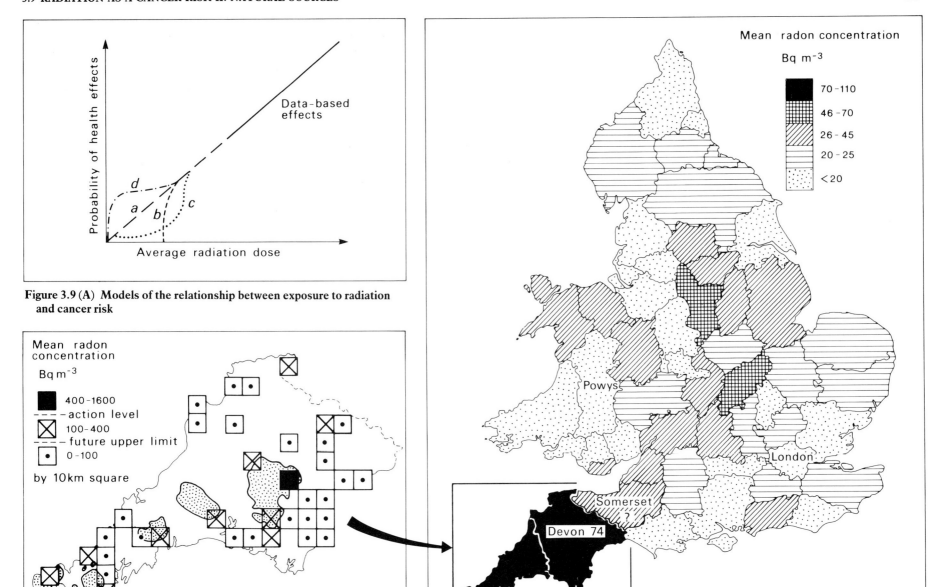

Figure 3.9 (A) Models of the relationship between exposure to radiation and cancer risk

Figure 3.9 (C) Distribution of radon intensity in dwellings in Bq m^{-3} by 10 km grid squares in Devon and Cornwall

Figure 3.9 (B) Distribution of radon intensity in dwellings in Bq m^{-3} for counties of England and Wales

3.9 RADIATION AS A CANCER RISK II: NATURAL SOURCES

The public health hazards posed by ionizing radiation are classified under ICD E926 (see Figure 2.1), **EXPOSURE TO RADIATION**. Such radiation changes the physical state of atoms which it strikes causing them to become electrically charged or ionized. In certain circumstances the presence of such ions in living tissues can disrupt normal biological processes. Ionizing radiation may therefore represent a health hazard to mankind. Some exposure to ionizing radiation cannot be avoided and sources include naturally occurring radionuclides in the earth, a few building materials, water and cosmic rays. The most important man-made sources of exposure are X-rays and radioisotopes used in medical diagnosis and treatment, fallout from nuclear explosives testing, nuclear accidents (see Figure 5.3) and radionuclides emitted from nuclear installations in the course of normal operation (see Figure 3.8). Absorbed radiation creates an increased risk of cancer (ICD 140–208 and 230–239) while irradiation of the reproductive organs may increase the risk of hereditable (genetic) damage.

A relatively new category of hazards to human health is presented by the growing exposure to ionizing radiation. As noted in the accompanying box, a certain amount of ionizing radiation occurs naturally in the environment and we examine one such source, radon-222 in this plate.

Radon-222

Commonly called radon, radon-222 is a natural radioactive gas which is created in all earth materials by the decay of trace quantities of uranium and, along with radon-220 from thorium, accounts for nearly 70 percent of the average annually received natural radiation dose in mid-latitudes which runs at about 40 Bq m^{-3}. Radon is transferred through the pores of the rock, soil and masonry and emerges at the surface. It accumulates indoors to a degree determined by the rate of entry from the ground and the rate of loss from the dwelling. Thus the presence of chimney flues, double glazing and so on in dwellings can produce enormous variability in contiguous dwellings.

The four immediate decay products of radon-222, commonly called radon daughters, are radioactive isotopes of solid elements with short half-lives, two of which decay by emitting alpha particles. Radon daughters form a radioactive aerosol which is inhaled. They are deposited in the respiratory tract causing the epithelial cells to be irradiated by alpha particles, especially in the bronchial region of the lung and so may increase the risk of lung cancer (ICD 162). The National Radiological Protection Board has recommended an action level which corresponds to a mean indoor activity concentration of radon gas (where the mean is taken over one year) of 400 Bq m^{-3} for existing dwellings and an upper bound of 100 Bq m^{-3} per annum for future dwellings.

Risk evaluation: epidemiological evidence

The induction of lung cancers by radiation has been deduced from epidemiological studies, principally of atom bomb survivors in Hiroshima and Nagasaki, and of underground miners exposed to elevated concentration of radon daughters. The incidence of lung cancer observed experimentally in animals exposed to radon daughters is proportional to their exposure and is consistent with risk estimates from human epidemiological studies. The range of exposures for which an excess of lung cancer has been observed in underground miners overlaps exposure in dwellings. The epidemiological experience can therefore be applied with appropriate adjustment to the domestic situation at high levels of exposure. For example, a study by Muller et al. (1985) shows that 82 cases of lung cancer were observed in a population of about 13,000 uranium miners from Ontario in Canada, with a mean equilibrium activity exposure of 42 MBq h m^{-3}, compared with 57 expected cases. This cancer mortality and exposure provides a crude illustration of the risk from the lifetime exposure that would accrue if exposed at approximately 100 MBq h m^{-3}.

The theoretical basis of radiation protection

Several models are available and are illustrated in diagram (A). The simplest reflects the assumption that exposing a population to radiation will affect their health and that the number of people affected will be in proportion to the total radiation dose, no matter how small the dose is. In this model, the known effects on human health, calibrated mainly from Japanese atomic bomb survival data, is straightforwardly linear through the origin of the graph [curve a in diagram (A)]. Some researchers postulate a threshold below which the risk is effectively zero (curve b). Other models argue that, as the dose becomes lower, the risks are disproportionately lower (curve c) or higher (curve d) than the linear model. Most researchers work to the linear model.

Indoor radon concentrations in England and Wales

Diagram (B) shows the mean indoor activity concentration in Bq m^{-3} of radon gas on a county basis in England and Wales. The data are given in O'Riordan *et al.* (1987). The sample sizes collected were relatively small, averaging 35 per county and ranging from 3 in Powys to 187 in outer London. No county exceeds the recommended action level; however, Cornwall (19 observations) exceeds the limit for future dwellings. Devon (43 observations) is also substantially higher than most other counties.

These averages conceal great local variability, and there are many dwellings which do exceed the established thresholds. For example, selective surveys in Devon and Cornwall conducted by O'Riordan *et al.* yielded 24 and 19 percent of dwellings sampled which exceeded the action level. The variation in radon concentrations in the two counties was virtually identical and could be represented approximately by a lognormal distribution with a median of 160 Bq m^{-3} and a geometric standard deviation of about three.

Relationship to rock types in Devon and Cornwall

The level of radon gas concentration is related to the subsurface geology and, while sedimentary rocks are weakly implicated, the areas of the United Kingdom underlain by igneous rocks yield the highest levels because they contain substantial traces of uranium. Of the 81 dwellings built on granite in the O'Riordan study, about 35 percent exceeded the action level of 400 Bq m^{-3}, compared with 21 percent in the survey at large. Diagram (C) shows this relationship for Devon and Cornwall by plotting the mean indoor radon concentration on a 10km square grid basis. The Hercynian granite is relatively rich in trace uranium and is extensively faulted and fissured which increases radon emanation from the ground.

On the basis of the study, O'Riordan *et al.* estimate that some 20,000 dwellings in the United Kingdom exceed the recommended action level of 400 Bq m^{-3} and some 2,000 may exceed 1000 Bq m^{-3}, mostly located in southwest England.

Sources and Further Reading

Diagram (A) is redrawn from the International Atomic Energy Agency (1986), *Facts about Low-level Radiation*, Vienna: IAEA. Diagrams (B) and (C) are based on M.C. O'Riordan, A.C. James, B.M.R. Green and A.D. Wrixon (1987), *Exposure to Radon Daughters in Dwellings*, Publication no. NRPB-GS6, Chilton, Oxfordshire: National Radiological Protection Board , pp.14–15 and Figure 2.

The relationship between lung cancer and the ionizing effects of radiation are considered in a rapidly growing set of publications. These include: National Council on Radiation Protection and Measurements (1984), *Exposures from the Uranium Series with Emphasis on Radon and its Daughters*, NCRP Report no. 77, Washington, DC: Government Printing Office; United Nations Scientific Committee on the Effects of Atomic Radiations (1982), *Ionizing Radiations: Sources and Biological Effects*, New York: United Nations; and International Commission on Radiological Protection (in press), *Lung Cancer Risk from Environmental Exposure to Radon Daughters*, ICRP Publication no. 50 Oxford: Pergamon Press. The report on uranium miners in Ontario is by J. Muller, W.C. Wheeler, J.F. Gentleman, J.F. Suranyi, G. and R.A. Kusiak (1985), 'Study of mortality of Ontario miners', in *Occupational Radiation Safety in Mining*, vol. 1, Toronto: Canadian Nuclear Association, pp. 335–43.

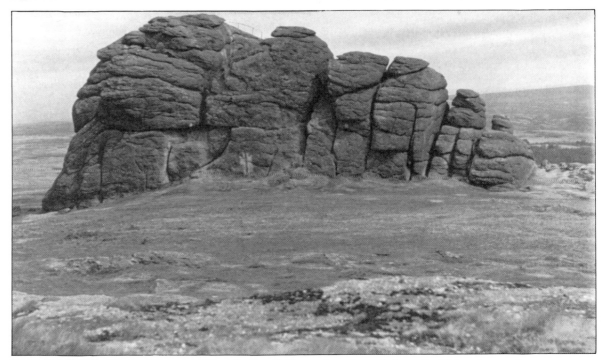

Figure 3.9 (D) Hay Tor on Dartmoor. Note the heavily fissured granite rock through which radon gas rises (Source: L.A. Harvey and D. St. Leger-Gordon (1953), *Dartmoor*, London: Collins, Plate IVa, opp. p.15. Photograph by courtesy of Humphrey and Vera Joel.)

3.10 ISCHAEMIC HEART DISEASE IN ICELAND

ISCHAEMIC HEART DISEASE (ICD 410–414; see Figure 2.1) refers to those conditions of the heart in which localized tissue ischaemia is produced because of the obstruction of arterial blood flow. It includes, *inter alia*: acute (ICD 410) and old (ICD 412) myocardial infarction, which is the localized death of some of the tissue of the middle muscular layer of the heart wall usually resulting from the obstruction of the local circulation by a thrombosis or embolus; angina pectoris (ICD 413), a disease condition marked by brief paroxysmal attacks of chest pain precipitated by deficient oxygenation of the heart muscles, and which may be a symptom of artherosclerosis. Ischaemic heart disease is a leading cause of death in developed countries and appears to be increased by, among other things, polysaturated fat diets accompanied by lack of exercise.

Mapping observed deaths from ischaemic heart disease

This figure examines regional variations in the distribution of deaths in Iceland from all forms of ischaemic heart disease in the five years from 1966 to 1970 and illustrates how areas with significantly high and low incidence may be identified. The cartographic techniques of *proportional circles* and *squares*, in which the area of the circle or square is made proportional to the value mapped, are used to display the data in diagrams (A)–(C); see Figure 1.3 for details. *Adjusted residuals*, defined in Figure 1.8, are the means employed to isolate areas of high and low incidence in diagram (D).

Diagram (A) shows the total number of deaths recorded from ischaemic heart disease for the eight regions of Iceland in the quinquennium, 1966–70. The regions are identified by Arabic numbers in diagram (D) as follows: (1) Reykjavík, (2) Reykjanes, (3) Vesturland, (4) Vestfirðir, (5) Norðurland Vestra, (6) Norðurland Eystra, (7) Austurland, and (8) Suðurland. The total for Iceland appears in the southeast corner of the map.

The map given in diagram (B) relates the number of deaths from ischaemic heart disease to the resident population of each region by plotting the data as an observed death rate per 100,000 population. The area of each square is proportional to the crude death rate, which has not been adjusted to allow for regional variations in the demographic composition of the resident population.

Mapping expected deaths from ischaemic heart disease

The map given in diagram (C) shows the expected number of deaths from ischaemic heart disease in each region. These expected values were computed in the following way:

Step 1 The Icelandic death rate per 100,000 population from this cause was calculated for each of 13 age groups of both males and females. The age groups chosen were: under 1 year, 1–4, 5–9, 10–14, 15–19, 20–29, 30–39, 40–49, 50–59, 60–69, 70–79, 80–84, and 85 years and above.

Step 2 For each region, the resident population in each of these age–sex categories was determined from the Census of Iceland for 1970.

Step 3 The expected deaths in a given region were generated by taking the rates calculated in step 1 and multiplying them by the population totals determined in step 2. Finally, the result was divided by 100,000 to give the number of deaths in each region.

Thus the values on map (C) give the number of deaths from ischaemic heart disease which we would expect in each region on the basis of the experience of Iceland as a whole, but corrected for the age and sex composition of the local population. The procedure is very similar to calculating standardized mortality ratios as described in Figure 2.7.

Maps (A) and (C) together enable us to address the question of whether there is marked regional variation in the observed incidence of ischaemic heart disease. Map (D) plots the differences or residuals between maps (A) and (C) as (observed–expected) deaths. One square is used to denote a unit difference. Negative differences are stippled and correspond with a deficit of deaths from this cause in the particular region. Positive differences have a grey tint and correspond with an excess of deaths.

Interpreting regional variations

The issue of whether the observed excesses and deficits are significant in a statistical sense is tackled by calculating, as described in Figure 1.8, the adjusted residuals between observed and expected deaths. If there is no significant regional variation, the adjusted residuals should lie approximately on the straight line on the probability chart in diagram (D). The numbers 1 to 8 in bold face on this chart correspond with the regions as numbered on the map. The other numbers in each region are the adjusted residuals calculated from the (observed–expected) deaths using equation (1.8.3). The adjusted residuals are approximately Normally distributed, so that scores ≥ 1.96 indicate, with 95 percent confidence, regions with significantly high mortality, while scores ≤ -1.96 mark regions with significantly low mortality. The scores also represent the values of the adjusted residuals plotted

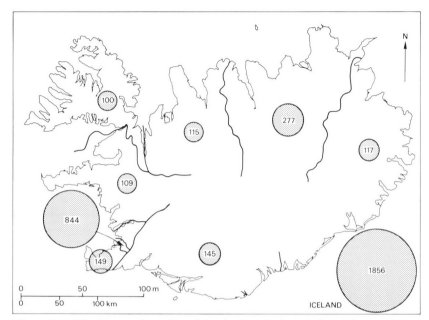

Figure 3.10 (A) Observed number of deaths from ischaemic heart disease, by region

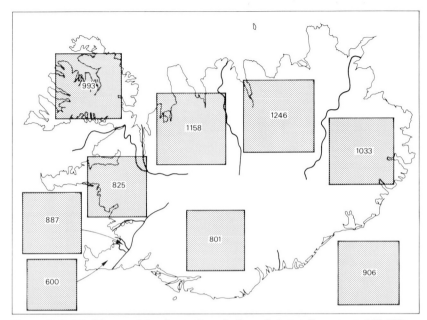

Figure 3.10 (B) Observed death rate from ischaemic heart disease per 100,000 population, by region (unadjusted)

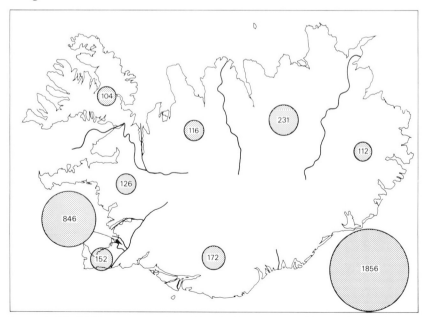

Figure 3.10 (C) Expected number of deaths from ischaemic heart disease, by region (age/sex adjusted)

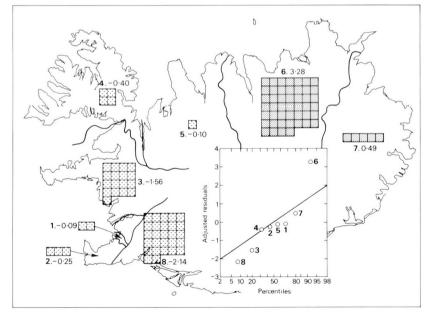

Figure 3.10 (D) Significance of regional variations in number of deaths from ischaemic heart disease

against the percentiles of the Normal distribution on the inset chart. For example, one of the northern areas, region 6, has an adjusted residual of 3.28, implying a significant regional excess of deaths from ischaemic heart disease compared with the general Icelandic experience. No other region has an excess, but region 8 in southwest Iceland has a significant deficit. There is no obvious geographical explanation of these extrema known to the authors and further investigation is required.

Sources and Further Reading

The medical data used for the Icelandic maps shown here were taken from the volumes of *Heilbrigðisskýrslur* (Public Health in Iceland) 1966–70, and the demographic data from *Mannfjöldaskýrslur árin 1961–70* (Population and Vital Statistics, 1961–70). The same source was used for Figures 3.13–3.15 in this chapter of the Atlas.

For a discussion of world variations in heart disease, see G.M. Howe, L. Burgess and P. Gatenby (1977), 'Cardiovascular disease', in *World Geography of Human Diseases*, edited by G.M. Howe, London: Academic Press, pp.431–76. Two relevant studies on spatial variations at other scales in this group of diseases are N.D. McGlashan and N.K. Chick (1974), 'Assessing spatial variations in mortality: ischaemic heart disease in Tasmania', *Australian Geographical Studies*, 12, pp.190–206, and G.F. Pyle (1971), *Heart Disease, Cancer and Stroke in Chicago*, Department of Geography, University of Chicago, Research Papers no. 134, Chicago: Chicago University Press. See also M.S. Meade (1983), 'Cardiovascular disease in Savannah, Georgia', in *Geographical Aspects of Health: Essays in Honour of Andrew Learmonth*, edited by N.D. McGlashan and J.R. Blunden, London: Academic Press, pp.175–96. A national atlas of cardiovascular diseases is given in Daiwa Health Foundation (1980), *Atlas of Cardiovascular Disease for Cities, Towns and Villages in Japan, 1969–74*, Tokyo: Daiwa Health Foundation, while national maps of ischaemic heart disease are included in M.J. Gardner, P.D. Winter, and D.J.P. Barker (1984), *Atlas of Mortality from Selected Diseases in England and Wales, 1968–1978*, Chichester: John Wiley, pp.18–19, 45.

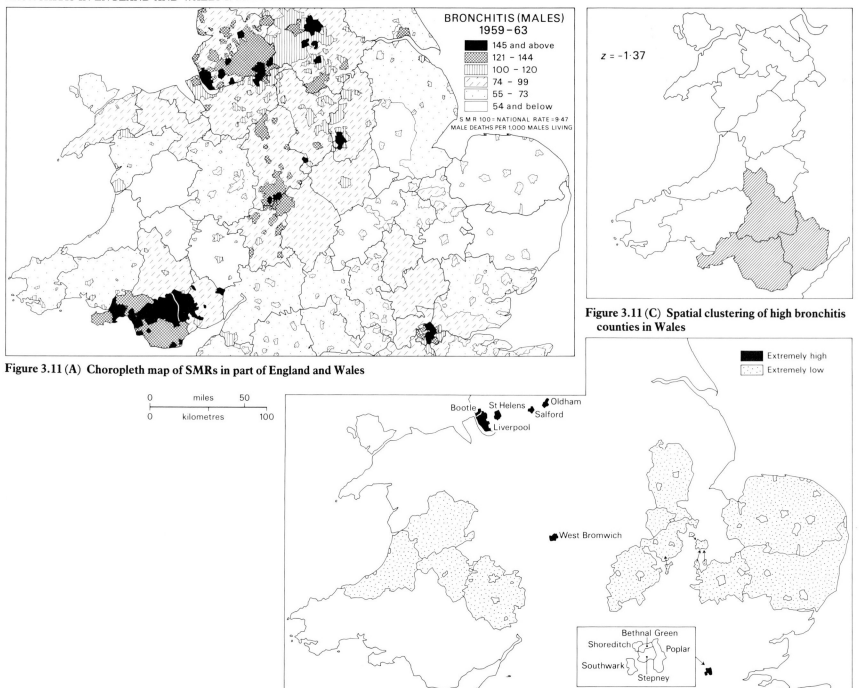

BRONCHITIS (MALES) 1959–63

145 and above
121 – 144
100 – 120
74 – 99
55 – 73
54 and below

S M R 100 = NATIONAL RATE = 9·47
MALE DEATHS PER 1,000 MALES LIVING

Figure 3.11 (A) Choropleth map of SMRs in part of England and Wales

0   miles   50
0   kilometres   100

$z = -1·37$

Figure 3.11 (C) Spatial clustering of high bronchitis counties in Wales

Extremely high
Extremely low

Oldham
Bootle   St Helens   Salford
Liverpool

West Bromwich

Bethnal Green
Shoreditch   Poplar
Southwark   Stepney

Figure 3.11 (B) Districts on Map (A) which are significantly high or low at the 95 per cent confidence level

3.11 BRONCHITIS IN ENGLAND AND WALES I: MESO SCALE PATTERNS

BRONCHITIS is an inflammation of the bronchial tree and may be either acute or chronic. In **ACUTE BRONCHITIS** (ICD 466; see Figure 2.1) chemical, physical or infectious irritation of the bronchial tree results in short-term inflammation of the bronchi and excess mucous production. The mucous is carried upwards by the cilia, with which the mucosa of the major bronchi are lined, onto cough-sensitive areas to initiate the two most common symptoms of bronchitis, cough and expectoration of mucous. Chemical and physical irritation of the bronchi can result from exposure to a variety of agents including hot and toxic gases and irritant dusts. Acute bronchitis refers also to a more specific disease commonly found as a complication of upper respiratory tract infections and influenza. Additionally, the clinical features of acute bronchitis may occur as prodromal symptoms of viral infections such as influenza. The causative viruses seem to break down the resistance of the bronchial mucosa to invasion by a variety of pyogenic bacteria and, if not treated, may lead to pneumonia.

CHRONIC BRONCHITIS (ICD 491; see Figure 2.1) refers to long-standing inflammation of the bronchi and is often associated with fibrosis, emphysema, asthma and chronic sinusitis. In this condition, the mucosa of the bronchi is permanently injured, ciliary action is reduced or absent, chronic infection is present and there is hypersecretion of mucous by glands. The most common symptoms are again cough and expectoration. Chronic bronchitis results from continued exposure to aggravating physical and chemical agents, and is almost always made worse by damp and cold in the winter months.

Sources and Further Reading

See under Figure 3.12.

Geographical distribution

Diagrams (A)–(C) examine the geographical distribution of deaths from bronchitis as defined in ICD 466 and 491. Map (A) shows the distribution of deaths for males by local authority areas in the five-year period between 1959 and 1963. The map covers Wales and the central part of England from Lancashire in the north to London in the south. The data are mapped as standardized mortality ratios (SMRs), thus allowing for the local age composition of the male population. The computation of standardized mortality ratios is discussed in Figure 2.7. The national average has been given an SMR of 100 and corresponds to a death-rate of 9.47 per thousand males living. The cartographic technique used is that of the choropleth map (see Figure 1.5). The styles of shading have been chosen to become darker as mortality increases. It appears from diagram (A) that the areas of excess deaths are concentrated in parts of the London region, and in the older industrial and coalfield regions of Lancashire, the West Midlands, Nottinghamshire and South Wales. We are seeing on the map evidence of the classic association of chronic forms of the disease with prolonged exposure to coal-dust, asbestos and other air-borne chemical and physical irritants common in industrial England and Wales up to this period.

Statistical significance of extremes

To examine this pattern in more detail, the map shown in (B) has been prepared from (A) by applying the idea of statistical significance discussed in Figure 1.7(C). It has been assumed that the SMRs have been drawn from a Normal population. We have *stippled* on map (B) those areas with standard Normal scores less than or equal to -1.64 (significantly low at the 95 percent level in a one-tailed test) and shaded *black* those areas with SMRs greater than or equal to 1.64 (significantly high). The map highlights the stark contrast between regions of high and low mortality. The former includes southern Lancashire (the dock areas of Liverpool and the chemical industry and coalfield areas of St Helens, Salford and Oldham), part of the West Midlands industrial area focused on West Bromwich and some East-End London boroughs. The latter includes the clean-air rural areas of mid-Wales, the East Midlands and East Anglia. It is interesting to note that, although South Wales undoubtedly has high mortality compared with the national average, it is still not sufficiently high to be statistically significant at the probability level chosen.

Spatial autocorrelation

Map (C) looks at the question of regional concentration of mortality from bronchitis in Wales using the spatial autocorrelation methods discussed in Figure 1.9. On the map, the Welsh counties have been diagonally shaded (called black, B) if their average annual number of deaths from bronchitis in males exceeded the average for the United Kingdom in the period considered; counties were left white, W, otherwise. The BW statistic defined in Figure 1.9 was evaluated, yielding a standard Normal score (z-score) of -1.37. Although suggestive of spatial clustering of the high mortality counties, this z-score is not significant at the conventional 95 percent probability level, a result which is consistent with map (B). However, it is important to remember that, since there are only 13 Welsh counties on map (C), the sample size is small and this will reduce the confidence we can place statistical conclusions.

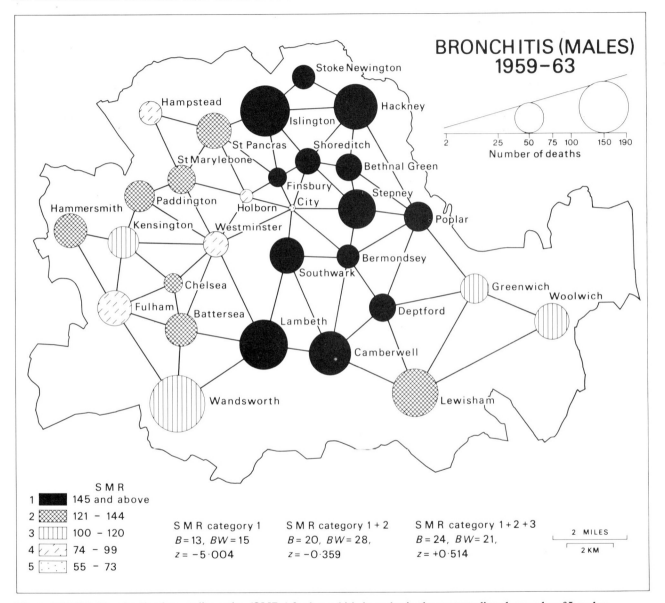

BRONCHITIS (MALES)
1959–63

Number of deaths

SMR
1 █ 145 and above
2 ▨ 121 – 144
3 ▥ 100 – 120
4 ▤ 74 – 99
5 ▦ 55 – 73

SMR category 1
$B = 13$, $BW = 15$
$z = -5.004$

SMR category 1 + 2
$B = 20$, $BW = 28$,
$z = -0.359$

SMR category 1 + 2 + 3
$B = 24$, $BW = 21$,
$z = +0.514$

2 MILES
2 KM

Figure 3.12 (A) Standardized mortality ratios (SMRs) for bronchitis in males in the metropolitan boroughs of London, 1959–1963

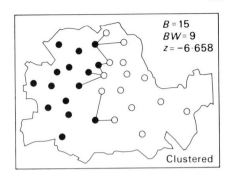

$B = 15$
$BW = 9$
$z = -6.658$

Clustered

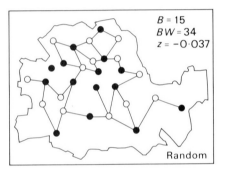

$B = 15$
$BW = 34$
$z = -0.037$

Random

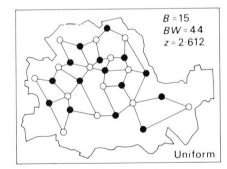

$B = 15$
$BW = 44$
$z = 2.612$

Uniform

Figure 3.12 (B) Representative join-count patterns, with *BW* joins marked

3.12 BRONCHITIS IN ENGLAND AND WALES II: MICRO SCALE PATTERNS

In the previous figure, geographical variations in male deaths from acute and chronic bronchitis (ICD 466 and 491) between 1959 and 1963 were examined at the coarse geographical scale of England and Wales (for disease description see box in Figure 3.11). Compared with the national death rate, several of the London boroughs stood out as having excess mortality comparable with the older industrial areas of northern England and South Wales.

London distributions

In the present figure, the geographical scale is increased to examine the same bronchitis data in more detail for the spatial cross-section formed by the 29 London boroughs. At the period to which these data refer, the insidious and disabling effects of bronchitis constituted one of the main problems of industrial life in Britain and were responsible for the loss of some 25 million working days per annum. During the period 1954–58, bronchitis was the third most important cause of death in men.

Diagram (A) maps the number of male deaths from bronchitis between 1959 and 1963 as standardized mortality ratios (SMRs; see Figure 2.7), thus adjusting the data to allow for any variations from borough to borough in the age composition of the population. A combination of different cartographic techniques has been used to display the data. The number of deaths in each borough is shown using *proportional circles* (see Figure 1.3) in which the area of the circles is made proportional to the number of deaths recorded. The visual impact has been enhanced by dividing the range of values into six classes and then shading the circles to produce a *choropleth* effect. To define the classes, 'natural breaks' in the data were selected as described in Figure 1.6. Finally, although the geographical location of the boroughs with respect to each other has been retained, the boroughs have been translated onto a *graph* (see Figure 1.9). The boroughs are represented by the proportional circles and form the nodes on the graph. Links have been drawn between nodes if the two boroughs concerned shared a common section of borough boundary.

The national average male death rate from bronchitis in the period studied was 9.47 per thousand males living and has been given an SMR of 100. Bearing in mind that the data refer to a period in which legislation to control air pollution was in its infancy, diagram (A) tells a dramatic story for this major industrial city with its great dockland. Only four boroughs (Fulham, Westminster, Holborn and Hampstead) had SMRs below the national average. A high degree of spatial grouping in the boroughs with the highest SMRs is evident, focused upon the industrial and (then) inner dockland areas in the East End and boroughs to the north and south.

Spatial autocorrelation tests

The geographical pattern formed by the borough-to-borough variations in SMRs may be assessed quantitatively using the spatial autocorrelation techniques described in Figure 1.9. Diagram (A) was reduced to three two-colour maps by coding boroughs black, B if they had SMRs of (a) 145+, (b) 121+ and (c) 100+. For each of these three cases, the remaining boroughs were coded white, W and the BW join count statistic was evaluated to yield the Normal score (z-score) given by equations (1.9.1), (1.9.2), (1.9.6) and (1.9.7). The results obtained appear in the key to diagram (A) which shows, *inter alia*, the number of boroughs coded black, the number of BW joins and the z-score for each of the cases, (a), (b) and (c), outlined above.

The extreme geographical concentration of the 13 boroughs with SMRs of 145 or more is confirmed by the z-score of -5.004, indicating a deficit of BW joins which is significant at any conventional probability level. When, however, cases (b) and (c) are considered, the values of z are non-significant. There is a statistical reason for this which is outlined in the technical appendix.

Clustered and uniform distributions

To illustrate the range of values for the BW statistic which can be obtained from different kinds of spatial patterns, we have coded in diagram (B) the 29 metropolitan boroughs with 15 B and 14 W in such a way that the B and W zones form distinct regional blocks (clustered), are randomly mixed (random) and, finally, have the W zones uniformly distributed among the B as on the rows and columns of a chessboard (uniform). As discussed in Figure 1.9, spatial clustering yields a small BW count, so that for the clustered pattern a large negative z-score results. Conversely, uniform mixing of B and W zones produces a large number of BW links compared with random expectation and, as shown in the uniform pattern, a significant positive z-score of 2.612. If the B and W boroughs are randomly mixed, the observed number of BW links will approximate expectation and produce a z-score close to zero (-0.037 in this example).

Sources and Further Reading

Detailed maps of the distribution of bronchitis in Britain are included in G.M. Howe, editor (1970), *National Atlas of Disease Mortality in the United Kingdom*, second edition, London: Royal Geographical Society, pp.58–61. See also the maps of bronchitis and emphysema in M.J. Gardner, P.D. Winter, and D.J.P. Barker (1984), *Atlas of Mortality from Selected Diseases in England and Wales, 1968–1978*, Chichester: John Wiley, pp.30–1, 51. For further discussion of the data used in Figures 3.11 and 3.12 see A.D. Cliff and P. Haggett (1981), 'Mapping respiratory disease', in *Scientific Foundations of Respiratory Medicine*, edited by J.G. Scadding, G. Cumming and W.M. Thurlbeck, London: Heinemann, pp.30–43.

A parallel study of the distribution of bronchitis in another mid-latitude country is given in D.O. Anderson (1968), 'Geographic variations in deaths due to emphyema and bronchitis in Canada', *Canadian Medical Association Journal*, 98, pp.231–41. For a description of world-wide variations in bronchitis, see J.C. Young (1977), 'Bronchitis', in *World Geography of Human Diseases*, edited by G.M. Howe, London: Academic Press, pp.319–37.

The spatial ecology of bronchitis is examined in I.T.T. Higgins (1973), 'The epidemiology of chronic respiratory disease', *Preventive Medicine*, 2, pp.14–33, in J.R.T. Colley (1982), 'Chronic non-specific lung disease (CNSLD) and asthma', in *Epidemiology of Diseases*, edited by D.L. Miller and R.D.T. Farmer, Oxford: Blackwell Scientific, pp.163–75, and C. Fletcher and R. Peto (1976), *The Natural History of Chronic Bronchitis and Emphysema*, Oxford: Oxford University Press.

The methods of analysis employed in Figures 3.11 and 3.12 are discussed further in A.D. Cliff and J.K. Ord (1981), *Spatial Processes: Models and Applications*, London: Pion, pp.1–33.

Technical appendix

Cliff and Ord (1981, chapter 6) have considered the relative performance of a wide variety of measures of spatial pattern in geographical cross-sections. We have opted here, as in Figure 1.9, to use the number of BW joins as our test statistic. It can be shown that the BW test is most efficient at detecting pattern when either the probability, p of an area being coloured B is 0.5 (free sampling) or half of the areas are B (non-free sampling). The terms, free and non-free sampling, are defined in the technical appendix to Figure 1.9. The efficiency falls quite rapidly when these conditions are not met. For the three cases (a), (b) and (c) in diagram (A), the number of boroughs coded B is 13, 20 and 24 respectively, yielding corresponding values of p as 0.45, 0.69 and 0.83. Hence the test readily detects the patterning in the B boroughs in case (a) but is confounded in (b) and (c) by the disproportionate number of boroughs coded B.

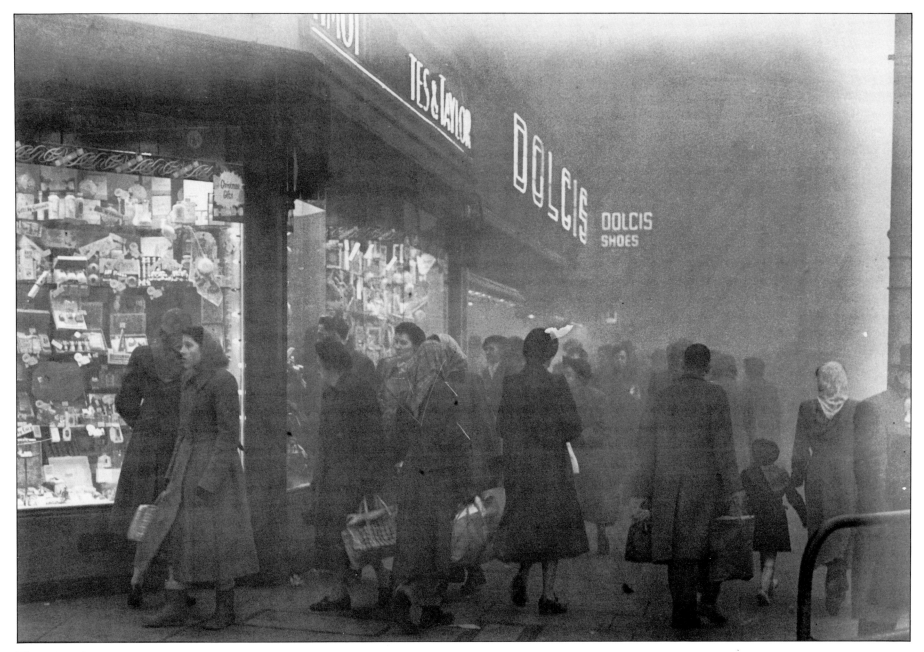

Figure 3.12 (C) London smog of 1952
(Source: The Keystone Collection, London.)

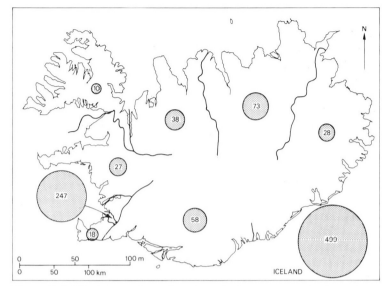

Figure 3.13 (A) Observed number of deaths from pneumonia, by region

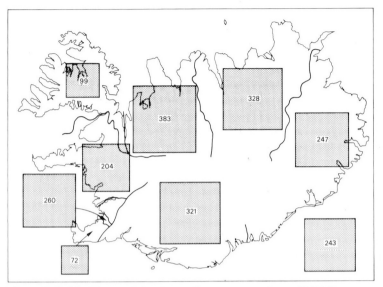

Figure 3.13 (B) Observed death rate from pneumonia per 100,000 population, by region (unadjusted)

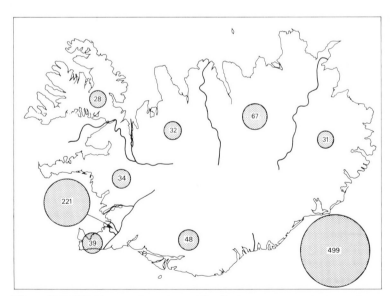

Figure 3.13 (C) Expected number of deaths from pneumonia, by region (age/sex adjusted)

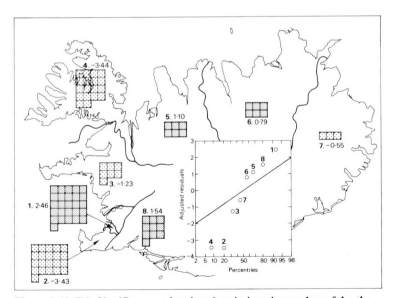

Figure 3.13 (D) Significance of regional variations in number of deaths from pneumonia

3.13 PNEUMONIA IN ICELAND

PNEUMONIA (ICD 480–486; see Figure 2.1) is the term used to describe inflammation of the lung. Pneumonias may be grouped as follows: (a) primary, that is those caused by pathogenic cocci, bacilli, viruses and fungi which primarily attack the lung; (b) pneumonias which occur in more or less specific forms as part of systemic infections such as tuberculosis; (c) pneumonias caused through physical or mechanical injury of the lung such as shock, aspiration of foreign bodies or fluids, and trauma which predisposes the lungs to infection by organisms that would normally be of low virulence; and (d) pneumonias caused, for example, by the aspiration of oil, chemicals, exposure to X-rays and allergic reaction. The disease is a common complication of virus diseases which affect the upper respiratory tract, such as influenza. Untreated, mortality can be high with the young, elderly and infirm particularly at risk.

Mapping observed pneumonia deaths

This figure examines regional variations in the distribution of deaths in Iceland from all forms of pneumonia in the five years from 1966 to 1970 and illustrates how areas with significantly high and low incidence may be identified. The cartographic techniques of *proportional circles* and *squares*, in which the area of the circle or square is made proportional to the value mapped, are used to display the data in diagrams (A)–(C); see Figure 1.3 for details. *Adjusted residuals*, defined in Figure 1.8, are the means employed to isolate areas of high and low incidence in diagram (D).

Diagram (A) shows the total number of deaths recorded from all forms of pneumonia for the eight regions of Iceland in the quinquennium, 1966–70. The regions are identified by Arabic numbers in diagram (D) as follows: (1) Reykjavík, (2) Reykjanes, (3) Vesturland, (4) Vest-fiðir, (5) Norðurland Vestra, (6) Norðurland Eystra, (7) Austurland, and (8) Suðurland. The total for Iceland appears in the southeast corner of the map.

The map given in diagram (B) relates the number of deaths from pneumonia to the resident population of each region by plotting the data as an observed death rate per 100,000 population. The area of each square is proportional to the crude death rate, which has not been adjusted to allow for regional variations in the demographic composition of the resident population.

Mapping expected pneumonia deaths

The map given in diagram (C) shows the number of deaths from pneumonia which we would expect in each region on the basis of the experience of Iceland as a whole, but corrected for the age and sex composition of the local population. The computational procedure is described in Figure 3.10.

Maps (A) and (C) together enable us to address the question of whether there is marked regional variation in the observed incidence of pneumonia. Map (D) plots the differences or residuals between maps (A) and (C) as (observed–expected) deaths. One square is used to denote a unit difference. Negative differences are stippled and correspond with a deficit of deaths from this cause in the particular region. Positive differences have a grey tint and correspond with an excess of deaths.

Interpreting regional variations

The issue of whether the observed excesses and deficits are significant in a statistical sense is tackled by calculating, as described in Figure 1.8, the adjusted residuals between observed and expected deaths. If there is no significant regional variation, the adjusted residuals should lie approximately on the straight line on the probability chart in diagram (D). The numbers 1 to 8 in bold face on this chart correspond with the regions as numbered on the map. The other numbers in each region are the adjusted residuals calculated from the (observed–expected) deaths using equation (1.8.3). The adjusted residuals are approximately Normally distributed, so that scores ≥ 1.96 indicate, with 95 percent confidence, regions with significantly high mortality, while scores ≤ -1.96 mark regions with significantly low mortality. The scores also represent the values of the adjusted residuals plotted against the percentiles of the Normal distribution on the inset chart. For example, region 4 in northwest Iceland has an adjusted residual of -3.44 implying a significant deficit of deaths from pneumonia, compared with the general Icelandic experience, in this region. The only other region with a significant deficit is region 2 in southwest Iceland. A significant excess of deaths appears in region 1, the capital, Reykjavík. This excess almost certainly reflects the concentration of the highest-level medical care, along with the University medical school, in the capital to serve the whole island. This results in a focus of the elderly and the seriously ill upon Reykjavík for treatment, and such individuals are particularly susceptible to certain forms of pneumonia. Because these patients are not normally resident in Reykjavík, they do not appear in the demographic composition data for the capital used to generate the expected levels of deaths. By the same token, the 'drain to the capital' of such individuals may account, in part, for the deficits in other regions.

Sources and Further Reading

For sources of data for maps see Figure 3.10.

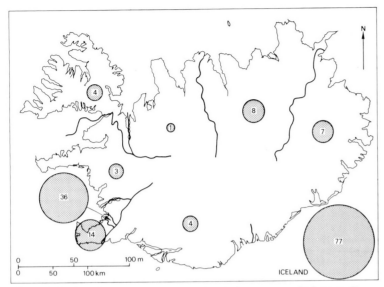

Figure 3.14 (A) Observed number of deaths from congenital anomalies, by region

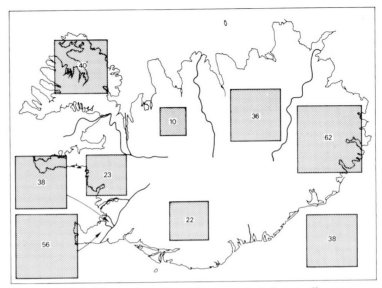

Figure 3.14 (B) Observed death rate from congenital anomalies per 100,000 population, by region (unadjusted)

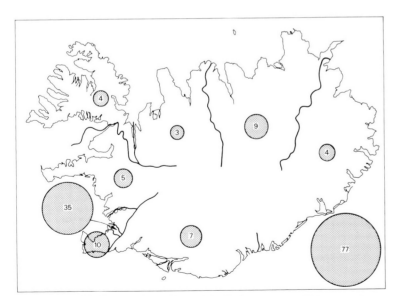

Figure 3.14 (C) Expected number of deaths from congenital anomalies, by region (age/sex adjusted)

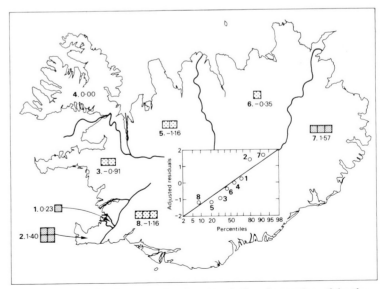

Figure 3.14 (D) Significance of regional variations in number of deaths from congenital anomalies

3.14 CONGENITAL ANOMALIES IN ICELAND

The diseases collectively known as **CONGENITAL ANOMALIES** appear as numbers 740–759 in the ICD list (see Figure 2.1). *Inter alia* they include diseases ranging from syphilis and congenital cataracts acquired *in utero* as a result of maternal disease, through well-known anomalies such as spina bifida and cleft palate and lip, to malformations of the heart and blood vessels, all parts of the skeleton, the gastrointestinal tract and the nervous system. Much progress has recently been made in the early diagnosis (frequently *in utero*) and treatment of these disorders, which represent an increasingly important branch of paediatric medicine.

Mapping observed deaths from congenital anomalies

This figure examines regional variations in the distribution of deaths in Iceland from all forms of congenital anomalies in the five years from 1966 to 1970 and illustrates how areas with significantly high and low incidence may be identified. The cartographic techniques of *proportional circles* and *squares*, in which the area of the circle or square is made proportional to the value mapped, are used to display the data in diagrams (A) – (C); see Figure 1.3 for details. *Adjusted residuals*, defined in Figure 1.8, are the means employed to isolate areas of high and low incidence in diagram (D).

Diagram (A) shows the total number of deaths recorded from congenital anomalies for the eight regions of Iceland in the quinquennium, 1966–70. The regions are identified by Arabic numbers in diagram (D) as follows: (1) Reykjavík, (2) Reykjanes, (3) Vesturland, (4) Vestfirðir,

(5) Norðurland Vestra, (6) Norðurland Eystra (7) Austurland, and (8) Suðurland. The total for Iceland appears in the southeast corner of the map.

Mapping expected deaths from congenital anomalies

The map given in diagram (B) relates the number of deaths from congenital anomalies to the resident population of each region by plotting the data as an observed death rate per 100,000 population. The area of each square is proportional to the crude death rate, which has not been adjusted to allow for regional variations in the demographic composition of the resident population.

The map given in diagram (C) shows the number of deaths from congenital anomalies which we would expect in each region on the basis of the experience of Iceland as a whole, but corrected for the age and sex composition of the local population. The computational procedure is described in Figure 3.10.

Maps (A) and (C) together enable us to address the question of whether there is marked regional variation in the observed incidence of congenital anomalies. Map (D) plots the differences or residuals between maps (A) and (C) as (observed–expected) deaths. One square is used to denote a unit difference. Negative differences are stippled and correspond with a deficit of deaths from this cause in the particular region. Positive differences have a grey tint and correspond with an excess of deaths.

Interpreting regional variations

The issue of whether the observed excesses and deficits are significant in a statistical sense is tackled by calculating, as described in Figure 1.8, the adjusted residuals between observed and expected deaths. If there is no significant regional variation, the adjusted residuals should lie approximately on the straight line on the probability chart in diagram (D). The numbers 1 to 8 in bold face on this chart correspond with the regions as numbered on the map. The other numbers in each region are the adjusted residuals calculated from the (observed–expected) deaths using equation (1.8.3). The adjusted residuals are approximately Normally distributed, so that scores ≥ 1.96 indicate, with 95 percent confidence, regions with significantly high mortality, while scores ≤ -1.96 mark regions with significantly low mortality. The scores also represent the values of the adjusted residuals plotted against the percentiles of the Normal distribution on the inset chart. For example, region 1, the capital Reykjavík, has an adjusted residual of 0.23.

The geographical distribution of deaths from congenital anomalies is random and it is obviously encouraging to find such a result.

Sources and Further Reading

The sources of data for the congenital anomaly maps of Iceland are as set out in Figure 3.10 of this Atlas. Comparable data for England and Wales are available in *Congenital Malformation Statistics*, London: DHSS, 1976. The epidemiology of congenital defects is described in D.T. Janerich, R.G. Skalko and I.H. Porter (1974), *Congenital Defects*, New York: Academic Press; D.T. Janerich and A.P. Polednak (1983), 'Epidemiology of birth defects', *Epidemiologic Reviews*, 5, pp.16–37; and C. Peckham, R.D.T. Farmer and E.M. Ross (1982), 'Congenital malformations', in *Epidemiology of Diseases*, edited by D.L. Miller and R.D.T. Farmer, Oxford: Blackwell Scientific, pp.452–66.

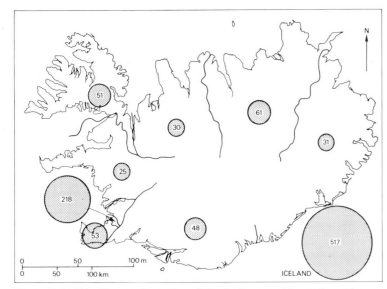

Figure 3.15 (A) Observed number of deaths from accidents, by region

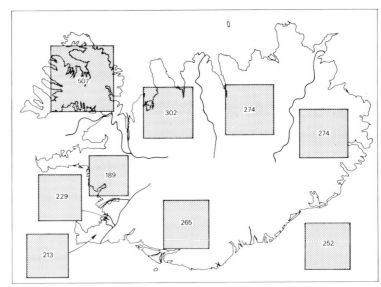

Figure 3.15 (B) Observed death rate from accidents per 100,000 population, by region (unadjusted)

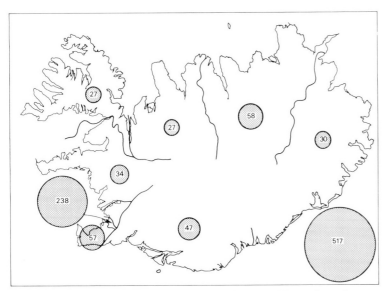

Figure 3.15 (C) Expected number of deaths from accidents, by region (age/sex adjusted)

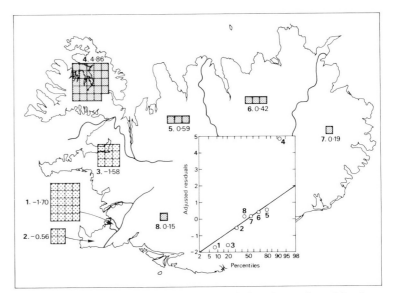

Figure 3.15 (D) Significance of regional variations in number of deaths from accidents

3.15 ACCIDENTS IN ICELAND

The regional Icelandic data aggregated under this heading include ICD classes E810–E823 (**MOTOR VEHICLE ACCIDENTS**) and E825–E949 (**ALL OTHER ACCIDENTS**). See Figure 2.1.

Mapping observed accident deaths

This figure examines regional variations in the distribution of deaths in Iceland from all forms of accidents in the five years from 1966 to 1970 and illustrates how areas with significantly high and low incidence may be identified. The cartographic techniques of *proportional circles* and *squares*, in which the area of the circle or square is made proportional to the value mapped, are used to display the data in diagrams (A)–(C); see Figure 1.3 for details. *Adjusted residuals*, defined in Figure 1.8, are the means employed to isolate areas of high and low incidence in diagram (D).

Diagram (A) shows the total number of deaths recorded from accidents for the eight regions of Iceland in the quinquennium, 1966–70. The regions are identified by Arabic numbers in diagram (D) as follows: (1) Reykjavík, (2) Reykjanes, (3) Vesturland, (4) Vestfirðir, (5) Norðurland Vestra, (6) Norðurland Eystra, (7) Austurland, and (8) Suðurland. The total for Iceland appears in the southeast corner of the map.

The map given in diagram (B) relates the number of deaths from accidents to the resident population of each region by plotting the data as an observed death rate per 100,000 population. The area of each square is proportional to the crude death rate, which has not been adjusted to allow for regional variations in the demographic composition of the resident population.

Mapping expected accident deaths

The map given in diagram (C) shows the number of deaths from accidents which we would expect in each region on the basis of the experience of Iceland as a whole, but corrected for the age and sex composition of the local population. The computational procedure is described in Figure 3.10.

Maps (A) and (C) together enable us to address the question of whether there is marked regional variation in the observed incidence of accidents. Map (D) plots the differences or residuals between maps (A) and (C) as (observed–expected) deaths. One square is used to denote a unit difference. Negative differences are stippled and correspond with a deficit of deaths from this cause in the particular region. Positive differences have a grey tint and correspond with an excess of deaths.

Interpreting regional variations

The issue of whether the observed excesses and deficits are significant in a statistical sense is tackled by calculating, as described in Figure 1.8, the adjusted residuals between observed and expected deaths. If there is no significant regional variation, the adjusted residuals should lie approximately on the straight line on the probability chart in diagram (D). The numbers 1 to 8 in bold face on this chart correspond with the regions as numbered on the map. The other numbers in each region are the adjusted residuals calculated from the (observed–expected) deaths using equation (1.8.3). The adjusted residuals are approximately Normally distributed, so that scores ≥ 1.96 indicate, with 95 percent confidence, regions with significantly high mortality, while scores ≤ -1.96 mark regions with significantly low mortality. The scores also represent the values of the adjusted residuals plotted against the percentiles of the Normal distribution on the inset chart.

As an example, region 4 in northwest Iceland has adjusted residual of 4.86, indicative of a very significant excess of deaths from accidents in this region. Northwest Iceland is one of the main fishing areas in the country, with its ports facing extensive banks in the Denmark Strait between Iceland and Greenland. As an industry, fishing has traditionally had a high accident rate which is reinforced here by working in severe winter weather on the fringes of the Arctic Circle.

To develop this theme, we note that the negative residuals on diagram (D) all occur in the southwest of the island. This area is more generally urbanized than the rest of Iceland and has an economic base involving manufacturing and service industries as well as fishing and farming. The economy in the remainder of the island is dominated by fishing and farming and their associated industries, all of which tend to have high accident rates.

Sources and Further Reading

The sources of data for the accident maps of Iceland are as set out in Figure 3.10 of this Atlas.

An epidemiological description of accidents is given in R.D.T. Farmer, A. Nixon and J. Connolly (1982), 'Accidents', in *Epidemiology of Diseases*, edited by D.L. Miller and R.D.T. Farmer, Oxford: Blackwell Scientific, pp.369–86, while the standard work on accidents is W.H. Rutherford (1980), *Accident and Emergency Medicine*, Tunbridge Wells: Pitman Medical. A recent account of accidents in the home in Iceland is contained in E.A. Friðriksdóttir and Ó. Ólafsson (1987), *Rannsókn á 7562 slysum byggð á gögnum Slysadeildar Borgarspítalans árið 1979* (An analysis of 7562 home accidents in the greater Reykjavík area, 1979), Special Publication Number 2 of *Heilbrigðisskýrslur* (Public Health in Iceland), Reykjavík: Office of the Director General of Public Health.

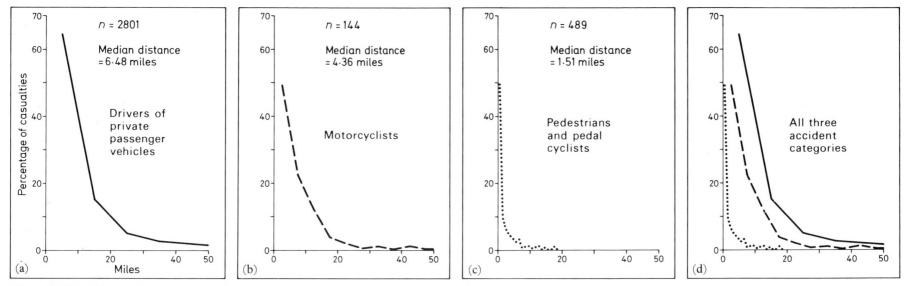

Figure 3.16 (A) Distance between place of accident and residence for three categories of victim

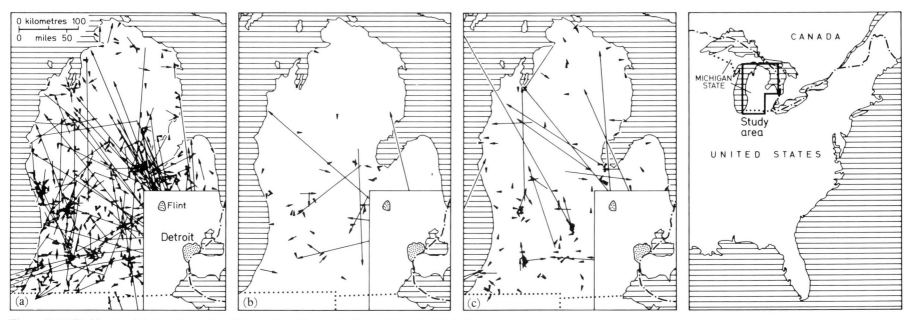

Figure 3.16 (B) Vectors joining place of accident and residence for three categories of victim

3.16 ROAD TRAFFIC ACCIDENTS I: MICHIGAN

ROAD TRAFFIC ACCIDENTS (ICD E810–E819 and E826–E829; see Figure 2.1) are a major drain upon the health services of the developed nations, resulting in casualties who require immediate medical attention and, frequently, long-term care. In this and the next figure, we look at the geographical distribution of road traffic accidents at two spatial scales, the meso and the micro.

Mapping accidents at the meso scale

The data from which the diagrams have been prepared relate to fatal road traffic accidents in the state of Michigan in 1969. They are analysed in Moellering (1974), upon which the following account is based. The location of the study area is shown on the last map in (B). It covers an area approximately 200 miles from east to west and about 300 miles from north to south.

The data have been presented in two ways. The graphs in (A) plot the percentage of casualties (on the vertical axis) against distance in miles (on the horizontal axis) from the victim's place of residence to the location of the accident. Graph (a) relates to private passenger vehicle drivers, graph (b) to motorcyclists and graph (c) to pedestrian and pedal cyclists. The three line traces have been superimposed on graph (d). In each case, the number of observations, n, from which the graph has been prepared has been given, along with the median distance between place of residence and site of the accident; half the observations lie above and half below the median. The maps in (B) positioned below each graph of (A) use vectors to link place of residence to location of the accident for each of the casualties. The arrow heads are at the site of the accident.

Interpreting accident maps

There are several striking features about the graphs. The rank order of the median distances is as expected; cars give the greatest personal mobility and have the biggest median distance from home to accident site. The least mobile group, pedestrians and bicyclists, have the smallest median. Yet even for passenger vehicle drivers the median distance is only 6.48 miles. As a set, the graphs clearly imply that most road traffic accidents occur within a relatively short distance of home. This reflects the large proportion of local-area trips for journey-to-work, shopping, and so on in the total number of trips made, and it means that the percentage of accidents falls off exponentially with distance in all the graphs plotted (cf. Figures 3.3 and 3.4).

The vector map of all private passenger vehicle drivers who were killed in Michigan seems chaotic. To bring order to the map, Moellering used *regression analysis* to relate the trip distances (the *dependent* or *effect variable*) between place of residence and site of accident to a large number of traffic and demographic variables (called the *explanatory variables*). See Figure 1.14 for a discussion of regression maps. The traffic variables included whether the residence was in an urban or a rural area, whether the accident site was urban or rural, the type of road, the date and time of the accident and weather conditions. The demographic variables included age, race, sex, occupation and whether the driver had been drinking or taking drugs. If we regard variation in the length of the journey to death as a function of the various explanatory variables, then step-wise regression analysis may be used to decide which of the explanatory variables is most important in accounting for the observed variation in the length of the final journey. Moellering found the journey length was overwhelmingly determined by the traffic variables, particularly whether the trip was urban or rural and on major or minor roads; characteristics of the individual played only a minor part.

Age and traffic accidents

For pedestrians and bicyclists, the regression analysis yielded slightly different results. Although the traffic variables remained important, age of the casualty turned out to be critical. Most of the short journeys to death involved the under 20s and the over 50s. Obviously pedestrians and bicyclists are vulnerable in traffic and, whereas the young frequently exercise insufficient care, the elderly respond to danger less rapidly, especially as sight and hearing fail.

In the case of motorcyclists, the analysis was restricted by the small sample size. All the casualties were young males. Time of day was an important explanatory variable. Most of the short final journeys occurred between midnight and 8.00 a.m., reflecting the risks of driving at night when tired or intoxicated.

The study of road traffic accidents usually considers four basic groups of explanatory variables: vehicle characteristics; road layout and weather conditions; human physical characteristics; and driver behaviour. The impact of weather conditions upon the distribution of road traffic accidents throughout the year is considered later [Figure 4.5 (C)] in an Icelandic context and a winter excess of deaths is found. Moellering's study ignores vehicle characteristics, but it does show road characteristics to be more important than human variables in producing short journeys to death.

Sources and Further Reading

See under Figure 3.17.

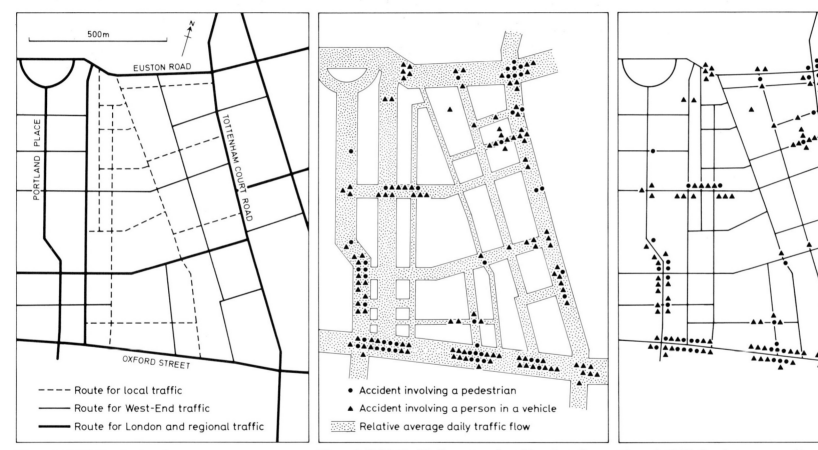

Figure 3.17 (A) Road network

Figure 3.17 (B) Traffic flow on roads and location of accidents

Figure 3.17 (C) Road structure and locations of accidents

3.17 ROAD TRAFFIC ACCIDENTS II: LONDON

ROAD TRAFFIC ACCIDENTS (ICD E810–E819 and E826–E829; see Figure 2.1) place a significant burden upon any area's medical services. The emergency procedures which have to be mobilized in the event of an accident are not only costly in their own right but, because they interrupt the normal routine of hospital and ambulance services, have a hidden opportunity cost to public health authorities. As we saw in the preceding figure, most road traffic accidents occur within a short distance of place of residence and therefore within urban areas. Existing street layouts in most towns date from the days when traffic was essentially on foot and they cater poorly for the frequently conflicting needs of pedestrians, cars and cyclists.

In this figure, we examine the geographical distribution of road traffic accidents in an area of central London to show that some of the simple solutions proposed by planners to reduce accidents often simply relocate them and, in some cases, actually increase the number occurring. The example is based upon data contained in the classic report by Colin Buchanan *et al.* (1963), *Traffic in Towns*.

Central London

The data and maps taken from Buchanan relate to an area approximately 500 metres from east to west and 1000 metres from north to south in central London bounded by Portland Place, Euston Road, Tottenham Court Road and Oxford Street [see diagram (A)]. At the date of the study (July–December, 1962), this was an area of mixed land use on densely developed sites within which 9,000 people lived and 50,000 worked. It contains the great Oxford Street shopping centre, and the major part of its industry was devoted to the clothing trade. The road network is shown in skeleton form in diagram (A). Tottenham Court Road had been made one-way in 1961. It is readily seen that the network consists of a complex, awkwardly arranged set of streets with a mass of intersections within the four bounding arterial roads. These intersections are an obstruction to the flow of traffic and are potential accident sites.

In diagram (A), the roads have been drawn in three different line types to distinguish routes which handle (a) traffic passing through the area either on its way to other parts of London or else away from London altogether (heavy solid lines) from (b) those roads serving the West End in general (light solid lines) and the study area in particular (pecked lines). Virtually all the roads gave direct access to properties in addition to their function for passage. Obviously there is no need for the through traffic using routes (a) to be in the area at all. It is bad practice to mix such vehicles with local traffic and it generally results in a high accident rate from flow conflicts and lack of awareness by the through traffic of local conditions.

Accidents and traffic flow

Diagram (B) illustrates the relative average daily traffic flow on each of the routes. The width of the stippled bands is in direct proportion to the flow level, a cartographic technique employed and discussed in Figure 3.3. As expected, the diagram shows that the routes carrying through traffic are the most heavily used. Oxford Street and Tottenham Court Road are those where both pedestrian and traffic flows are greatest. At the time of the study, Oxford Street had a normal two-way peak hour flow of 2,200–3,000 vehicles per hour, while counts showed 4,200 pedestrians per hour crossing Oxford Street both ways at its centre and 2,700 per hour crossing at the junction of Oxford Street and Tottenham Court Road. Diagram (B) also plots the location of accidents involving pedestrians (solid circle) and those involving a passenger vehicle (solid triangle) in relation to flow levels.

The majority of accidents of all kinds are seen to occur on the four main through routes where both traffic and pedestrian flows are heaviest.

Accidents and street geometry

Although there is a clear correlation between traffic and pedestrian flow levels and the frequency of accidents, street geometry also plays a part. The relationship of accidents to the topological structure of the network is shown in diagram (C). Here the knots of accidents in the vicinity of intersections are very evident, but in many cases with some considerable tail-back from the four main routes into the local-area and West-End networks. That is, the accidents are bunched close to the points at which either the local area roads intersect with the through routes or where the heavy traffic flows intermingle with much-used pedestrian routes. Most of the accidents to pedestrians occur on the busiest traffic routes or at junctions.

A common response to the delays caused at the intersection of main roads is for the traffic to seek alternate routes which by-pass the bottlenecks. Such re-routing may be by design; the temporary reduction in congestion achieved by signposting alternate routes is a cheap way for the traffic engineer to buy time. Sometimes the re-routing occurs as drivers learn quicker routes for themselves. In both cases, the effect is to introduce through traffic into the heart of frequently residential local areas where neither the road system nor the residents are equipped to cope. The consequences are the same under both models of the re-routing process; a redistribution in the number of accidents, especially involving pedestrians, away from intersections, to locations all along the new route. Examples are to be seen in diagram (C) on many of the roads cutting through the central part of the map between the four bounding arterial roads.

Current thinking on network design seeks to segregate vehicles and pedestrians as fully as possible. Through traffic is discouraged as far as possible from entering local areas and conflicting traffic flows are minimized by one-way streaming of traffic. The ultimate segregation of traffic and pedestrians is to ban cars from town centres altogether and this approach has been adopted in many western cities.

Sources and Further Reading

The diagrams in Figure 3.16 have been redrawn from H. Moellering (1974), *The Journey to Death: A Spatial Analysis of Fatal Traffic Crashes in Michigan, 1969*, Michigan Geographical Publication No. 13, Ann Arbor, Michigan: Department of Geography, pp.31, 46, 56 and 65.

The maps in Figure 3.17 are based on diagrams given in C. Buchanan (1963), *Traffic in Towns*, London: Her Majesty's Stationery Office.

Much of the basic work on network design and road safety is carried out by the Road Research Laboratory of the Department of Transport. A basic reference is Road Research Laboratory (1963), *Research on Road Safety*, London: Her Majesty's Stationery Office. See also *Traffic Accidents in Hertfordshire: Black Sites Before and After Survey*, Hertfordshire County Council, 1981, and W.L. Cresswell and P. Froggart (1963), *The Causation of Bus Driver Accidents: An Epidemiological Study*, London: Oxford University Press. The distribution of road vehicle accidents by local authority areas is given in M.J. Gardner, P.D. Winter and D.J.P. Barker (1984), *Atlas of Mortality from Selected Diseases in England and Wales, 1968–1978*, Chichester: John Wiley, pp.34–5, 54. Regular reports on UK traffic accidents are given in the Department of Transport's annual *Road Accidents Casualty Report*, London: Her Majesty's Stationery Office.

General questions on the epidemiology of traffic accidents are addressed in L.G. Norman (1962), *Road Traffic Accidents: Epidemiology, Control and Prevention*, Geneva: World Health Organization.

CHAPTER FOUR
TIME-SERIES

Figure over   Icelandic fever hospital ward
Source   Lyósmyndir Sigfúrsar Eymundssonar, Reykjavík: Almenna bókafélagið, 1976, Figure 51, p.77.

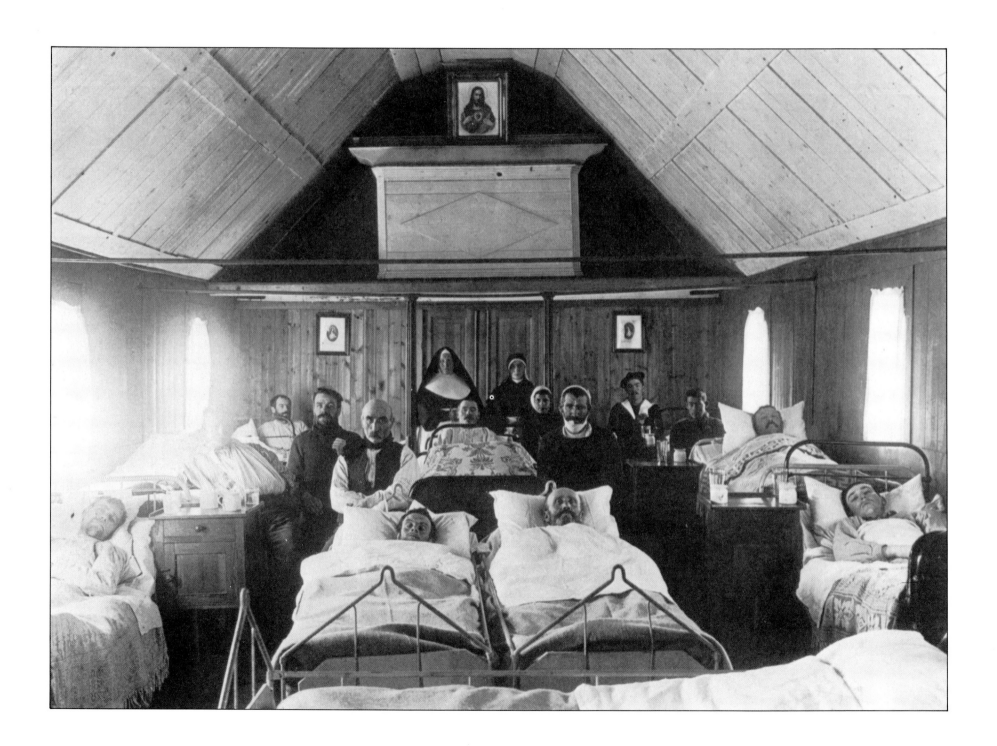

TIME-SERIES

INTRODUCTION

In the previous chapter we focused upon ways of analysing data collected at a set of geographical locations. We now consider the analysis of observations which have been recorded at different points in time to create a *time-series*. In one fundamental respect data which have been measured at either geographical or temporal locations are the same. In both, the relative position of any particular observation with respect to the other members of the series is unique to it; the members of space and time-series cannot be translocated without destroying the natural *serial ordering* imposed upon the data by time and space. Just as the city of London has a unique location in the United Kingdom which places it north of Southampton and south of Birmingham, so the year 1965 has a particular time position which places it later than 1964 and earlier than 1966.

In the same way that the ordering of events in space creates patterns which, as we saw in chapter 3, frequently give clues about the aetiology of disease, so the patterns formed by observations in time may contain similar evidence for the medical scientist. It is thus important to be able to characterize and to analyse time-series of observations, and it is towards these goals that this chapter is directed. We begin by providing a formal definition of a time-series and by illustrating some of the basic types of time-series which may be encountered. Methods of analysis are considered in the remainder of the chapter.

4.1 TYPES OF TIME-SERIES

Sample time-series

For a brief historical period between 1925 and 1935, quarterly data on the incidence of a series of infectious diseases were collected by the Health Committee of the League of Nations for the major cities of the world. Although the bulk of the data relate to Europe, all settled areas of the world are represented. Inevitably, the data are of variable quality as judged by levels of reporting so that, to aid comparability, the data are best standardized by their own internal means and variation as described in Figures 2.7 and 2.10 (technical appendix). Figure 4.1 shows the quarterly time-series so obtained for the number of reported cases of measles per thousand population in the cities of Frankfurt-am-Main (Germany), London (England), Trieste (Italy) and Paris (France). For a description of measles as a disease see the boxed definition in Figure 3.3.

We formally define a time-series as a set of ordered observations on a quantitative characteristic (here, reported cases of measles) taken at different points in time. Although it is not essential, it is common for these points, as here, to be equidistant apart. The essential quality of a time-series is the ordering of the observations according to the time-variable, as distinct from observations which are not ordered at all (for example, chosen simultaneously) or which are ordered according to their own internal properties (for example, by magnitude).

Components in time-series

It is evident from diagrams (A) – (D) that time-series may assume many different shapes. We may usefully consider a general time-series to be a sum of four components which will be present in varying degrees in any observed series. These components are

(a) *trend* or long-term movement;
(b) *seasonality*;
(c) *cyclical* fluctuations about the trend, over and above any seasonal effects, of greater or lesser regularity;
(d) a *residual*, irregular, or random effect.

Trend

The essential idea of *trend* is that it is the smooth rising or falling of a series. The measles series for Frankfurt-am-Main shown in (A) exhibits trend. Although the number of reported cases goes up and down, over the entire length of the series from 1925 to 1935 the general trend is for the number of reported cases to fall. In technical terms, the smoothness of trend, either up or down, implies that it may be represented by a

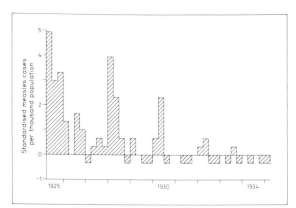

Figure 4.1 (A) Frankfurt-am-Main (Germany): secular trends in series

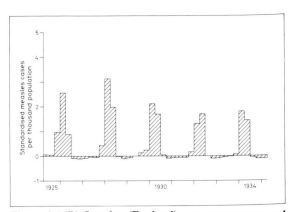

Figure 4.1 (B) London (England): strong two-year cycle

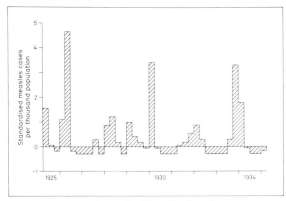

Figure 4.1 (C) Trieste (Italy): mixed cycles

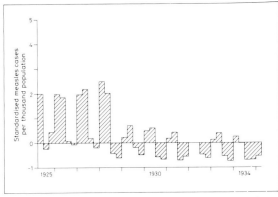

Figure 4.1 (D) Paris (France): discontinuity in series

continuous and differentiable function of time. The time-series for the other three cities shown in diagram (B) – (D) do not exhibit trend, in that the average number of reported measles cases does not rise or fall smoothly through time.

Seasonality

All the series exhibit fluctuations in the number of cases reported; that is, the case-load is not constant through time. Perhaps the easiest of these fluctuations to understand are those which are due to some cyclical generator associated with periodic astronomical phenomena. In the case of measles, for example, it is well known that, in northern temperate latitudes, measles cases peak in the winter season of the year and that they are at a minimum in the summer. That is to say, there is marked *seasonal* variation in measles incidence. This seasonality is not generally ascribed to the direct effect on the measles virus of temperature, but to the effect of temperature on the population at risk from the disease. For the childhood disease of measles, winter produces crowding in heated classrooms and homes. This results in frequent and close contact between individuals, leading to increased virus transmission. The series for Paris [diagram (D)] shows the seasonal component most distinctively, with peaks of cases in the first half and troughs in the second half of most years.

Cycles

We must be careful to distinguish between seasonal effects and fluctuations of a *cyclical* kind unrelated to astronomical phenomena. Thus the time-series for London [diagram (B)] does not display an annual rhythm of peaks and troughs but instead a very marked upswing every two years. The series for Frankfurt [diagram (A)] shows a similar two-year cycle, falling in size through time; that is, the cyclical component itself has trend. The series for Trieste [diagram (C)] is altogether more complicated, with major peaks about every four years and lesser peaks in between; the size of peaks thus forms an alternating series of a high peak followed by a low peak, and so on.

In the case of measles where a single attack generally confers lifelong immunity, the spacing of these cyclical epidemic peaks, as opposed to the seasonal rhythm of events, is generally related to the birth rate of the local population and the frequency with which it is exposed to the virus. Small populations and isolatedness result in widely spaced epidemics, and vice versa. These features are seen in the series for Trieste which had a population of around a quarter of a million at the time, compared with the half million of Frankfurt, the three millions of Paris and the eight millions of Greater London. The series become steadily more regular with increasing population.

Residual effects

If we can determine the trend, seasonal and cyclical components in any time-series and abstract them from the data, we are commonly left with a fluctuating series which may, at one extreme, be purely random or, at the other, a smooth oscillatory movement. Usually, it is somewhere between the two. This represents the *residual* component, (d), above.

Discontinuities

Some time-series exhibit features which may not be attributed to any of the four components of trend, seasonal, cyclical or random effects so far discussed. Most common are series which exhibit marked discontinuities or *shifts* in their temporal behaviour. That for Paris [diagram (D)] after 1928 provides an example. These discontinuities generally reflect a change in data recording practices. They make the comparison of time-series behaviour either side of the shift very difficult unless some form of correction is applied.

It is one of the aims of time-series analysis to separate time-series into the components discussed in this figure and we consider some appropriate techniques in Figure 4.2.

Sources and Further Reading

The quarterly data for measles cases for the four cities are taken from the League of Nations, Health Section, *Quarterly Report*, published in Geneva between 1925 and 1935. Data are available for 61 cities, mostly European but with a world-wide distribution.

A good introduction to time-series analysis is provided in C. Chatfield (1980), *The Analysis of Time Series: An Introduction*, second edition, London: Chapman and Hall. See also J.M. Gottmann (1981), *Time Series Analysis*, Cambridge: Cambridge University Press, and J.D. Cryer (1986), *Time Series Analysis*, Boston: Duxbury Press. Geographical applications of time-series methods are discussed in L.W. Hepple (1981), 'Spatial and temporal analysis: time series analysis', in *Quantitative Geography*, edited by N. Wrigley and R.J. Bennett, London: Routledge and Kegan Paul, pp.92–6.

4.2 DECOMPOSING A TIME-SERIES

Trends in time-series

Time-series may be regarded as a sum of four components, namely: (a) *trend*, or long-term movement, either up or down; (b) *seasonal effects*; (c) *cyclical fluctuations* about the trend over and above any seasonal effects; (d) a *residual*.

Diagram (A) shows the quarterly time-series of reported measles cases per thousand population between 1925 and 1935 in the city of Johannesburg, South Africa (population about half a million at the time). A description of measles appears in Figure 3.3. It is evident that the number of reported cases rose slowly over the study period, a long-term trend which may reflect improved recording rates as medical services increased. Regression techniques provide the simplest way of defining the straight-line trend in the data and the solid line in diagram (A) shows this for the Johannesburg data.

An alternative approach is to fit a *moving average* to each point in the series. Because the data are quarterly, a five-point average may be used; that is, each quarterly value in the series is replaced by an average of the five surrounding quarters of which it is the centre. This moving average is drawn as a solid line in diagram (B). While, like the regression trend-line illustrated in (A), it progresses generally upwards and eliminates local detail, it permits the broader fluctuations in the series to be modelled. Again, computational details are given in the technical appendix. The detrended series is obtained by subtracting the moving average values from the

corresponding original data points. This produces the stippled bar-graph illustrated in diagram (C). Comparison with the bar-graph of (B) shows that the detrended series now fluctuates around a constant level.

Seasonal components and decomposed series

Once trend has been eliminated, we can turn our attention to the seasonal component. Provided that there is no trend in the seasonal component itself, we expect seasonal effects over a year to be roughly self-cancelling and to sum to zero. That is, an excess of cases in one quarter will be offset by a deficit in another and so on. This notion lies at the heart of procedures for determining seasonal effects. The seasonal weights for the Johannesburg data which meet this zero sum requirement are plotted as the solid line in (C). Each year, there is an excess of cases in first and fourth quarters and a deficit in second and third quarters. To remove seasonal effects, the seasonal weights are subtracted from the data series.

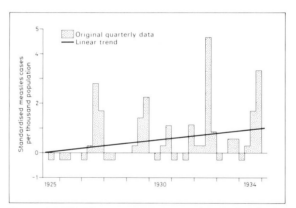

Figure 4.2 (A) Linear trend in quarterly measles data for Johannesburg (South Africa)

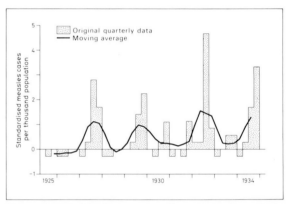

Figure 4.2 (B) Moving average (five quarters) applied to Johannesburg series

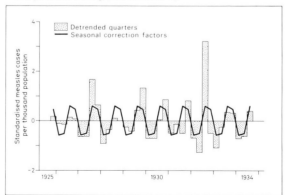

Figure 4.2 (C) Detrended Johannesburg series with seasonal cycles identified

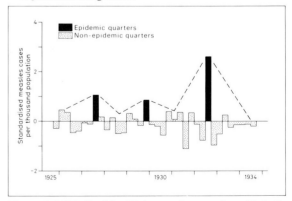

Figure 4.2 (D) Residual Johannesburg series with both trend and seasonal components removed

Diagram (D) shows the Johannesburg series after the removal of both trend and seasonal components. We are left with cycles of major measles epidemics (in black) about every two to three years separated by relatively quiet periods.

Sources and Further Reading

The data source for the Johannesburg series plotted in (A) is given in Figure 4.1 of this Atlas.

The principles of decomposition are set out in C. Chatfield (1980), *The Analysis of Time Series: an Introduction*, second edition, London: Chapman and Hall, pp.12–55, and their implementation with MINITAB procedures for analysis are given in J.D. Cryer (1986), *Time Series Analysis*, Boston: Duxbury Press, pp.9–73.

Technical appendix

Trend removal

The simplest way of removing **trend** from a time-series is to use regression analysis. Let y_t denote the reported number of measles cases per thousand population in the t-th quarter of a T-element time-series. Then the model,

$$y_t = b_0 + b_1 t + e_t, t = 1, 2, \ldots, T, \quad (4.2.1)$$

fits a linear time-trend to the data. If we use m_t to denote the value of y_t given by the fitted model, it follows that the differences $(y_t - m_t)$ represent the *detrended* time-series. The solid line in diagram (A) gives the trend-line obtained from model (4.2.1) for the Johannesburg data. The trend accounts for just over 7 percent of the total variation in the series while, using ordinary least squares, $\hat{b}_0 = -0.008$ and $\hat{b}_1 = 0.026$.

The regression approach has several deficiencies as a method for separating out the trend component in any time-series. Unless a fairly complex polynomial in time is fitted, only very simple trends may be modelled. It is troublesome to update when new observations arrive since estimation of the model uses the whole of the series.

Finally, the observations in the detrended series are intercorrelated in a way which reflects the model fitted.

The preferable procedure is to fit a moving average to the series since any smooth function can be represented locally by a polynomial to a fairly high degree of accuracy. The trend value at a given point is taken as the average of some set of points of which the given point is the centre. The set should contain an odd number of points to give symmetry about the centre point. If we denote the trend value by m_t at the centre point t, then

$$m_t = \sum_{j=-k}^{k} a_j y_{t+j} \quad (4.2.2)$$

for a $(2k + 1)$ point moving average. The $\{a_j\}$ are weights scaled to sum to unity. As discussed in Kendall (1973, chapter 3), the value of k is at choice. Common values are five and seven. Fitting a polynomial of order three is usually adequate for trend removal. The unscaled weights which should be used in equation (4.2.2) to achieve this are $[-3, 12, 17, 12, -3]$ when $k = 5$ and $[-2, 3, 6, 7, 6, 3, -2]$ when $k = 7$.

Other systems of weights may be used in equation (4.2.2). Many time spans over which we wish to average consist of an even number of points – the 24 hours of a day; as here, the four quarters of the year; 12 months, and so on. It is then highly desirable to bring the points of trend determination into line with the time-points of the observations. Taking as an example the quarterly Johannesburg data, a convenient procedure is to compute a five-point *centred* average with the unscaled weights $[1, 2, 2, 2, 1]$. There are two identical quarters in the average but each has only half the weight of the other quarters. Thus if the centre is the third quarter, the average will be of the first, second, third, fourth and fifth quarters. The fifth quarter is, of course, the first quarter of the next year and is taken as equivalent to the first quarter of the preceding year from a weighting viewpoint. This system of weights was used to calculate the trend line shown in (B).

Seasonal effect

The **seasonal effect** may be either additive or multiplicative. If m_t is the trend component, s_t is the seasonal and e_t is the residual, we may have, for example, either

$$y_t = m_t + s_t + e_t \quad (4.2.3)$$

or

$$y_t = m_t s_t e_t. \quad (4.2.4)$$

Multiplicative models are linear and additive on taking logarithms.

To estimate s_t in the additive model, we must first remove any trend, m_t, from the data to prevent it affecting our estimate of the seasonal component. Taking the quarterly data for Johannesburg as an example, we estimate the trend by a five-point moving average with scaled weights $1/8[1, 2, 2, 2, 1]$ and define the detrended series at all points t as $(y_t - m_t)$. We now impose the additional condition that

$$\sum_{t=1}^{4} s_t = 0. \quad (4.2.6)$$

That is, we require the seasonal effects to sum to zero. To articulate this condition, we take the detrended time-series of reported cases and calculate the mean value of all the first quarters of the detrended series, the mean value of all the second quarters and so on. The four means obtained are 0.42, −0.62, −0.50 and 0.65; the average of these means is −0.01. The seasonal effects are measured by subtracting the mean of means from the quarterly means to give values, subject to rounding, of 0.43, −0.61, −0.49 and 0.67 which sum to zero as required. These seasonal correction factors are plotted as the solid line in (C). To adjust the data for seasonality we should, for example, then subtract 0.43 from all first quarters and add 0.49 to all third quarters.

4.3 IDENTIFYING A TIME-SERIES MODEL

As we have seen in the previous two figures, any time-series may be viewed as a sum of four components namely long-term trend, seasonal effects, cyclical fluctuations reflecting the aetiology of the disease and random variation. For example, many countries have experienced steady changes or *trends* upwards as reporting levels of infectious diseases have improved; downwards as the quality and scope of medical protection has increased. It is also well known that many infectious diseases such as influenza have a winter or *seasonal* peak of cases.

Sample time-series

The time-series shown in graph (A) records the number of reported measles cases per 1000 population on a quarterly basis between 1925 and 1935 for the city of Manchester (population nearly three-quarters of a million at the time) in the United Kingdom. A description of measles as a disease is included in the boxed definition accompanying Figure 3.3. Using the methods described in Figure 2.10 (technical appendix), the series has been standardized by its median and inter-quartile range before plotting. The diagram shows the strong *cyclical* fluctuations found when the number of reported measles cases in large cities is plotted against time. As discussed later in section 6.5, the population size of Manchester has been sufficiently large throughout the twentieth century for measles to be endemic in the city. Since an attack of measles confers life-long immunity, the approximately two-year cycle of major measles epidemics shown in chart (A) may be related to the time required

for a population not previously exposed to the virus to build up sufficiently by births to sustain an epidemic.

Autocorrelation functions (ACFs)

In Figure 4.2, moving average techniques were utilized as a basis for decomposing a time-series into the component parts discussed above. Other

approaches exist which may be employed to determine the percentage contribution of each of the components to the total variation in a time-series. The most important are those based upon the *autocorrelation* (ACF) and *partial autocorrelation* (PACF) functions, and transformations of them. In the time-series literature the use of these methods to recognize the components in a series, with a view to modelling them, is referred to as model *identification* and graphs

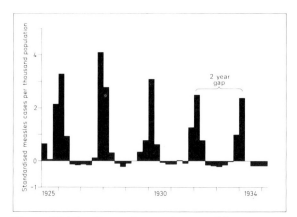

Figure 4.3 (A) Quarterly measles record for Manchester (England) on a standardized basis

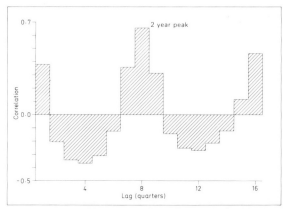

Figure 4.3 (B) Autocorrelation function (ACF) of the Manchester series

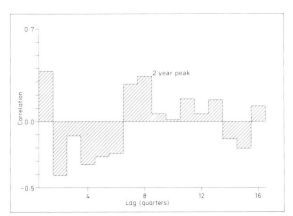

Figure 4.3 (C) Partial autocorrelation function (PACF) of the Manchester series

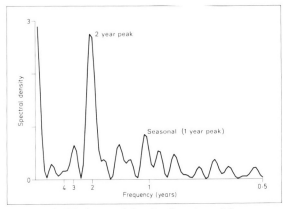

Figure 4.3 (D) Spectral density function of the Manchester series

(B) – (D) illustrate the methodology involved.

In diagram (B), we have plotted the ACF of the time-series shown in (A). In order to compute the ACF, the degree of correlation between all pairs of quarterly observations which are 1,2,3 . . . quarters apart in the series is calculated; technical details are given in the appendix to this figure. The greater the degree of association between all such pairs of observations, the bigger will be the correlation. Perfect positive association yields a value of 1.0, a perfect inverse relationship a value of -1.0, while no association yields a value of zero. The number of quarters which separate any pair of observations is termed the lag. This is plotted on the horizontal axis, while the correlation appears on the vertical axis. Thus diagram (B) shows that the Manchester series has high positive correlations at lags 1, 7–9, and finally at lags 15–16. The highest association of nearly 0.7 occurs at lag 8.

These results may be interpreted as follows.

(a) The high correlation at lag 1 implies that similar levels of measles cases are recorded in consecutive quarters; this is apparent from inspection of the original time-series. Although it is not the case here, we note that, if a time-series has a time-trend, then a high correlation will also be produced at lag 1. As the time-trend line plotted on Figure 4.2(A) shows, a linear time-trend implies that adjacent months in the series have similar levels of reported cases, yielding high correlations at lag 1. In fact, large correlations are commonly found at lag 1 in most time-series and simply reflect the smooth rise and fall of disease incidence over continuous time.

(b) The peak correlation at lag 8 is a result of the strong association between time periods which are eight quarters apart and reflects the clearly marked biennial cycle in the Manchester data.

(c) The secondary peak at lag 16 provides no new information but arises as a harmonic of the basic two-year cycle in the data.

(d) The large negative values at lags 4 and 12 reflect the fact that a winter of high measles incidence is followed in the succeeding winter by low measles incidence. This again reflects the two-year cycle in the data.

Partial autocorrelation functions (PACFs)

Graph (C) is a plot of the PACF (on the vertical axis) against lag (on the horizontal axis) for the Manchester data. Whereas the ACF makes no allowance at lags greater than 1 for any interaction effects between quarters which intervene between the lag of interest, the PACF filters out such effects. As a result the signal is slightly less distinctive but still shows the features of substantial correlation at lag 1 and the biennial cycle (large negative correlation at lag 4 and large positive correlation at lag 8). Notice that, because interaction effects are allowed for, the high correlation at lag 16 on the ACF has disappeared in the PACF because it is simply a multiple of the basic harmonic at 8 quarters.

Spectral density function

Graph (D) uses spectral analysis to examine the structure of the time-series by fitting cosine curves of different wavelengths and amplitudes to the data. The percentage of the total variation in the series accounted for by a cosine curve of a particular wavelength and amplitude is called the *spectral density*; technical details are given later in Figure 5.12. Density is plotted on the vertical axis of (D) against a function of the wavelength called the frequency (wavelength per unit time).

Again, the very marked biennial cycle in the Manchester data is detected; cosine curves with a frequency of two years account for the greatest proportion of the total variation in the series. The second highest density value occurs at one year and reflects the annual winter upswing of reported cases of measles (the seasonal component).

All three diagrams, (B), (C) and (D), describe the characteristic 'signatures' of the original data in a way which allows the basic components of the time-series to be determined. The ACF and PACF, through the high correlations at lags 1 and 8, point to the smoothly varying two-year cycles of measles epidemics, while the spectral density highlights not only the biennial cycle but also the seasonal upswing of cases in every winter.

Note that, in interpreting the diagrams, the horizontal axes for the ACF and PACF increase in lag with distance away from the origin of the axis. In the case of the spectral density the longest wavelengths are towards the left and the shortest towards the right.

Sources and Further Reading

The data source for the Manchester series plotted in (A) is given in Figure 4.1 of this Atlas.

A standard work on model identification in a spatial context is R.J. Bennett (1979), *Spatial Time Series: Analysis, Forecasting and Control*, London: Pion. See also C. Chatfield (1980), *The Analysis of Time Series: an Introduction*, second edition, London: Chapman and Hall, pp.60–81, and J.M. Gottmann (1981), *Time Series Analysis*, Cambridge: Cambridge University Press, pp.125–60. The principles of identification with MINITAB procedures for analysis are given in J.D. Cryer (1986), *Time Series Analysis*, Boston: Duxbury Press, pp.9–73.

Technical appendix

Let y_t denote the value of some variable at time t and y_{t-k} denote its value at a time period k lags removed from t. Then the k-th lag autocorrelation, r_k, can be conveniently computed from

$$r_k = [\sum_{t=1}^{T-k} (y_t - \bar{y})(y_{t+k} - \bar{y})] / \sum_{t=1}^{T} (y_t - \bar{y})^2. \qquad (4.3.1)$$

The partial autocorrelations, b_{kk}, denote the correlation between y_t and y_{t-k}, given $y_{t-1}, \ldots y_{t-k+1}$, where

$$b_{k+1,k+1} = (r_{k+1} - \sum_{j=1}^{k} b_{kj} r_{k+1-j}) / (1 - \sum_{j=1}^{k} b_{kj} r_j) \quad (4.3.2)$$

and

$$b_{k+1,j} = b_{kj} - b_{k+1,k+1} b_{k,k+1-j}, j = 1, 2, \ldots, k. \quad (4.3.3)$$

Here, $\bar{y}$ is the mean of a T-element time-series and, additionally, $b_{11} = r_1$. The ACF is a plot of r_k against k while the PACF is a plot of b_{kk} against k. The spectral density is the fast Fourier transformation of the ACF.

4.4 LONG-TERM TRENDS IN MORTALITY IN ICELAND

Numbers and rates

Time-series of morbidity and mortality data published by public health organizations appear in two basic forms. Sometimes the *number* of cases or the number of deaths from a particular disease is given. On other occasions, the data are expressed as a *rate*; that is, the number of cases or deaths per unit of population. Both kinds of data need to be analyzed with care. A rising or falling trend in the number of cases or deaths may simply reflect the fact that the population total itself is rising or falling, rather than be evidence of a trend of medical significance.

Expressing the data as a rate per unit of population by-passes the above problem, but introduces another. It then becomes impossible to be sure of the absolute number of cases or deaths since the shape of the resulting time-series will again depend on whether or not a trend is present in the population data. Thus five deaths in a population of 100 yields the same rate as 500 in a population of 10,000. It is only when population size is constant through time that trends in the level of cases or deaths can be readily determined from data expressed as rates.

Arithmetic and logarithmic plots

Hence when interpreting time-series of morbidity and mortality which have been plotted as either numbers or rates, it is important to have some information about the demographic history of a population if a sound assessment of the significance of the patterns in such data is to be

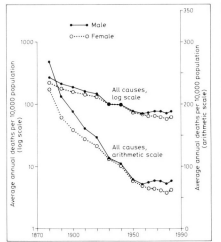

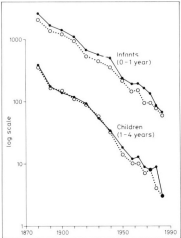

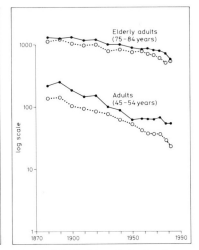

Figure 4.4 (A) Trends in death rates for Icelandic population, 1876–1985

Figure 4.4 (B) Trends in death rates for Icelandic infants and children, 1876–1985

Figure 4.4 (C) Trends in death rates for Icelandic adults and elderly adults, 1876–1985

made. The issues are illustrated in the present figure by examining the time-series of deaths from all causes in Iceland over the 110-year period between 1876 and 1985.

Diagram (A) gives the average annual number of deaths per 10,000 population from all causes. In this and parts (B) and (C) of the figure, male and female deaths have been separated. The data in diagram (A) have been plotted using both arithmetic and logarithmic scales on the vertical axis, while a logarithmic scale alone has been used in diagrams (B) and (C). On a logarithmic scale, death rates between one and ten occupy the same plotting distance as rates between ten and a hundred, or between a hundred and a thousand. Using logarithms therefore stretches out the scale of numbers as it descends towards zero. It is thus a particularly useful transformation to employ with data which contain both very large and very small numbers, and it will have the effect of producing straight-line plots from data which rise or fall exponentially. This can be seen by comparing the arithmetic and logarithmic curves on diagram (A); it implies that the graphs in (B) and (C) fall exponentially when plotted on an arithmetic scale.

Trends in the overall Icelandic population

As in all developed countries, the long-term trend in mortality in Iceland shown in diagram (A) has been steadily downwards from well over 200 per 10,000 population in the last quarter of the nineteenth century to around 70 in the mid-1980s. This pattern reflects improved standards of living and medical care. Man's lack of immortality means that such a downward trend cannot persist indefinitely, and it is evident from the graphs in (A), especially when plotted on an arithmetic scale, that the decrease in death rates flattened out markedly in 1950 and has been

effectively constant since then. Again, as in other Western nations, the death rate among males has been consistently higher than that among females except between 1930 and 1950 when the rates were substantially the same for both sexes. The Icelandic economy has always been dominated by fishing and farming and the excess of male deaths, especially in the first half of the period, reflects the large number of occupational deaths in these industries (cf. Figure 3.15).

As seen in Figure 2.12, the fall in death rates shown in diagram (A) has taken place in a total population which has grown rapidly and constantly throughout the period considered from about 70,000 at the beginning to around 230,000 in the mid-1980s. This rapid population growth stands in marked contrast to most other developed nations, and it is all the more remarkable that the dramatic fall in death rates should have taken place as the total population grew so quickly.

Trends in the young Icelandic population

Diagrams (B) and (C) show how the decline in death rates over study period has been distributed in the population. Mortality among infants and among children aged between one and four years fell steadily over the whole period, producing the steeply descending graphs in (B). Among infant males, for example, it was over 2,600 per 10,000 population in 1876, but around 70 by the 1980s. The graphs in diagram (B) show some irregularity in the downward progression between 1950 and 1970. Figure 6.5(C), later, indicates that this 20-year window coincides with dramatic and unusual changes in the Icelandic birth rate. It had been constant for the preceding 75 years but then, about 1940, it exploded dramatically for some 20 years before settling down on a new and higher plateau.

Trends in the adult elderly Icelandic population

In contrast to the rapidly falling infant mortality, diagram (C) shows that, although the death rate among adults aged 45–54 years also declined over the period, it was not nearly so marked as that for the very young. The mortality curves for the elderly in diagram (C) indicate that the death rate there scarcely changed over the 110 years considered, fluctuating around 2,000 per 10,000 population. Male mortality exceeded female mortality in all the age groups considered, although the differences are slight in the one to four age group.

Mortality in Iceland thus displays the patterns familiar in all the developed nations namely, a general decline in death rates which is concentrated primarily among the very young. Our understanding of these patterns is, however, deepened when we bear in mind that the demography of the country has been very different from that in most other Western nations. Iceland experienced rapid population growth and high birth rates over the period considered, whereas declining birth rates and stagnant population totals have been the norm in other Western nations.

Sources and Further Reading

The medical data used for the Icelandic maps shown here were taken from the volumes of *Heilbrigðisskýrslur* (Public Health in Iceland), 1966-70, and the demographic data from *Mannfjöldaskýrslur árin 1961–70* (Population and Vital Statistics, 1961–70).

4.5 SEASONAL INCIDENCE OF DISEASE I: CIRCULAR CHART METHODS

Seasonal variation in mortality and morbidity

An important aspect of time-series analysis is detecting the changing rhythm throughout the year – the seasonal variability – of disease mortality and morbidity. So, for example, an increase in the incidence of common infectious diseases like influenza and measles is a familiar feature of the winter months in the countries of North America and Europe. Other infectious diseases strike most frequently in the northern summer. As we saw in Chapter 1, the visitations of cholera in the nineteenth century to the cities of northern Europe provide an example. Although we may be familiar with the idea of changing seasonal incidence for infectious diseases, it may be that non-infectious causes of death also display seasonal changes. Do road traffic accidents, for example, peak in the winter in northern latitudes because of the poorer weather conditions and icy roads?

Circular charts

A cartographic device used by meteorologists to study variability is the wind-rose, in which the frequency with which winds are observed to blow from particular compass directions is plotted around the circumference of a circle. We may employ essentially the same device to study variations in the seasonal incidence of disease mortality and morbidity.

To illustrate the method, consider diagram (A) which plots the monthly variability in deaths from all causes in Iceland between 1961 and 1970. Over this ten-year period, a total of 13,494 deaths was recorded at an average of 112 per month. A circle is drawn at any convenient scale with twelve radiating spokes representing the months of the year. The length of each spoke denotes, to scale, the average value of 112. Taking January as an example, the observed average annual death rate in Iceland from all causes in January between 1961 and 1970 was, in fact, 119.8. This value is obtained by dividing the total number of deaths observed in all ten Januaries of the time-series (1198) by ten.

Using the scale already fixed, we can then plot at the appropriate position on the radiating spoke for January a point whose value is 119.8. This procedure is repeated to define the locations of the points which represent the observed average annual death rates for the other eleven months of the year. The twelve points are then joined to define a polygon which has been stippled in each of the diagrams (A) – (F). We can then readily

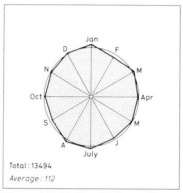

Figure 4.5 (A) Deaths from all causes in Iceland, 1961–1970

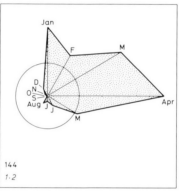

Figure 4.5 (B) Deaths from influenza in Iceland, 1961–1970

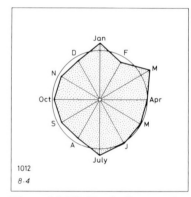

Figure 4.5 (C) Deaths from road traffic accidents in Iceland, 1961–1970

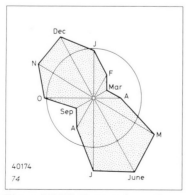

Figure 4.5 (D) Reported measles cases in Iceland, 1900–1944

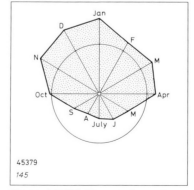

Figure 4.5 (D) Reported measles cases in Iceland, 1945–1970

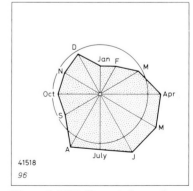

Figure 4.5 (F) Reported measles cases in Fiji, 1946–1981

identify those months of the year in which the death rate exceeds the average and lie outside the reference circle, and those months which are below average and which are contained within the reference circle. In the case of deaths from all causes diagram (A) shows, as might be expected, that there is very little seasonal variability; January has the greatest excess.

Contrasts in seasonal mortality

Diagram (B) illustrates the seasonal pattern of reported deaths from influenza in Iceland between 1961 and 1970 (for disease description see boxed definition in section 6.4). Over the period, a total of 144 deaths were directly attributed to the disease at an average of 1.2 per month. This average, however, conceals enormous seasonal variability. All the deaths were effectively concentrated in the first quarter of the year, with a three-month period in the autumn months from September to November when no deaths at all were reported.

In contrast, when we consider the changing monthly incidence of deaths from road traffic accidents in Iceland over the same period [diagram (C)], a similar marked lack of variability from month to month is found as with deaths from all causes. Nevertheless, it is noticeable that, although the monthly fluctuations are not great, the months in the second half of the year are below average while, with the exception of February, those in the first half of the year are at or above average. This difference is almost certainly attributable to driving conditions in the Icelandic winter, with the combination of long nights, dirt roads, and snow and ice until June in many areas.

Contrasts in seasonal morbidity

So far in this figure, seasonal variations in mortality have been considered. In contrast, diagrams (D) – (F) focus upon morbidity from a single disease – measles. A description of measles as a disease is included in the boxed definition accompanying Figure 3.3. The standard accounts of measles incidence ascribe to it a strong seasonal pattern. Thus Ball (1976, pp. 245–6) describes measles as having 'a higher incidence in the colder months, reaching a peak in January and February which is most marked in an epidemic year.' This generalization is based on northern temperate countries and so we should expect the corresponding months to be July and August in southern temperate countries. Diagram (D) shows the monthly pattern of reported cases in Iceland from 1900–44, while diagram (E) illustrates the Icelandic pattern between 1945–70. Diagram (F) plots the monthly variation in cases in the southern Pacific island of Fiji, 1946–81.

In Iceland, there is a stark contrast in the seasonal patterns between the pre- and post-war periods. From 1900–44, the distribution is clearly bimodal with above average measles incidence from October–December and again from May–July. In the post-war period, the seasonal pattern familiar throughout Europe and North America is found, with an excess of cases concentrated in the winter half of the year from November to April. Variations in levels of infection in measles from month to month are not generally ascribed in the literature to the effects of temperature and humidity on the virus itself, but rather to the impact of such conditions on the population at risk from this childhood disease. The crowding of the under-fifteen

population into heated rooms at home and school in northern winters, creating ideal conditions for virus transmission, accounts for the winter peak observed in Iceland throughout the period 1900–70. The late spring and early summer peak in the pre-war period reflects a significant feature of the Icelandic economy at the time. The haymaking season in Iceland peaks in June and this traditionally communal activity was significant in spreading the virus through the island's farming communities in a period when farming was the most important segment of the economy (Cliff, Haggett, Ord and Versey, 1981, pp. 127–28).

When we move to the southern hemisphere and to the island of Fiji at latitude 18 degrees south [diagram (F)] then, allowing for the fact that April to August corresponds with the winter half of the year, the traditional pattern of a winter excess of cases is once more found.

Sources and Further Reading

Data on deaths for Iceland (A, B and C) are based on *Heilbrigðisskýrslur* (Public Health in Iceland) 1966-70, and the demographic data are taken from *Mannfjöldaskýrslur árin 1961–70* (Population and Vital Statistics, 1961–70). Measles cases in Iceland (D and E) are taken from the data tables in A.D. Cliff, P. Haggett, J.K. Ord and G.R. Versey (1981), *Spatial Diffusion: An Historical Geography of Epidemics in an Island Community*, Cambridge: Cambridge University Press, pp.201–29. Measles cases in Fiji (F) are drawn from the World Health Organization's *World Health Statistics Annual*, Geneva, 1946 to 1981.

The circular graphing method is described in F.J. Monkhouse and H.R. Wilkinson (1971), *Maps and Diagrams*, third edition, London: Methuen, pp.241–7. Statistical analysis of circular distributions is treated in K.V. Mardia (1972), *Statistics of Directional Data*, London: Academic Press.

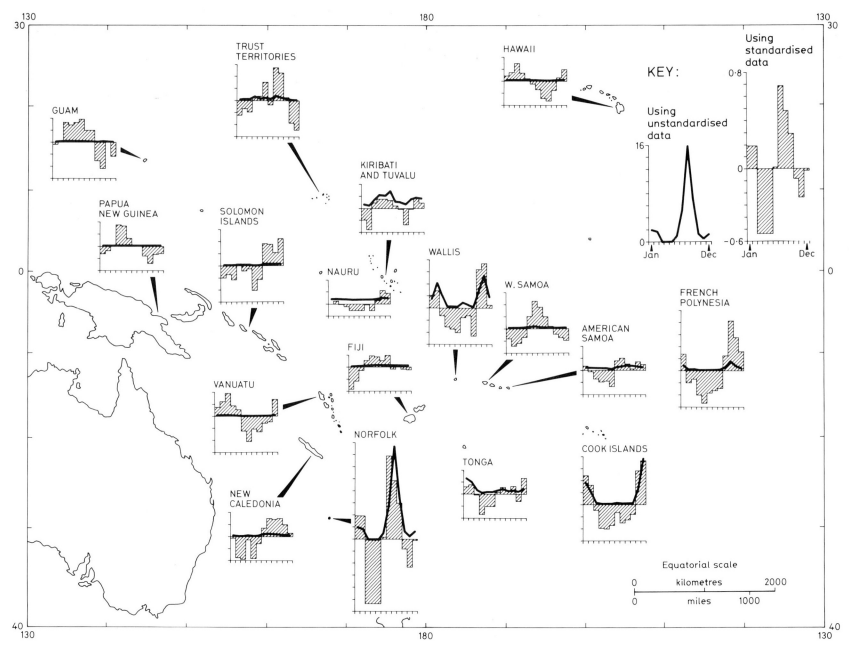

Figure 4.6 (A) Monthly incidence of measles in eighteen Pacific island groups 1946–1981

4.6 SEASONAL INCIDENCE OF DISEASE II: CLIMAGRAPHS

Global variations in seasonality

The relationship between the incidence of different diseases and seasonal rhythms tends to be most commonly associated with high latitude countries where there is a marked contrast between summer and winter weather. In these regions, the differences between the external environment (for example, air temperature) and the internal environment (for example, degree of crowding of individuals within buildings) can be clearly identified. Thus there is no doubt that, in the case of the common infectious diseases, the cold northern winters and the resulting congregation of people into heated rooms increases virus transmission between individuals and helps to account for the upturn in reported cases each winter.

However, fluctuations in disease incidence may also occur in tropical and sub-tropical countries where the association with environmental change is more difficult to establish. In this figure, we show how the problem may be tackled by examining seasonal patterns of measles cases in some Pacific island groups and by using *climagraphs* to relate the patterns to two obvious climatic variables, temperature and precipitation.

Measles incidence in the Pacific

Map (A) shows the average monthly incidence of reported measles cases per thousand population in eighteen Pacific island groups between January 1946 and December 1981 (for disease description see box in Figure 3.3). The structure of each graph is given by the keys located in the northeast corner of the map. The average monthly incidence using unstandardized data (solid line trace) and standardized data (diagonally shaded histograms) is plotted on the vertical axis. The standardization is described in Figure 2.10 (technical appendix) and computational formulae are given in the technical appendix to the present figure. The horizontal axis gives the months of the year running from January to December.

In small communities like Norfolk Island, which experienced only two epidemics in the period considered, the average case rate for any single month is more likely to reflect the accident of the month in which a measles carrier visited the island than any recognizable seasonal cycle related to rhythmic changes in either the physical or the demographic environment. Nevertheless, there are regularities which can be detected. Fiji, with the fullest data record, exhibits a clear seasonal difference between the high measles months from April to August (the southern hemisphere winter) and the low months from September to March (the southern hemisphere summer). This Fijian pattern is repeated in Western Samoa, the Trust Territories of the Pacific and Guam, and it mirrors the seasonal experience of northern latitudes for measles epidemics.

In contrast in Hawaii, which is not much further north than Guam, this pattern is reversed; the months of high measles incidence very obviously follow the trend common in northern mid-latitude countries, running from November to April. One possible explanation for this clear reversal is that Hawaii is one of the states of the United States, with regular airline traffic linking the two. The United States has a seasonal measles regime similar to other northern countries, and the link to Hawaii may result in the North American pattern dominating the island's regime.

We must be cautious in tropical oceanic environments like this part of the Pacific basin when using terms such as 'winter' and 'summer'. Some island groups display a complex pattern with double peaks of measles incidence (for example, Wallis), and the onset of wet and dry seasons may well play a more important role than the relatively minor contrasts in temperature.

Seasonal incidence and climatic variation

We may examine the relationship between seasonal incidence of disease and the climatic variables of precipitation and temperature using climagraphs. As shown in diagram (B), each graph plots the monthly averages for precipitation (horizontal axis) and temperature (vertical axis) for the capital cities of six of the island groups, using climatic data taken from Wernstedt (1972). Connecting the monthly plots in temporal order gives a characteristic trace. All occupy the warmer parts of the graphs and show a very small temperature range but major contrasts in precipitation. The seasonal cycles in these tropical islands are dominated by precipitation changes and, since the alternation of wind and pressure belts may give more than one wet season during the year the tracks, like that of American Samoa, can be complex and overlapping.

The seasonal incidence of measles has been superimposed upon the monthly tracks. To simplify plotting, average measles incidence for each month has been coded in terms of positive and negative deviations from the annual mean. Excess months have been defined as those with positive scores on the measles incidence graphs of diagram (A) drawn from standardized data; deficit months are those with negative scores.

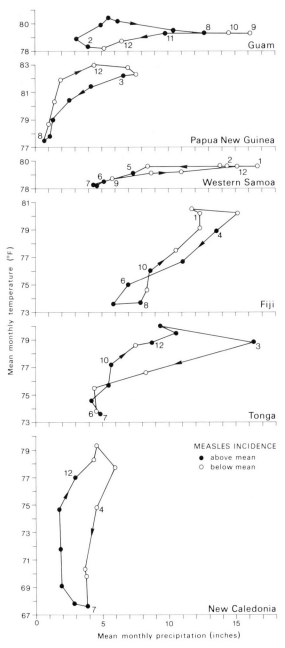

Figure 4.6 (B) Climagraphs of monthly incidence of measles in six Pacific island groups, 1946–1981

Inspection of the climagraphs shows there is no simple association of measles incidence with the relatively cooler months. All have excess measles cases in some of the hottest and wettest months of the year but a common pattern is for the measles season either to start or to be substantially concentrated in the relatively cooler and drier months.

Thus if climatic influences play a part in determining month by month variation in measles incidence in the Pacific (and, as the map shows, these variations certainly arise) then these are considerably more subtle than those in higher latitudes. Perhaps the climatic effect may be operating through an intermediate demographic factor (for example the movements of seasonal migrant workers in the Pacific) rather than in a direct aetiological manner.

Sources and Further Reading

The map is taken from A.D. Cliff and P. Haggett (1985), *The Spread of Measles in Fiji and the Pacific: Spatial Components in the Transmission of Epidemic Waves through Island Communities*, Publication HG18, Canberra: Australian National University, Research School of Pacific Studies, Department of Human Geography, Figure 17, p.78. The climatic data in (B) is based on F. Wernstedt (1972), *World Climatic Data*, Lamont, Penn.: Climatic Data Press.

The demography and epidemiology in the region are described in N. McArthur (1967), *Island Populations in the Pacific*, Canberra: Australian National University Press, and the environmental variation in J.-H. Chang (1968), 'Rainfall in the tropical southwest Pacific', *Geographical Review*, 58, pp.142–4.

Technical appendix

Let x_t denote the observed average incidence in month t of reported measles cases per thousand population. The unstandardized data is a plot of x_t against months. Now let $x_t' = \log(1 + x_t)$ and $z_t = (x_t' - \bar{x}')/s_{x'}$, where $\bar{x}'$ is the mean and $s_{x'}$ is the standard deviation of the $\{x_t'\}$. Then the standardized data are a plot of z_t against months.

4.7 INTERNATIONAL VARIATIONS IN MEASLES SERIES

When plotted as a time-series, the reported numbers of cases of most common infectious diseases propagated by person-to-person transmission display two common characteristics. First, most are recorded in the intense *epidemic* phases of the disease which appear to recur at regular intervals. These epidemic episodes are separated by relatively quiet inter-epidemic periods when either few or no cases of the disease occur. Second, the time gap between the epidemics appears to be a function of the population size of the community within which the disease is studied. In this figure, the characteristic signature formed by these recurring waves of disease is examined for measles (for disease description see box in Figure 3.3).

Measles time-series for four countries

Diagrams (A) – (D) plot the time-series of reported cases between 1945 and 1970 for four countries, arranged in decreasing order of population size. Diagram (A) shows that in the United States, with a population of 210 millions in 1970, epidemic peaks arrived every year. The dramatic reduction in the amplitude of the waves after 1964 was due to the introduction of systematic vaccination programmes (cf. Figure 4.9). In Britain [diagram (B)], with a 1970 population of 56 millions, peaks occurred every two years. Denmark [diagram (C)], with a population of 5 millions, had a more complex pattern with some evidence of a three-year cycle in the latter half of the period. Iceland (0.2

millions) stands in contrast to the other countries illustrated in that only eight waves occurred in the 25-year period, and no cases were reported in several years. The Icelandic case is considered in detail in section 6.5.

Measles epidemiology

An understanding of why measles occurs in epidemics and is propagated as a wave-train can only be achieved by considering the virus itself. The explosive growth in the number of cases which characterizes the upswing of a major epidemic implies that the virus is being passed from one host to many others. The sequence of measles virus infection in an individual host normally involves three stages. First, a *latent period* occurs, extending from initial exposure to the virus, to the first appearance of cold-like

symptoms. The length of this period is 8–12 days. This is followed by a prodromal period of some 2–4 days in which the patient shows upper respiratory catarrhal disorder and fever. It culminates in the third stage or external rash period which lasts on average 4–7 days. The infected host is able to transmit the virus in both the prodromal and external rash conditions, and we refer to this as the *infectious period*, lasting on average some 7–9 days. The prodromal period is the most critical for virus spread since the host is infectious and still only displays cold-like symptoms.

These ideas enable us to view transmission of the disease as a chain structure. Diagram (E) shows the chains resulting from virus transmission between a host i and a susceptible j where the open circles denote the onset of infection. In the shortest chain (8 days), the host i makes contact with j on day 1 of the infectious period,

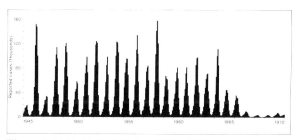

Figure 4.7 (A) United States, 1945–1970

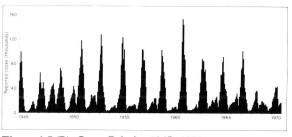

Figure 4.7 (B) Great Britain, 1945–1970

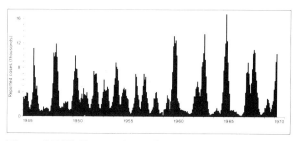

Figure 4.7 (C) Denmark, 1945–1970

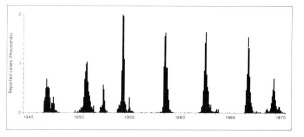

Figure 4.7 (D) Iceland, 1945–1970

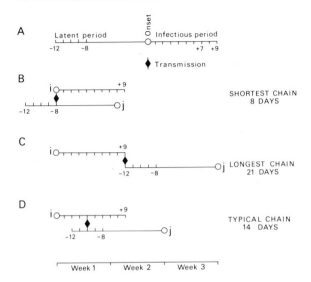

Figure 4.7 (E) Measles transmission chain

and *j* is latent for as short a time as possible. The longest chain (21 days) arises when *i* transmits on the last day of the infectious period and *j* is latent for as long as possible. The average chain length is about 14 days.

The chain mechanism described accounts for the continued existence of the measles virus under endemic conditions. For an epidemic to occur, we must assume that a host has access to a large number of susceptibles. Burnet and White (1972, pp.15–16) describe measles as

a typical childhood disease in which a single attack is followed by lifelong immunity ... [Of] all infections, its ecology is simplest to understand. A child becomes infected perhaps by someone from another city. From this child a number of five-, six-, or seven-year-olds are infected perhaps at school and a fairly rapid spread occurs to all exposed children not yet insusceptible by virtue of a previous attack. Almost every susceptible child exposed to contact ... will contract the disease. The epidemic will spread progressively through a city, twelve or fourteen days between successive crops of infectives. As each child passes through his infection he becomes immune and the virus finds greater and greater difficulty in spreading. Eventually measles disappears from the community.

With time, another crop of susceptible children is born and 'sooner or later, the measles virus re-enters the community and the cycle is repeated' (Burnet and White, 1972, p.16).

International variations and epidemiological behaviour

It is this basic process of (a) a build-up by births of individuals who have not been exposed to the disease, (b) the spread of infection by the chain-process described, (c) the exhaustion of the stock of susceptibles through contraction of measles and (d) the renewed build-up of the pool of susceptibles by births, which accounts for the repeating measles waves shown in all four countries of diagrams (A) – (D). As discussed later in section 6.5, the size and spacing of the epidemics depends upon the size of the community studied. In subcontinental areas with large populations, like the United States, enough births occur for the chains of infection never to be broken. Hence measles was endemic in the United States throughout the period considered, with peaks in every winter when susceptibles crowded into heated rooms at school and home. Conversely, in Iceland with a small total population and an island location, births failed to renew the susceptible pool rapidly enough for the chain transmission process to continue uninterrupted.

In the period considered, measles thus disappeared from the island between epidemics, and the susceptible pool then built up again in a measles-free environment to await reintroduction of the virus from the outside world.

While both the time-series plots and the virus-transmission mechanism described in this figure have been illustrated using measles epidemics, the same features are to be found in most infectious diseases spread by person-to-person transmission. Examples include whooping cough, German measles and influenza.

Sources and Further Reading

The time series in (A) are taken from A.D. Cliff, P. Haggett, J.K. Ord and G.R. Versey (1981), *Spatial Diffusion: an Historical Geography of Epidemics in an Island Community*, Cambridge: Cambridge University Press, Figure 3.1, p.38. See also A.D. Cliff and P. Haggett (1980), 'Geographical aspects of epidemic diffusion in closed communities', in *Statistical Applications in the Spatial Sciences*, edited by N. Wrigley, London: Pion, pp.5–44.

4.8 TIME-SERIES AND GEOGRAPHICAL SCALE

PERTUSSIS (ICD 033) is an acute infection of the respiratory tract caused by the coccobacillus *Haemophilus pertussis*. It is most contagious before the cough becomes severe and usually remains contagious for at least one month after the onset of the spasmodic attacks. The incubation period varies from 5–20 days. During the following 7–14 day *catarrhal stage* which follows, the disease may simulate the common cold. The cough usually gets progressively worse, especially at night. This *spasmodic stage* is marked by an increase in the severity, frequency and duration of cough attacks. When a spell terminates in a characteristic whoop, the diagnosis is certain. It is seldom heard, however, during the early weeks of the disease. Bronchopneumonia is the most frequent serious complication. Under adverse circumstances, 10 percent mortality can occur, mainly among infants. Pertussis vaccine has high protective value.

A very high proportion of geographically related medical data are available only for irregular territorial units (cf. Figure 1.4) and are likely to remain so for some decades to come. In this figure we therefore look at the implications of these irregular collecting areas for statistical analysis at different geographical scales. The problem is studied in the context of time-series methods but the results hold for the analysis of any area-based data.

Whooping cough and vaccination

A common feature of medical care in the developed nations in the post-war period has been the increasing use of vaccination to control the spread of infectious disease. One disease so treated is whooping cough. It is a particularly interesting disease to study from a time-series point of view. Public concern at the possible side effects of vaccination means that levels of vaccination often fall quite sharply between whooping cough epidemics, so that the number of vaccinations displays response cycles which wax and wane in close sympathy with the epidemic curve. In this figure, using annual data for Iceland for the period between 1951 and 1970, the relationship between the number of vaccinations performed and the number of reported cases of whooping cough, both per thousand population, is examined at three different geographical scales. The collecting areas studied are first, Iceland as a whole; second, the five standard regions of the country; and, finally, the smallest geographical units for which data are available, namely the country's 50 medical districts (cf. Figure 2.11).

Correlation at the national level

Diagram (A) plots against time for Iceland both the number of vaccinations performed and the reported number of cases of whooping cough. The time-series of vaccinations displays a marked upwards time-trend which reflects increased medical care. To prevent this time-trend confounding any analysis, the data for vaccinations have been detrended using the methods given in Figure 4.2, and then also plotted in diagram (A). Comparison of the detrended vaccination curve with that for cases of whooping cough shows that there is a positive association. Vaccination rates rise in epidemics and fall in the inter-epidemic periods. The degree of association between the two series may be measured using the correlation coefficient. This ranges between +1 (perfect positive association) and −1 (perfect inverse association); a value of 0 means that there is no relationship between the variables. A correlation coefficient of +0.60 exists between the case rate and the detrended vaccination data.

Correlation at the regional level

In diagram (B), the association between case rates and vaccinations is studied for the five standard regions of Iceland. The data have been plotted in a different way from those in diagram (A). The scattergrams forsake the natural time-ordering of the data and give the matching case rate/vaccination pairs for each of the twenty years in the time-series irrespective of their time position. When interpreting the graphs, we must remember that the vaccination data have been detrended, so that a value of 0 on the horizontal axis indicates a vaccination rate equal to the average rate prevailing around the years of the point in the time-series. Values less than zero represent below-average vaccination rates; values greater than zero correspond to above average rates. Regression trend-lines have been fitted and the values of the correlation coefficients between case and vaccination rates in each region are shown.

The scattergrams have several features of interest. The points for which case rates are zero (and which therefore sit on the *x*-axis of the scattergrams) represent the years between epidemics when whooping cough was largely absent from Iceland. Many of these points are grouped around the zero position on the *x*-axis, implying that rates of vaccinations were average in these years. If these points are discounted, then there is a tendency in all regions for rates of vaccinations to increase when case rates increase, a pattern which is reflected in the positive correlation coefficients and positive-gradient trend-lines. The relationship is most clearly seen in the South. It is also important to note that

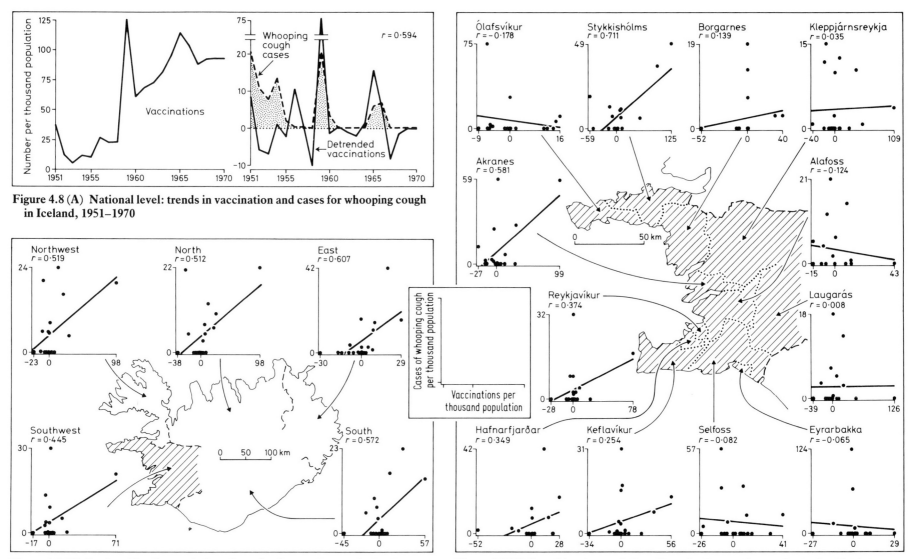

Figure 4.8 (A) National level: trends in vaccination and cases for whooping cough in Iceland, 1951–1970

Figure 4.8 (B) Regional level: correlation of vaccinations and cases for the five Icelandic regions

Figure 4.8 (C) Local level: correlation of vaccinations and cases for twelve districts within the Southwest region

only in the East does the regional correlation coefficient exceed that for Iceland as a whole given in diagram (A).

Correlation at the local level

Diagram (C) plots the scattergrams for each of the twelve medical districts which comprise the Southwest region. At this geographical scale, there is great variety in the relationship between case and vaccination rates. Some medical districts (for example, Hafnarfjarðar and Akranes) mirror the regional and national patterns while others (such as Selfoss and Laugarás) bear no resemblance. Again notice that in only two of the twelve medical districts does the correlation coefficient exceed the Southwest regional value plotted in diagram (B).

Linking results at different geographical scales

In each of the diagrams, (A), (B) and (C), the same time period has been considered. In addition the data for each of the regions has been obtained by adding together the data relating to its constituent medical districts, while the national series was generated by adding together the data for each of the five regions. In all instances, the additions were performed prior to scaling by population totals. Thus in diagrams (A) – (C) we have examined the same data at different geographical scales and we have witnessed the fact that the association between case and vaccination rates, as measured through the correlation coefficient, generally increases as the geographical scale becomes coarser. The dependence of the correlation coefficient upon the territorial base is well known to statisticians and it is just one example of the general yoking of statistical quantities to the size of the collecting areas. Many attempts have been made, without success, to solve the problem. But it is inherently unsolvable because collecting areas or territories are man made and therefore arbitrary rather than 'natural' units. The same comment applies to time-series. Days, weeks, months and quarters are equally arbitrary subdivisions of a year and the smaller units go to make up the larger.

We need to be aware of these problems if spurious associations are to be avoided. It is possible to get almost any value of association we choose just by juggling the boundaries of collecting areas. It is thus important to remember that detailed medical maps in which mortality indices have been most carefully standardized by age and sex still reflect their territorial bases in the patterns shown. For example, on the bronchitis mortality map of Figure 3.11, we need to be sure that some of the apparently 'unhealthy' areas owe nothing to the fragmented system of local government collecting districts. The dependence of statistical measures upon the data base makes inter-regional comparisons difficult and argues for the rapid and widespread adoption of Swedish and American practice in which data are collated for regular grid areas of agreed sizes so that the collecting unit effect is the same for all data. In the absence of such standardized data, we should try to develop models conditionally upon the structure of the data collecting units or restrict our comparisons to data gathered for the same- or similar-sized geographical units.

Sources and Further Reading

The data for whooping-cough cases and vaccination are taken from *Heilbrigdðisskýrslur* (Public Health in Iceland) 1951–70.

The technical problems of scale variation in statistical analysis are treated in A.D. Cliff and J.K. Ord (1981), *Spatial Processes: Models and Applications*, London: Pion, pp.118–40. See also S. Openshaw and P.J. Taylor (1981), 'The modifiable areal unit problem', in *Quantitative Geography*, edited by N. Wrigley and R.J. Bennett, London: Pion, pp.60–70.

4.9 DISCONTINUITIES IN TIME-SERIES: VACCINATION IMPACT

Measles has long been recognized as a potentially serious disease. Its ability to spread rapidly through susceptible populations, especially islands where the disease has been absent for many years, is well documented and is illustrated elsewhere in this Atlas (see Figures 5.4, 5.5 and section 6.5). Although the illness is typically mild, serious complications of the respiratory tract, the middle ear and central nervous system do occur and may result in death in malnourished populations. Thus in the developing countries, Walsh and Warren (1979) have estimated that 900,000 deaths occur annually as a result of measles infection (cf. Figure 2.5). In the United States, in the early years of the twentieth century, thousands of deaths were caused by measles each year (Hinman *et al.*, 1980) and, at mid-century, an annual average of more than half a million measles cases and nearly 500 deaths were reported in the decade from 1950–59.

It was against this background that the Centers for Disease Control, Atlanta, Georgia evolved in the United States a programme for the elimination of indigenous measles once a safe and effective vaccine was licensed for use in 1963. In this set of diagrams, the impact of this programme upon the time-series of reported measles cases in the United States from 1945–86 is examined.

The role of vaccination

As discussed later in section 6.5, it is estimated that a population of the order of 250,000–300,000 is required to maintain endemic measles. Work in Africa by McDonald in the early 1960s led him to suggest that one way of reducing the 'at risk' population in large countries below this endemicity threshold was by mass vaccination, so breaking the chains of measles infection illustrated in Figure 4.7(E). In the countries studied by McDonald, he argued that an annual mass vaccination campaign reaching at least 90 percent of the susceptible children would have the required effect. In 1966, Sencer *et al.* (reported in Sencer *et al.*, 1967) announced that the epidemiological basis existed for the eradication of measles from the United States using a programme with four tactical elements:

(a) routine immunization of infants at one year of age;
(b) immunization at school entry of children not previously immunized (catchup immunization);
(c) surveillance;
(d) epidemic control.

The immunization target aimed for was 90–95 percent of the childhood population. The high level of immunization needed to break infection chains has been confirmed by more recent theoretical calculations by Anderson and May (1982).

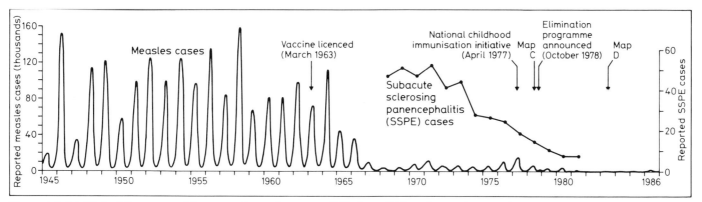

Figure 4.9 (A) United States monthly reported measles cases, 1945–June 1987, and annual cases of subacute sclerosing panencephalitis, (SSPE), 1968–1981

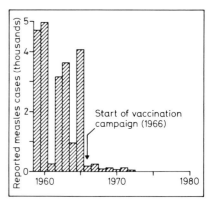

Figure 4.9 (B) Reported measles cases in the Hawaiian Islands, 1959–1981

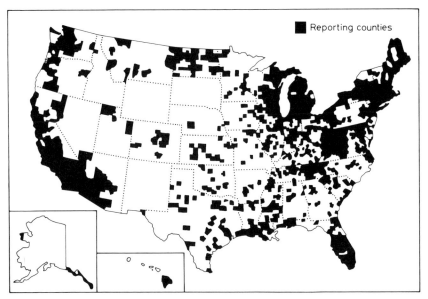

Figure 4.9 (C) US counties reporting measles, 1978

Figure 4.9 (D) US counties reporting measles, 1983

The United States time-series

Following the announcement of possible measles eradication, considerable effort was put into mass measles immunization programmes throughout the United States. Federal funds were appropriated and, over the three-year period from 1966 to 1968, an estimated 19.5 million doses of vaccine were administered. The discontinuity induced in the time-series of reported cases is shown for the United States as a whole in diagram (A) and, in diagram (B), for the Hawaiian Islands (the fiftieth state of the Union). In 1962, the year before measles vaccine was introduced, there were 481,530 cases of measles reported in the United States. By 1966 this number had been reduced by more than 50 percent to 204,136 and, by 1968, the reported incidence had plummeted to 22,231, less than 5 percent of the 1962 level.

In 1969, a vaccine against rubella (German measles) was licensed and all Federal funds were targeted against rubella; no Federal funds were allocated to the measles immunization programme from 1969–71. As a result, public sector vaccination declined. The susceptible population rose and, as diagrams (A) and (B) bear witness, the number of reported measles cases rose sharply, reaching 75,290 cases in 1971.

The Measles Elimination Program

By the mid-1970s, it was evident that the campaign against measles was running out of steam and that steady increases in incidence were occurring. To remedy this situation, a nation-wide childhood immunization initiative was launched in April 1977, followed by the announcement in October 1978 of a programme to eliminate indigenous measles from the United States by 1 October 1982. The immunization goal aimed for was again McDonald's 90 percent of the childhood population.

Geographical impact The impact of this second push against the disease is seen in the time-series (A) and (B). Geographically, the effects were equally dramatic. Maps (C) and (D) show the distribution of counties in the United States reporting measles cases at the start of the campaign (1978) and five years later in 1983. The contraction of infection from most of the settled parts of the United States in 1978 to restricted areas of the Pacific Northwest, California, Florida, the northeastern seaboard and parts of the Midwest is pronounced. The persistence of indigenous measles in many of these regions may be explained by the importation of cases from Mexico and Canada as mapped in Figure 3.3.

In 1983, twelve states and the District of Columbia reported no measles cases, and 26 states and the district of Columbia reported no indigenous cases. Four states (Indiana, 406; Illinois, 216; California, 181; Florida, 159) accounted for 64 percent of the 1,497 cases. Of the 3,139 counties only 168 (5 percent) reported any measles cases. In contrast, measles was reported from 195 counties in 1982 and from 988 in 1978 when the Measles Elimination Program began.

Unfortunately, total elimination still has not been achieved. Vaccination levels have fallen back and the continued importation of measles cases from overseas (Figure 3.3) has resulted in a resurgence of cases to 6,216 in 1986.

Subacute sclerosing panencephalitis (SSPE)

SUBACUTE SCLEROSING PANENCEPHALITIS (ICD 323.1; see Figure 2.1) is an important although infrequent complication of the measles infection. It is a slow-virus infection caused by the measles virus and is a degenerative neurological disorder characterized by the onset of mental deterioration and myoclonic seizures. It usually occurs late in childhood or in adolescence, approximately 7–10 years after acute measles illness. Although spontaneous improvement can occur, the vast majority of patients develop spacity, rigidity and continued intellectual deterioration which leads to death over a period which varies from months to years.

While there is some dispute as to whether the SSPE virus is classical measles virus or a variant, it is generally agreed that it is a complication of severe measles attack and that measles vaccine is protective against it. The epidemiological evidence for the United States is shown in diagram

(A) where the number of reported SSPE cases is plotted on an annual basis against the time-series of reported measles cases. The decline in the reported SSPE cases has paralleled the decline in measles occurrence. In addition, studies by Detels *et al.* (1973) and Halsey *et al.* (1978, 1980) show from case-control studies that SSPE patients are less likely to have received measles vaccine than controls, while cohort analysis indicates that, in the United States since 1966, there has been a progressive decrease in the incidence of SSPE in cohort groups born in succeeding years.

Prospects for measles eradication

The global prospects for measles eradication are discussed by Yekutiel (1980) and Fenner (1986). Comparison of the biological and sociopolitical features of measles and smallpox suggest factors that make global eradication of the former much more difficult than smallpox (see figure 6.2). Nevertheless, the United States experience shows that vigilant efforts to maintain high vaccination levels, strong surveillance and, as implied by the flows shown in Figure 3.3, an aggressive response against imported cases in measles-free zones can pin the disease back into diminishing areas of the world.

Sources and Further Reading

The sources of the measles time-series in (A) and maps (C) and (D) are data in the *Morbidity and Mortality Weekly Reports* published by the Centers for Disease Control, Atlanta. The SSPE data in (A) are from A.R. Hinman, W.A. Orenstein, A.B. Bloch, K.J. Bart, D.L. Eddins, R.W. Amler and C.D. Kirby (1982), 'Impact of measles in the United States', Paper to International Symposium on Measles Immunization, Washington, DC, March 1982, p.12. The Hawaiian data in (B) are given in A.D. Cliff and P. Haggett (1985), *The Spread of Measles in Fiji and the Pacific: Spatial Components in the Transmission of Epidemic Waves through Island Communities*, Publication HG18, Canberra: Australian National University, Research School of Pacific Studies, Department of Human Geography, Figure 16, p.77.

The measles eradication campaign in the United States is described in A.R. Hinman, A.D. Brandling-Bennett and P.I. Nieburg (1979), 'The opportunity and obligation to eliminate measles from the United States', *Journal of the American Medical Association*, 242, pp.1157–62 and in A.R. Hinman, A.D. Brandling-Bennett, R.H. Bernier, C.D. Kirby and D.L. Eddins (1980), 'Current features of measles in the United States: feasibility of measles elimination', *Epidemiologic Reviews*, 2, pp.153–70. The relationship to reduction in SSPE is referred to in R. Detels, J.A. Brody, J. McNew and A.H. Edgar (1973), 'Further epidemiological studies of subacute sclerosing panencephalitis', *Lancet*, 2, pp.11–14, and in N.A. Halsey, J.F. Modlin and J.T. Jabbour (1978), 'Subacute sclerosing panencephalitis (SSPE): an epidemiological review', in *Persistent Viruses*, edited by J.G. Stevens, G.J. Todoro and C.F. Fox, ICN–UCLA Symposia on Molecular and Cellular Biology, vol. 11, New York: Academic Press, pp.101–14. The possible link between measles and other neurological conditions is explored in J.D. Mayer (1981), 'Geographical clues about multiple sclerosis', *Annals of the Association of American Geographers*, 71, pp.28–39.

General epidemiological aspects of virus eradication in relation to population thresholds are discussed in D.J. Senser, H.B. Dull and A.D. Langmuir (1967), 'Epidemiological basis for the eradication of measles', Centers for Disease Control, *Public Health Report*, 82, pp.253–6, and in D.A. Griffiths (1973), 'The effects of measles vaccination on the incidence of measles in the community', *Journal of the Royal Statistical Society A*, 136, pp.441–9.

CHAPTER FIVE
SPACE–TIME METHODS

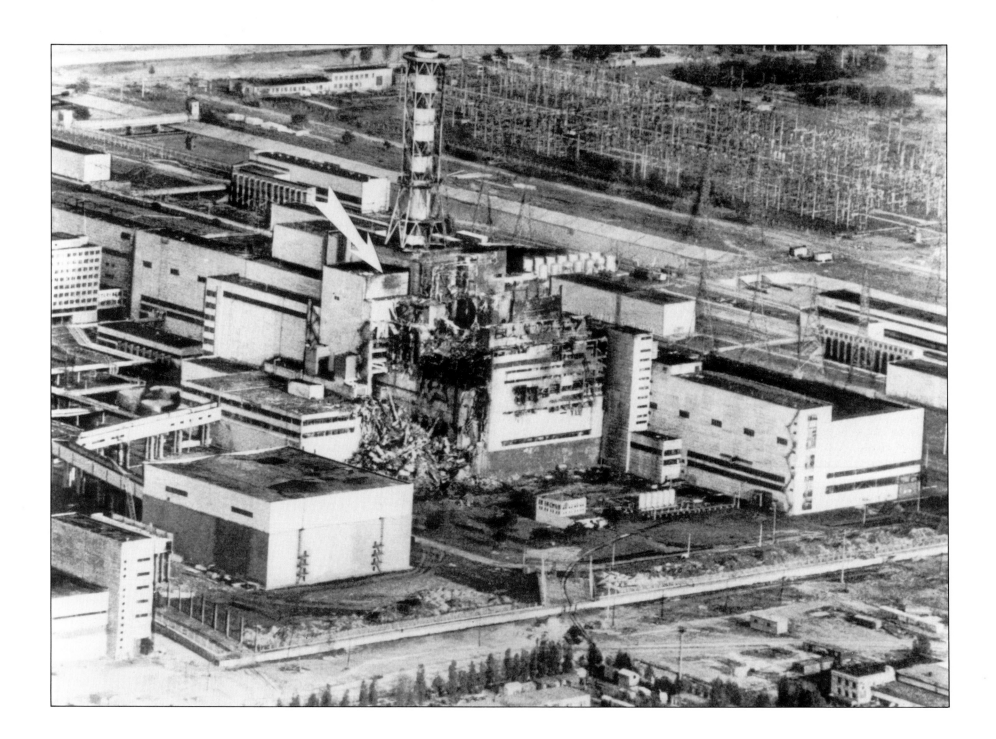

SPACE–TIME METHODS

INTRODUCTION

In Chapter 3, some methods were presented which enable the variability of disease over space to be examined. Recognition of the fact that the incidence of disease changes greatly from one region of the earth's surface to another raises naturally the complementary issue of whether similar variability exists in the time domain, and appropriate techniques for the analysis of single-region time-series were presented in Chapter 4.

However, the separation of space and time made in these two chapters produces but a partial understanding of the dynamics of disease processes. Regions do not operate as isolated units and the incidence of disease varies simultaneously in both the spatial and the temporal domains. Indeed, it is the interdependence of time and space which, as Gould (1970, p.444) has noted, 'allows us to substitute pattern, and therefore predictability and order, for chaos and apparent lack of independence – of things in time and space.'

The linking of time and space units is readily illustrated by the many infectious diseases such as influenza which arrive in one part of the globe from another and are then passed on after an interval of time to further areas, supporting the remark of the statistician, Stephan (1934), that 'data of geographic units are tied together like bunches of grapes, not separate like balls in an urn.' The analysis of the relationships in such linked space–time systems is the theme of this chapter.

5.1 SPACE–TIME FRAMEWORKS AND CHOLERA EPIDEMICS

The examples of cholera and the nineteenth-century public health movements

It is the transmissibility of many diseases between geographical regions, with varying time intervals between steps in the transmission chain, which glues time and space together. The key role played by transmission in this respect is shown in diagrams (A) and (B). These illustrate the diffusion of a mid-twentieth century cholera pandemic (for disease description see box in Figure 1.1).

The examples of cholera spread discussed in Chapter 1 were all based upon the geography of classical Asiatic cholera (*Vibrio cholerae*) in the nineteenth century. In 1905, a different cholera strain, *cholera El Tor*, was identified for the first time in the bodies of six Muslim pilgrims at the El Tor quarantine station outside Mecca. By the 1930s the new strain had become endemic in the Celebes; these islands have a largely Muslim population. Map (A) shows, at a continental scale, the subsequent spread of *cholera El Tor* from its initial main focus in the Celebes across Eurasia. Vectors are used to plot the general directions of movement, and the position of the disease front at different dates is also marked.

Up to 1960 spread had remained localized in southeast Asia. Most of India became involved [map (B)], again largely through the role of Muslim pilgrim movements. In 1961, however, the disease burgeoned. It began to diffuse out with devastating speed from the Celebes and India where it had replaced the classical cholera strain which had been endemic in the Ganges delta for centuries (see the last map in Figure

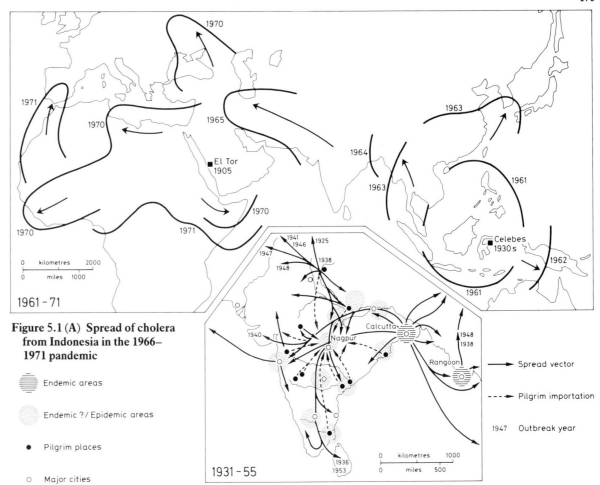

Figure 5.1 (A) Spread of cholera from Indonesia in the 1966–1971 pandemic

≡ Endemic areas

∴ Endemic ?/ Epidemic areas

● Pilgrim places

○ Major cities

Figure 5.1 (B) Main foci and spread lines for cholera epidemics within the Indian subcontinent, 1931–1955

1.1). By the early 1970s, it was pushing south into central Africa and west into Russia and Europe. Again, the great transport arteries familiar from the nineteenth-century waves seem to have been followed [cf. Figure 1.1 (D)]. It reached southern Spain in 1971 before finally receding.

The impact of one geographical area upon another after a time interval is also recognizable in the early attempts of many countries to restrict the effect of infectious diseases by both external and internal quarantine. The historical record suggests that, at least as far back as the Black Death, the inhabitants of one geographical area have seen the approach of disease from another as a wave about to engulf their own population. By the late nineteenth-century, the fears produced strong pressures in the industrialized countries for some kind of early-warning system for the approach of disease waves. For example, in 1888, Dr J. Tatham argued for a compulsory notification system for infectious diseases so that 'the sanitary authorities of one notification town may be warned in time of the approach of any infectious disease from other towns' (Benjamin, 1968, p.142).

Chapter organization

Thus a full understanding of disease-generating processes can only be obtained if time and space are considered simultaneously so that the complex interactions between regions and time-periods can be disentangled. As shown in Figure 3.1, earlier, we must be able to handle a three-dimensional data matrix. The methods required are sometimes complex and they form the subject matter of this chapter. Together they provide a powerful suite of techniques to characterize the main features of disease spread in the space–time matrix. As elsewhere in this book, most of the examples use human disease as illustrations but some departures from this trend are made. Hence we examine space–time patterns in two animal diseases which have important implications for man, namely rabies and fowlpest. We also trace the spread of the radiation cloud following the Chernobyl nuclear power station disaster to provide a further illustration of a new category of hazards to human health (cf. Figures 3.8 and 3.9).

We begin our study of space–time methods by examining time sequences of maps as the simplest way of adding a dynamic component to spatial cross-sections. We then consider the use of vectors to show the corridors of spread in space–time matrices. Where the landscape through which a disease is passing is approximately isotropic, wave-like motion is commonly observed. Examples of such disease waves are provided using epidemic data on the incidence of fowlpest and rabies.

If disease is transmitted from area to area, early warning is most easily obtained when the geographical units which are affected first can be identified and the velocity of spread from these units determined. Procedures for identifying both these leading units and speed of spread are given.

Although wave-like movement of disease is frequently observed in the space–time matrix, the presence of settlements of different sizes in a landscape often breaks up the flow into a series of spatially uneven components. Hence we also consider methods for assessing the impact of non-isotropic landscapes upon disease spread and velocity.

The chapter is concluded by a consideration of procedures for assessing the relative behaviour of temporal and spatial units. This permits the identification of those time periods and geographical areas in the space–time matrix which have suffered the impact of disease relatively more severely than other periods and areas.

Sources and Further Reading

The characteristics of cholera and its literature were surveyed in the opening chapter (see Figure 1.1). The global maps shown here have been taken from World Health Organization reports.

A detailed study of the spread of cholera in Africa is given in R.F. Stock (1976), *Cholera in Africa: Diffusion of the Disease 1970–75 with Particular Emphasis on West Africa*, African Environment Special Report No. 3, London: International African Institute.

5.2 MAPS SEQUENCED BY TIME I: MEASLES IN SOUTHWEST ENGLAND

The simplest way of breaking into the space–time data matrix shown in Figure 3.1 is by taking a series of cross-sectional slices through it. Each geographical slice may first be interpreted separately, and then viewed in relation to preceding and succeeding maps by regarding the space slices like a set of dinner plates stacked on top of each other to create the time-domain. The comparison in the time-domain is visual and is obtained by scanning the sequence like a movie.

Measles in southwest England

An example of such a set of maps sequenced by time is provided in this figure where we examine the pattern of measles incidence in southwest England for a four-week period spanning the year end and New Year, 1969–70. The maps have been taken from a 60-week sequence covering a major measles epidemic which affected southwest England between September 1969 and October 1970. A description of measles as a disease is provided in the box accompanying Figure 3.3.

Southwest England comprises the six counties of Cornwall, Devon, Dorset, Gloucester, Somerset and Wiltshire. It covers an area of some 9,000 square miles, slightly more than the state of Massachusetts. In 1970 the estimated civil population was 3.7 millions. For statistical purposes, the region is divided by central government into General Register Office (GRO) areas. The epidemiological data published regularly in the Registrar General's *Weekly Return* are col-

lected for this spatial framework of GRO areas, of which there were 179 in southwest England in 1970. The data recorded by the Registrar General include notifications of certain infectious diseases as supplied by the medical officer of health for each GRO area for the week (ending on a Friday). These returns are built up from the figures supplied by individual practitioners. Apart from variations in diagnosis, the level of reporting by different medical practitioners is not known, but multipliers of the order of two

may needed in the case of measles to increase the notifications actually recorded to the probable incidence level of the disease.

The choice of measles from the group of infectious diseases for which data are available for southwest England was determined by a number of factors. First, the high rate of incidence yielded a large number of notifications (over 250 a week during the sixty-week period between September 1969 and October 1970). Second, the transmission of the disease from

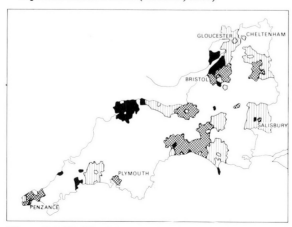

Figure 5.2 (A) Areas of southwest England with reported measles cases (week 52, 1969)

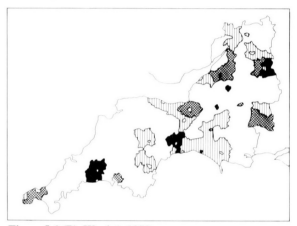

Figure 5.2 (B) Week 1, 1970

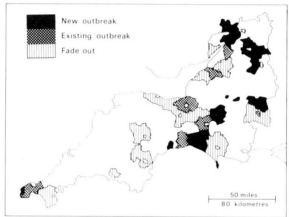

Figure 5.2 (C) Week 2, 1970

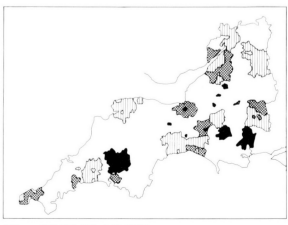

Figure 5.2 (D) Week 3, 1970

person-to-person without the presence of an intermediate host allowed demographic data to be combined directly into the analysis. Third, the highly contagious nature of the disease suggested that distance decay factors would operate strongly in guiding the spatial pattern of outbreaks. This point is reinforced by the prevalence of the disease among children, one of the most spatially-immobile age-groups in the population. Finally, measles has played a central role in the development of epidemiological theory (cf. section 6.5 and Figure 7.4).

For the southwest, 16,496 cases of measles were notified over 10,740 space–time recording units (179 areas × 60 weeks), an average of 1.54 notifications per area per week. Mapping of each week's returns showed that measles notifications were strongly clustered in both time and space. Nearly three-quarters of the 10,740 space–time recording units made zero returns. Maps (A) – (D) show a sequence of four weekly returns in mid-winter. The areas with measles are coded in one of three categories namely: *new outbreaks*, *existing outbreaks*, and *fade out*.

As shown in Figure 4.7(E), the average time between successive crops of measles cases in an epidemic is about two weeks, so that a GRO area was classified as a new outbreak if (a) in the week in question it returned a count of one or more cases to the Registrar General for inclusion in the *Weekly Return* and (b) it had made zero returns for three or more consecutive weeks before that. A GRO area was classified as an existing outbreak if (a) in the week in question it returned a count of one or more measles cases and (b) it made a non-zero return in any of the immediately preceding three weeks. After the last week with cases was recorded in a GRO area, we assumed that there was a period of two consecutive weeks (the fade out) during which further measles infections could have occurred and still be part of the same outbreak.

Location of new outbreaks

The location of 'new' outbreaks is of special interest since we can assume that (a) such outbreaks represent the reinfection of temporarily free areas from source GROs (located either inside or outside the southwest) where the epidemic was being maintained and (b) that, *ceteris paribus*, the probability of contact is higher for GRO areas adjacent to existing outbreaks than it is for distant areas. Of the 492 new outbreaks which occurred in the southwest during the study period, 76 percent were located in GROs which were either physically contiguous to existing outbreaks or to GROs in the fade-out category. As the distance from existing outbreaks increased so the probability of new outbreaks decreased. A further 20 percent of new outbreaks occurred with only one intervening quiescent GRO between the new outbreak and an existing outbreak, and a further four percent with only two intervening quiescent GROs. No new outbreaks were recorded four or more GRO areas away from an existing outbreak.

Location of persistent outbreaks

A second question raised by the maps concerns the location of persistent outbreaks. What characterized areas with a persistent pattern of notifications? For the 179 individual GRO areas, only the two with the largest populations (Bristol and Plymouth, named in diagram (C)) showed an unbroken record of measles cases over the sixty weeks from September 1969 to October 1970; conversely, nine of the areas recorded no cases over the entire period. Between these two extremes stood a sequence of intermediate GROs with a highly variable pattern of notifications. Reasons for the gradual change in the shape of

epidemics from the continuous succession of peaks and troughs of large towns to the spasmodic outbreaks of small communities are considered in section 6.5. The maps in the present figure show that, in the smaller communities outside the main population centres named on diagram (C), the virus will die out and require reintroduction from outside before another outbreak can occur. Communities of intermediate size tend to maintain the epidemic for extended (though not continuous periods). Two examples of GRO areas with outbreaks continuing over the period mapped are Penzance and Salisbury.

Sources and Further Reading

The maps shown in (A) are from P. Haggett (1972), 'Contagious processes in a planar graph: an epidemiological application', in *Medical Geography: Techniques and Field Studies*, edited by N.D. McGlashan, London: Methuen, pp.307–24 (Figure 22.2, p.310).

The epidemiology of measles is discussed in Figures 3.3, 4.7 and in Section 6.5 of this Atlas. In addition to the references given there see P. Stocks and M. Karn (1928), 'A study of the epidemiology of measles', *Annals of Eugenics*, 3, pp.361–98.

5.3 MAPS SEQUENCED BY TIME II: CHERNOBYL RADIATION INCIDENT

The Chernobyl accident

A dynamic element can be added to any mapped distribution by examining a sequence of maps, ordered over time, in which each map shows the distribution of the phenomenon of interest at a particular point in the time-series. The ordered series will create a movie-like picture of the distribution as it changes with time. One recent application of the method can be constructed from the maps of the spread of radiation over Europe following the explosion at the Chernobyl nuclear power station in the USSR which took place just after 01.00 hours local time on Saturday 26 April 1986. A wide range of fission products emitting ionizing radiation was released following the accident, especially since the graphite core of the reactor caught fire generating a vast amount of heat. The public health

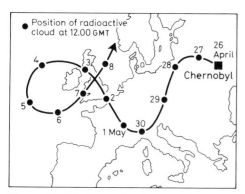

Figure 5.3 (A) General trajectory of Chernobyl radiation cloud, 26 April–8 May, 1986

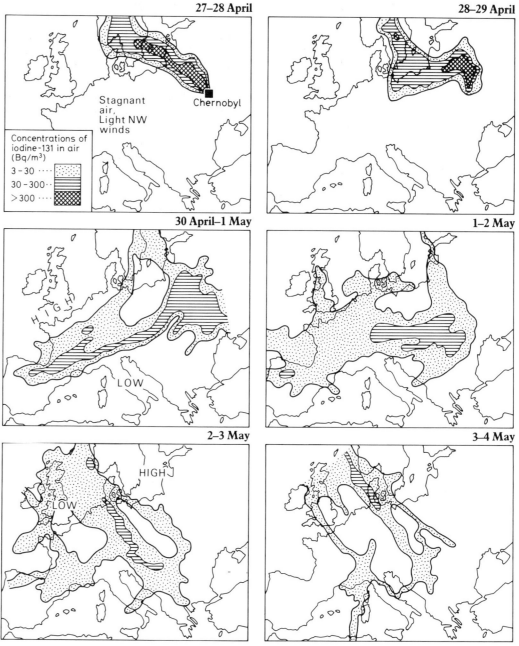

Figure 5.3 (B) Daily maps of the airborne concentration of iodine-131 radionuclide following the Chernobyl accident

[A more detailed account of this initial analysis may be found in ApSimon *et al.* (1987).]

hazards posed by ionizing radiation are classified in the ICD list under E926, **EXPOSURE TO RADIATION**; (see Figure 2.1). They are described in the box accompanying Figure 3.9.

One particular radionuclide whose airborne concentration was extensively measured to track the radiation cloud was iodine-131 (I-131) in becquerels per cubic metre of air. The measurements made across Europe have been collated by workers in the Air Pollution Group, Department of Mechanical Engineering, Imperial College of Science and Technology, London, and compared with a model of spread which enables a contoured surface of the concentration of I-131 to be produced. The following account is based primarily on their work. Diagram (A) gives the general trajectory followed by the radiation cloud between 26 April and 8 May, while the maps shown in diagram (B) are sequenced by time to illustrate the airborne concentration of I-131 in Bq/m^3 between 26 April and 4 May.

Spread of the Chernobyl cloud

The early part of the release spread up into Scandinavia on 27–28 April, passing close to the north-eastern corner of Poland as observed on the Sunday evening. On 29 April the release spread down southwards into Poland and East Germany, giving air concentrations over Poland of the order of 100 Bq/m^3 of I-131. This spreading persisted on 30 April, gradually clearing from Norway and Sweden. By 1 May the cloud was thrusting in a wedge across West Germany. At this point the cloud was almost splitting into two parts; one part blocked to the east by the anticyclone and one part which had flowed south of it. Air concentrations were higher in southern Germany than in the north which, like Denmark, had escaped the radioactivity, being protected by the anticyclone which also pushed the cloud away from northern Poland. The calculated arrival times of the southern section of cloud were a few hours ahead of observations and it subsequently overshot the observed area of exposure in Spain. There was a band of heavy rain giving high wet deposition over Bavaria, and stretching over Switzerland into southern France. There was also further rain over Sweden.

Between Thursday 1 May and Friday 2 May the cloud spread much more extensively, reaching up behind the anticyclone towards the UK. The later part of the release now led to contamination over southern Europe but there was little precipitation. By Friday 2 May to Saturday 3 May, material had largely cleared away from the source regions and Poland. Air now flowed northwards behind the anticyclone, with a band of more polluted air from Austria to the north coast of West Germany and much of Britain within the cloud. Rain led to some relatively high values of deposition in western Britain and then over Scotland on 3–4 May, although by this time the cloud was more dilute. Thereafter, the air circled round a depression just to the west of Britain and was drawn northwards from Europe, with frontal systems giving precipitation over the North Sea, Denmark and Norway. Until this time, Denmark had remained relatively free of the cloud. Trajectories and air concentrations in this second phase were difficult to estimate as material was carried aloft into the frontal systems.

The trajectory followed by the radiation cloud after 2 May is illustrated in diagram (A). It shows that, after that date, the cloud became caught up in the generally prevailing southwest to northeast flow of air over Britain to recross the country and head off again in the direction of Scandinavia.

Diagram (C) shows the relationship between ground level 'wet' deposition levels of radiation in becquerels per square metre and areas of heavy rainfall over Great Britain at 18.00 GMT

on 3 May. It is readily seen that many of the high radiation zones are closely associated with the areas of heavy rainfall. This was due to the washing action of the rain as it fell through the radiation cloud.

As the cloud moved across Europe and increased its geographical extent over the period shown in the map sequence, so levels of I-131 fell. It appears that fission products from the reactor were released at a fairly constant and high rate on days 1 and 2, but that levels decreased steadily after that as the Soviets brought the stricken reactor under control. This interpreta-

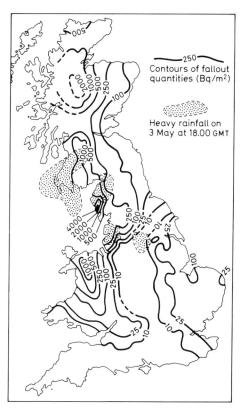

Figure 5.3 (C) Ground level deposition (recorded in grass) of radiation over Britain in relation to heavy rainfall

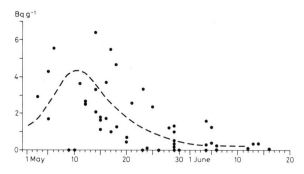

Figure 5.3 (D) Thyroid concentrations of iodine-131 against time

tion is reinforced by diagram (D). I-131 is concentrated in the thyroid and diagram (D) shows the I-131 activity in becquerels per gram as measured in 51 thyroid specimens in Italy during the period following the Chernobyl accident. There is an expected time lag between the accident on April 26 and peak thyroid concentration in the second week of May, but concentrations fell off exponentially after that.

Structure of the diffusion model

The maps shown in diagram (B) have been produced by a computer simulation model of geographical spread. The basic inputs to the model included:

(a) routinely collected data, such as wind speed, atmospheric pressure, rainfall and hours of sunshine, from weather stations in the international network; and

(b) gamma radiation measurements from stations throughout Europe.

To simulate the dispersal of the cloud, time was divided into three-hour blocks. The model then took levels of radioactive material estimated from surface measurements to have been present at the beginning of each three-hour block, and dispersed it over the map over the next three hours according to the pattern of surface atmospheric pressure. Rainfall measurements were included by smoothing out unevenly spaced measurements of precipitation over grid cells, each with an area of 10,000 square kilometres.

Sources and Further Reading

Map (A) is taken from F.B. Smith and M.J. Clark (1986), 'Radionuclide deposition from the Chernobyl cloud', *Nature*, 322, pp.690–1. The sequence of maps in (B) is from H. ApSimon and J. Wilson (1986), 'Tracking the cloud from Chernobyl', *New Scientist*, 17 July 1986, pp.42–5. A more detailed account of the initial analysis may be found in H.M. ApSimon, J.J.N. Wilson, S. Guirguis and P.A. Scott (1987), 'Assessment of the Chernobyl release in the immediate aftermath of the accident', *Nuclear Energy*, 26, pp.295–301. Map (C) is by D. Horrell of the Institute of Terrestrial Ecology, and is from the *Guardian*, 25 July 1986. The thyroid diagram (D) is from P. Orlando, G. Gallelli, F. Perdelli, S. de Flora and R. Malcontenti (1986), 'Alimentary restrictions and I-131 in human thyroids', *Nature*, 324, p.23.

The effects of radiation on health are described in E.J. Hall (1984), *Radiation and Life*, Oxford: Pergamon, and in the United Nations Scientific Committee on the Effects of Atomic Radiation (1982), *Ionizing Radiation: Sources and Biological Effects*, New York: United Nations.

5.4 VECTOR MAPS OF SPREAD I: GLOBAL LEVEL

Informal accounts of disease spread

Although much medical information is in the form of hard data and quantitative measurements, it is important to remember that a great deal of para-medical information about disease is available in a qualitative format through newspaper accounts and other ephemeral sources. For many of the epidemics of simple infectious diseases such as measles and influenza, these are an important source of information. In earlier decades, such accounts were often very detailed because the epidemics had a profound impact upon the economic and social lives of the areas they touched.

It is difficult to build precise space–time information from these data, but often the accounts are sufficiently informative that a general picture of the impact and spread of a disease can be reconstructed. With qualitative data, or for that matter unreliable quantitative data, it is misleading to add an air of precision by employing parametric methods for mapping and analysing the space–time patterns. It is much better to preserve the general feel of the source through use of cartographic techniques such as vector maps.

Introduction of measles into the Pacific islands

We illustrate the use of vector maps here by studying the spread of measles in the Pacific basin in the nineteenth century (see box accompanying Figure 3.3 for disease description). The account is based largely on the archival records of missionaries and colonial administrators, supplemented in the later part of the period by more formal medical records. Note that only recorded movements of the disease are plotted in Figure 5.4; there may have been other vectors for which records are not available.

The maps show the sequence of measles spread across the Pacific Basin. The patterns illustrated are not evident from the existing published literature but such evidence as is available suggests that the disease may have arrived in the Pacific somewhat later than other infectious viral diseases. For example, Samoa experienced its first influenza epidemic in 1830 (introduced by a missionary sailing ship), its first whooping cough epidemic in 1848 and its first mumps epidemic in 1850. Conversely, measles did not reach these islands until 1893.

The first world-wide survey of measles incidence was carried out by August Hirsch at the University of Berlin who concluded in his great *Handbook of Historical and Geographical Pathology* that the disease was, in all probability, widely diffused over Asia and Europe during the Middle Ages. At that time it was absent from the Americas and Australasia, while its position in Africa south of the Sahara is unclear.

The sequence of four maps employs vectors to show the generalized direction of measles spread in the Pacific Basin since 1800. The technique of vector mapping is straightforward. Dates of known occurrence are plotted and the likely corridors of movement between places are linked using vectors with the arrow heads denoting the direction of spread. The resulting maps differ from the flow maps in Figures 3.3 and 3.4 because no information about level of movement is provided.

Map (A) illustrates the most probable distribution of the disease around the rim of the Pacific Basin at the start of the nineteenth century. It was then endemic in the high-density population centres of south and east Asia, and was already established in eastern North America, central Mexico, Peru and central Chile.

Spread to Australia and Hawaii

The spread during the first half of the nineteenth century is shown in map (B). During this period, the 'virgin soil' state of many areas was broken down. As the vectors show, the attack came from two major directions. In the northern Pacific, the disease followed the westward movement of the colonists across North America. Measles was recorded in California in 1846 and two years later had started an epidemic in the Hawaiian islands. Still further north, measles was recorded in Alaska by 1848. The Californian and Alaskan routes are also closely related to the great gold rushes of the period on the Pacific seaboard of North America. In the southern Pacific, the main focus was on Australia. So far as newspaper records suggest, measles was unknown in Australia until the first outbreak in Sydney in 1828. Despite quarantine regulations, measles reappeared in Tasmania in 1842 and in Melbourne in 1850.

Map (C) shows the spread vectors during the critical decade from 1851 to 1860. The process of diffusion appears to have gone through two distinct phases. First, spread occurred from Victoria and New South Wales to the other Australian states; Queensland (1857), South Australia (1858) and West Australia (1860). In all three instances, the virus appears to have been carried by local shipping contacts, rather than directly introduced from Europe. The second phase saw the introduction of measles in 1854 into New Zealand, Tahiti and the Cook Islands.

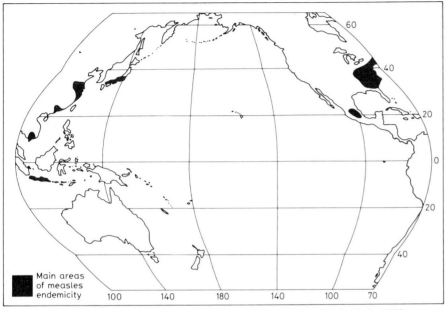

Figure 5.4 (A) Probable distribution of measles around the Pacific basin in 1800

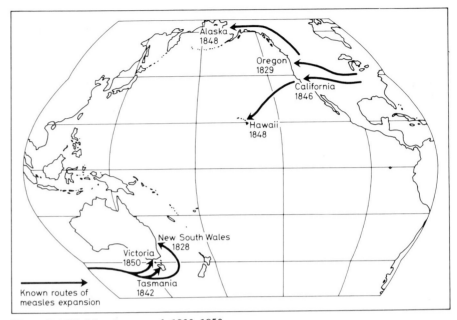

Figure 5.4 (B) Measles spread, 1800–1850

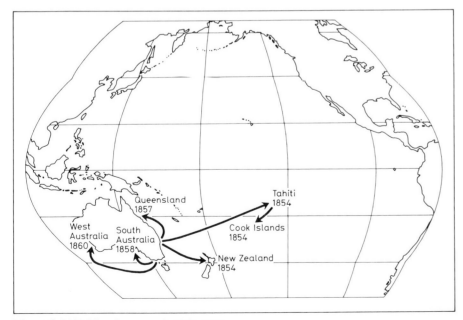

Figure 5.4 (C) Measles spread, 1851–1860

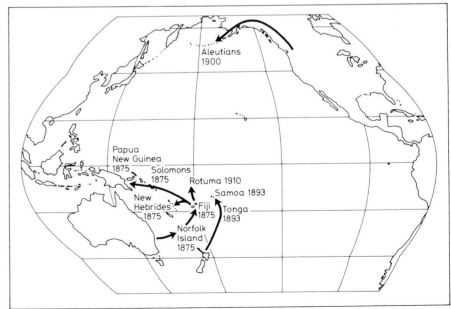

Figure 5.4 (D) Measles spread, 1861–1910

The impact on Fiji

The final map, (D), illustrates the closing stages of the invasion process from 1861 to 1910, by which date the present distribution of the virus in the Pacific had been largely established. The year 1875 was one of the most significant in the history of measles spread in the region since a major outbreak in Sydney was carried to a number of neighbouring islands in the southwest Pacific. The offending ship, HMS *Dido* [see photograph (E)], was returning the chief of Fiji and his royal party to Fiji via Norfolk Island after a state visit to New South Wales as the guests of the governor. A series of oversights, errors and a complete underestimate of the likely impact of measles in a virgin soil resulted in infection going ashore with the royal party. Devastation resulted. In Fiji, the number of deaths attributed to measles ranged from a lower limit of 28,000 to perhaps as many as 40,000 in a population of less than 150,000. The later spread, to Tonga and Samoa in 1893, to the Aleutians in 1900 and to Rotuma in 1910, all had much lower death rates of between 5 and 10 percent.

The maps show that the spread of measles into the island populations of the Pacific appears to have been a nineteenth-century phenomenon. In 1800, measles seems to have unknown in the basin; by 1900, it had visited most of the main island groups at least once. In this century, the increasing volume of contacts and the decreasing travel times have allowed the virus to be transmitted ever more readily (cf. Figure 7.2), particularly once the reservoir areas for measles had become established on the Pacific margins in the southwest (Australia and New Zealand) and in western North America.

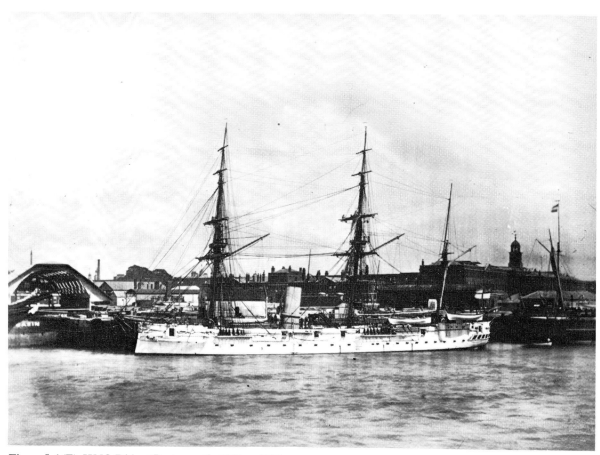

Figure 5.4 (E) HMS *Dido* at Portsmouth, 1871 or 1876

Sources and Further Reading

The map sequence (A) to (D) is taken from A.D. Cliff and P. Haggett (1985), *The Spread of Measles in Fiji and the Pacific: Spatial Components in the Transmission of Epidemic Waves through Island Communities*, Publication HG18, Canberra: Australian National University, Research School of Pacific Studies, Department of Human Geography, Figure 3, pp.22–3. The sources for these maps include A. Hirsch (1883), *Handbook of Geographical and Historical Pathology*, 3 volumes, translated from the second German edition by Charles Creighton, London: The New Sydenham Society,

together with original archives from missionary societies and local newspapers (such as Fiji's *Times* and *Argus*). The photograph of HMS *Dido* (E) is from the records of the National Maritime Museum, Greenwich.

For the spread of measles in the south Pacific see N. McArthur (1967), *Island Populations in the Pacific*, Canberra: Australian National University Press, and in the north Pacific, R.J. Wolfe (1982), 'Alaska's great sickness, 1900: an epidemic of measles and influenza in a virgin soil population', *Proceedings of the American Philosophical Society*, 126, pp.91–121.

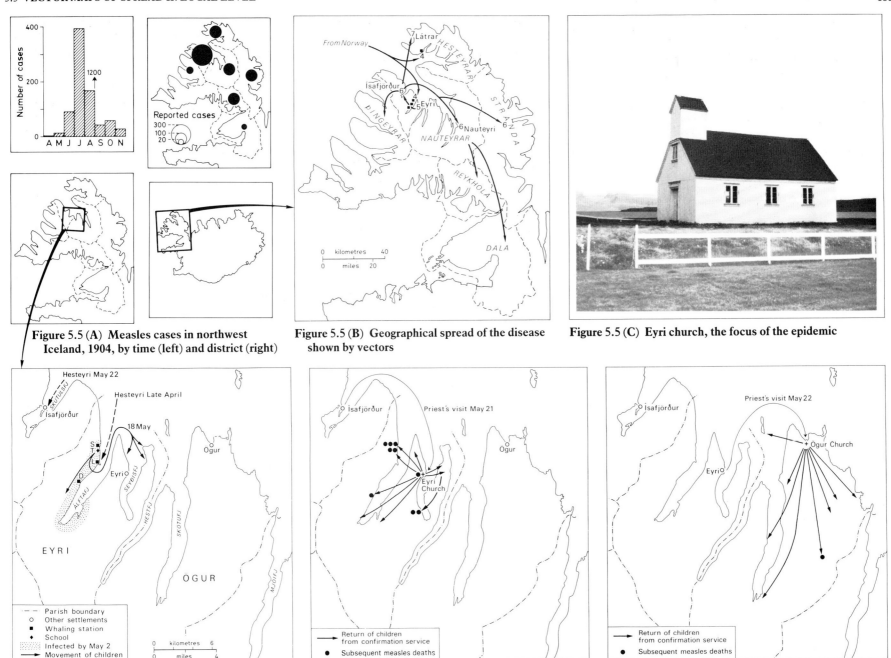

Figure 5.5 (A) Measles cases in northwest Iceland, 1904, by time (left) and district (right)

Figure 5.5 (B) Geographical spread of the disease shown by vectors

Figure 5.5 (C) Eyri church, the focus of the epidemic

Figure 5.5 (D) Introduction of the disease into Eyri parish, late April, 1904

Figure 5.5 (E) The spread from Eyri church after May 21, 1904

Figure 5.5 (F) The lack of spread from Ögur church after May 22, 1904

5.5 VECTOR MAPS OF SPREAD II: LOCAL LEVEL

Measles epidemic in northwest Iceland, 1904

Vector maps can be used to illustrate patterns of disease diffusion at a variety of different geographical scales. They are particularly useful when summarizing patterns reconstructed from documentary source material such as newspapers and church records [see diagram (G), later] where, as in Figure 5.4, much of the information is qualitative rather than quantitative. This set of six diagrams illustrates a case study in the historical reconstruction of the spatial and temporal links by which the infectious disease of measles spread through the local population in a remote corner of northwest Iceland in the summer of 1904 (see box in Figure 3.3 for disease description). The reconstruction has been made possible by the remarkable richness of the historical records for the events described. These include descriptive accounts in the form of doctors' reports and newspaper articles, as well as numerical evidence in the shape of morbidity and mortality data collected by both doctors and parish priests.

The general course of the epidemic in northwest Iceland, from its commencement in April 1904 until its demise in November of that year, is outlined in diagram (A), where location maps of the study area also appear. Some 2,000 cases of the disease were recorded in a population of less than 11,000, an attack rate of nearly 20 percent. As the graph of number of cases against month of reporting shows, more than two-thirds of the cases occurred in the months of July and August, when the three doctors in the region were overwhelmed and reported the epidemic as 'out of control'. The number of reported cases of measles by medical district is given using the method of proportional circles (cf. Figure 1.3). These indicate that the disease was focused upon the main town in the region, Ísafjörður. Of the 2000 cases of measles which occurred in the region as a whole, about 1500 were reported in Ísafjörður alone, where new cases occurred at the rate of some twenty a day for two months and involved half the population of the area.

The sequence of spread

Diagram (B) shows the geographical spread of the disease with a series of vectors, while the numbers by the arrowheads give the month of the year in which measles reached that particular location. The doctors' accounts relate how measles arrived in the northwest fjords of Iceland in late April when a Norwegian whaling ship visited the whaling station in Hesteyrar. It brought the disease from its home port of Haugesund near Bergen in Norway where an epidemic was in progress.

Despite attempts to contain the disease by quarantine, the crew members came into contact with the crew of a local shark-fishing vessel and both subsequently set sail for the town of Ísafjörður and the whaling stations near the local farm and church of Eyri, taking the disease with them. Quarantine succeeded in eliminating secondary cases in Ísafjörður but failed to quell the disease at the whaling stations near Eyri.

The role of Eyri church

A brief lull in events occurred until the 21 May when a Whitsuntide confirmation ceremony occurred at the church in Eyri illustrated in diagram (C). Most of the confirmed children were about fourteen years old. The church was packed with the families and friends of the confirmees. Many of the adults had been in contact with the crew members of the infected whaler and some of the crew members of the whaler itself were also present. The previous measles epidemic in the region occurred in 1882, so that many adults were susceptible as well as the children. As a result of this mixture of contacts, the epidemic was reinvigorated on the grand scale in the days that followed. The critical role of the church ceremony in this process is recognized in the following remark by the district's chief medical officer:

the spread of the disease was not out of hand until after Whitsun, 22 May; that day [sic] there was a service at Eyri, children were confirmed, and a large number of people were at the church. After that the disease spread very fast.

This sequence of events is illustrated on maps (D) and (E). As map (D) shows, in the early part of May, the general infection was restricted to the immediate vicinity of the whaling stations at Súðavík (S), Troð (T), Langeyri (L) and Dvergasteinn (D). By 18 May, and therefore immediately prior to the confirmation ceremony, the disease had spread from Álftafjörður into the neighbouring fjord of Seyðisfjörður in which the parish church of Eyri is located. The diffusion corridors are shown by vectors. After the confirmation ceremony, both the children and their families returned to their homes; one girl went back to Ísafjörður to go into domestic service, taking the disease with her to start the epidemic in the main town. The locations of the houses and the subsequent deaths among the local population which resulted from contact with the infected children are faithfully recorded by the Lutheran priest. They are plotted in (E).

Local parish comparisons

It so happened that on Whitsunday, 22 May 1904, the priest who had conducted the confirmation ceremony at Eyri moved on the neighbouring parish church at Ögur to hold a similar service. On that occasion no known measles cases were present. As can be seen from map (F), when the children returned to their homes from this ceremony (see vectors) only one subsequent measles death can be traced, as opposed to the nine that resulted from the Eyri ceremony on the preceding day. The contrast between the two churches underlines the fact that, at this local level, chance factors such as communal gatherings may play a critical role in 'supercharging' the rate of spread of disease. It is also worth noting that the initial infectives with measles were the crew of a whaling ship and therefore in a considerably older age group than would be associated with measles today.

Parish records

To illustrate the quality of the Lutheran church records as a data source for historical reconstructions of the sort undertaken here, photograph (G) shows a page from the register of deaths for Eyri parish in 1904. Entries 7–10 (white) refer to deaths from measles. A translation of these is provided. Other parts of the church records give on an annual basis births, marriages, confirmations, in and out migration, and a full census of each person, including occupation.

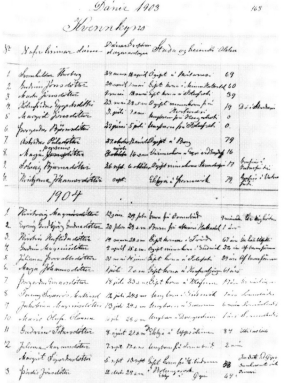

Figure 5.5 (G) Extract (above) and translation (below) from register of deaths, Eyri parish, 1904

Sources and Further Reading

The above account is based on A.D. Cliff, P. Haggett and R. Graham (1983), 'Reconstruction of diffusion processes at different geographical scales: the 1904 measles epidemic in northwest Iceland', *Journal of Historical Geography*, 9, pp.29–46. The contrast between this and Iceland's other measles epidemics is given in A.D. Cliff, P. Haggett, J.K. Ord and G.R. Versey (1981), *Spatial Diffusion: an Historical Geography of Epidemics in an Island Community*, Cambridge: Cambridge University Press, pp.55–91.

			Deaths (female)		
No.	Name of the deceased	Day of death	Day of burial	Standing and domicile	Age	
7	Þorgerður Einarsdóttir	18 July	23 same month	Married woman at Kleifar	19	of measles
8	Fanney Sigurrós Mattíasd.	12 July	24 same month	Infant at Súðavik	1	ditto
9	Jakobina Magnúsdóttir	13 July	24 same month	Infant at Saura	6 m.	ditto
10	Marie Ólafa Clausen	16 July	28 same month	Infant at Dvergasteinn	1	ditto

5.6 WAVES OF DISEASE SPREAD I: FOWLPEST IN ENGLAND AND WALES

Epidemics as waves

We have already seen earlier in this Atlas (Figures 4.1–4.3 and 4.7, for example) that virus-borne infectious diseases may occur as epidemics spaced regularly in time, separated by relatively quiet periods when few or no cases are reported. Thus, when the number of reported cases is plotted against time, the time-series appears as a wave-train, a feature which is characteristic of many of the diseases in ICD Group I (infectious and parasitic diseases). In this figure, we consider what happens to these waves as they move through time and space.

The diagrams given in (A) show how the shape of a disease wave may change when disease intensity (vertical axis) is plotted against time (horizontal axis). The waves illustrated differ in three important respects, namely:

(a) *amplitude*, as shown by the decreasing intensity from type 1 to type 3;

(b) *peakedness*, or degree of concentration of cases into the modal class. This also decreases from type 1 to type 3 so that the case load becomes more spread;

(c) *skewness*, or symmetry, which is strongly marked for type 1 but is progressively reduced so that type 3 conforms to a bell-shaped or Normal curve.

Much of our understanding of the relationships between such waves and epidemic processes is due to D.G. Kendall (1957) and we refer to the waves in (A) as Kendall waves. The association between the rate of infection, β, and the rate of recovery, μ, for any disease was shown by Kendall to be critical in determining which shape of wave will be observed at any time or in any place. Define $S_c = \mu/\beta$ and let S denote the total population at risk from the disease. The quantity, S_c, is known as the *relative recovery rate* and it defines a critical susceptible threshold population size whose magnitude compared with S determines the shape of the disease wave.

When S is substantially greater than S_c, a type 1

wave results. A high incidence of cases is recorded and, because there is a large S population, such waves peak sharply and early with most cases concentrated in the modal class. As a result, these waves have a marked positive skewness. Type 1 waves grow rapidly and move quickly through a population in their early stages. In contrast, type 3 waves are generated when the S population only slightly exceeds the threshold value, S_c. When an outbreak occurs in these circumstances, the low number of individuals at risk means that intensity is reduced, the wave is drawn out, and it both builds up and decays slowly. Type 2 waves occupy an intermediate position and are included to emphasize that the changing waveforms are examples from a continuum.

Kendall waves in time and space

The idea of systematic changes in the shape of a disease wave as it moves over both time and space is summarized in diagram (B), in which intensity is plotted against these two variables. The vertical shading illustrates the decreasing

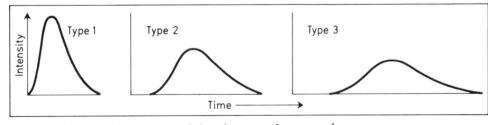

Figure 5.6 (A) Kendall's concept of changing wave shape over time

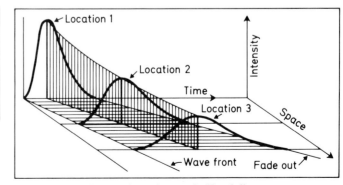

Figure 5.6 (B) Space–time changes in Kendall waves

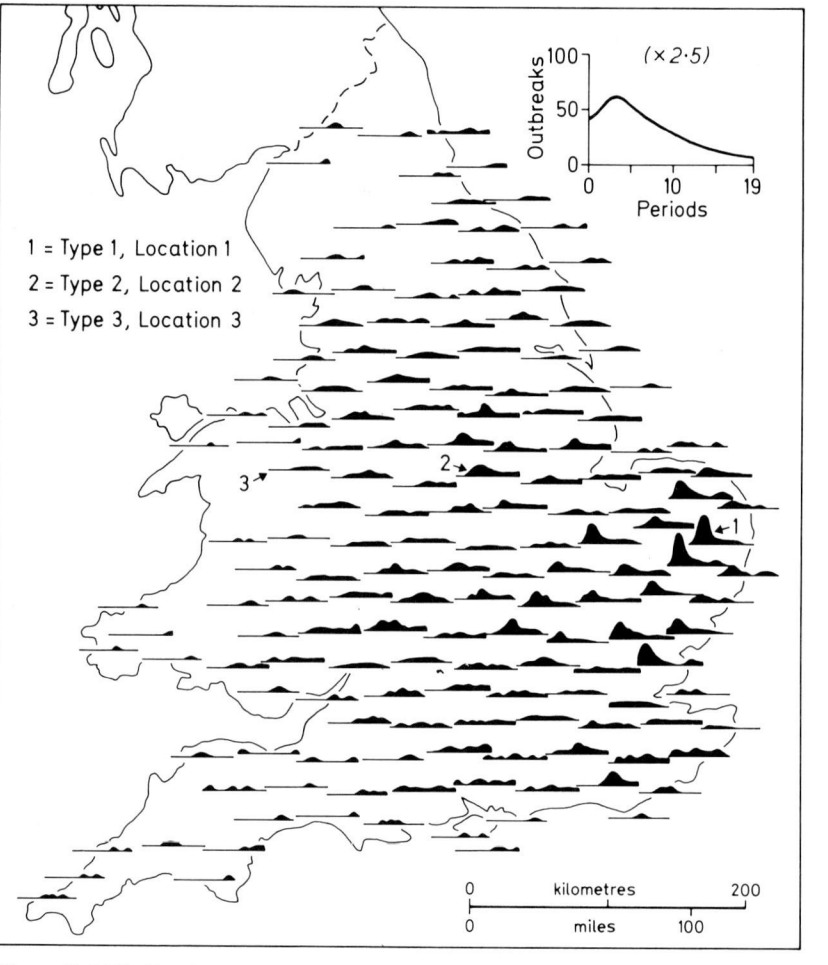

Figure 5.6 (C) Fowlpest epizootic of 1970–1971 in England and Wales

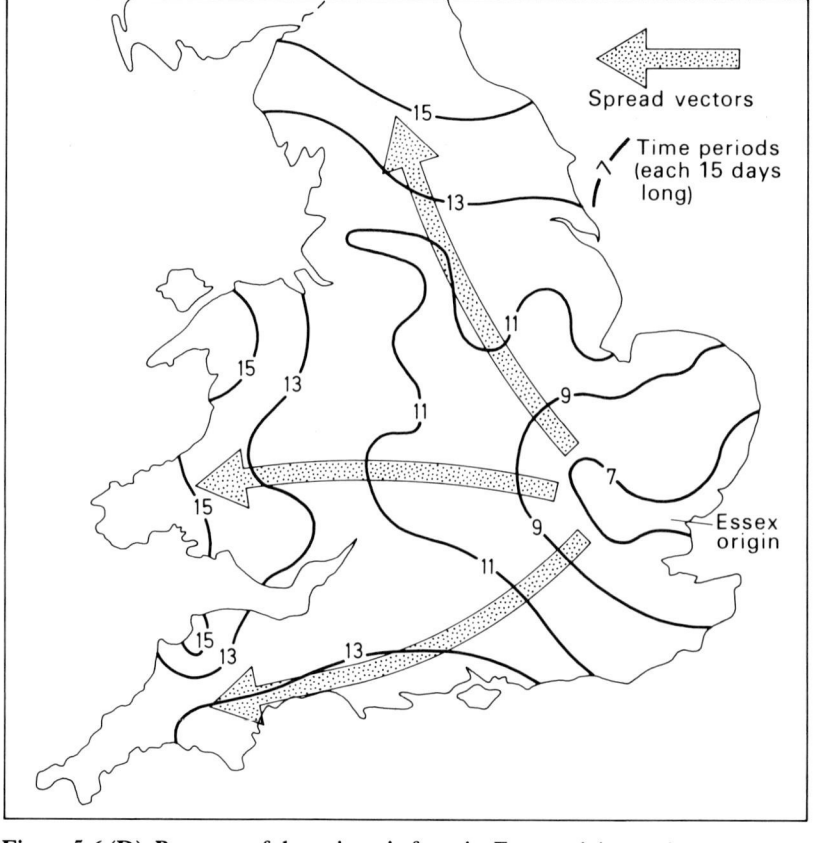

Figure 5.6 (D) Progress of the epizootic from its Essex origins to the rest of the country

height of the wave peak with distance from the centre of the outbreak, here taken as location 1. This diminution in wave height is exponential. The horizontal shading shows the steadily widening time interval between the passage of the wave front at a particular location, when the

first cases are recorded, and the last cases to occur (termed fade-out); that is, the wave fans out as it moves across space. The diagram implies that the energy of the wave is dissipated over time and space, ultimately to disappear.

If we relate diagram (B) back to diagram (A),

then we must assume that S/S_c is itself falling over space and time. This could occur in one of three ways: an increase in S_c, a reduction in S or both acting in combination. Increases in S_c could occur from either an increase in the recovery rate, μ, or from a decrease in the rate of infection, β. In practice, for a given disease, μ is likely to be roughly constant over time and we would have to look for temporally decreasing virulence or infectiousness of a disease to achieve the necessary threshold change by an increase in S_c. This is unlikely for many diseases.

It therefore seems preferable to account for the features shown in (B) by a reduction in S, rather than by an increase in S_c. This could stem from increasing knowledge of the epidemic over time, enabling S to be reduced by countermeasures such as isolation and vaccination. Such an explanation would, of course, only be applicable to human or domesticated animal populations.

The fowlpest epizootic in England and Wales

The causative virus of fowlpest or **NEWCASTLE DISEASE** (pneumoencephalitis) has a world-wide distribution in avian species. The disease is characterized first by respiratory and then nervous symptoms. Head twitching and lack of coordination may develop. Its main impact on man is economic when poultry flocks become infected and it is a major hazard in this respect. Egg production in affected birds drops markedly and seldom returns to normal, many eggs being deformed or soft-shelled. The incubation period is from three to ten days and the mortality rate is 90–95 percent.

Kendall's theoretical ideas are illustrated in maps (C) and (D), taken from Gilg (1973), where they are applied to the major fowlpest (Newcastle disease) epizootic which affected poultry populations in England and Wales in 1970–71. Fowlpest spreads very rapidly as an air-borne virus from one host to the next and from one geographical location to another. The disease is controllable by vaccination, but complacency since the last major epizootic in England and Wales, which occurred in 1964, had resulted in

protection levels falling to 53 percent. This is well below the 75 percent protection required to prevent major disease resurgence.

Both diagrams show the progress of the epizootic across England and Wales over a period from August 1970 to the end of May 1971. The disease was introduced into the Essex area in the late summer of 1970. From there it spread rapidly into East Anglia and thence in an irregular series of ripples across the rest of England and Wales. Time curves were plotted from Ministry of Agriculture data for some 6,500 recorded outbreaks. The data were aggregated onto a network of square grid cells of side 30 km for analysis. Map (C) gives, in their correct geographical locations, the time curves of the epizootic in the manner of diagrams (A) and (B), the number of outbreaks being plotted against nineteen fifteen-day periods. Fifteen days was chosen as a rough multiple of the average incubation period. The numbers 1, 2, and 3 on map (C) correspond directly with the theoretical curves illustrated in diagrams (A) and (B). Map (C) shows that the form of the wave changed with distance from the Essex hearth in roughly the manner hypothesized by the Kendall model. Thus the epizootic in East Anglia was in sharp decline some weeks before the first cases were reported in the north and west of the map, and the epizootic curves in the east were sharply peaked and skewed compared with those in the western and northern parts of the map. Isolated cases were reported in Scotland, with the furthest outbreak occurring in the Hebrides.

The main directions of spread of the epizootic are shown by vectors on map (D). The time contours give the mean date of passage of the wave. These are again in arbitrary fifteen-day periods, so that 7 is equivalent to early December 1970 and 15 to early April 1971. There is some evidence that the velocity of the epizootic slowed, at least temporarily, as it moved west-

wards; the spacing between the time-contours (9, 11 and 13) is greater than is the spacing up to 9 and after 13. Again this is in broad conformity with diagram (B) and almost certainly reflects the awareness of farmers in the west, increased vaccinations and Ministry restrictions on the movement of poultry.

Sources and Further Reading

Maps (C) and (D) are redrawn from A.W. Gilg (1973), 'A study in agricultural disease diffusion: the case of the 1970–71 fowl-pest epidemic', *Transactions of the Institute of British Geographers*, 59, pp.77–97. The change in waveforms is described in D.G. Kendall (1957), 'La propagation d'une épidémie ou d'un bruit dans une population limitée', *Publications of the Institute of Statistics, University of Paris*, 6, pp.307–31, and summarized in N.J.T. Bailey (1975), *The Mathematical Theory of Infectious Diseases and its Applications*, London: Griffin, pp.81–132. See also R.L. Morrill (1970), 'The shape of diffusion in space and time', *Economic Geography*, 46, pp.259–68.

5.7 WAVES OF DISEASE SPREAD II: RABIES IN EUROPE

RABIES (ICD 071; see Figure 2.1) is an acute illness which attacks the central nervous system. It is caused by a member of the rhabdoviruses, a group of bullet- or rod-shaped RNA viruses. All warm-blooded animals (mammal and bird) are susceptible, and the disease is spread to man when the saliva of the infected animal enters a wound or abrasion of the skin or mucous membrane. The incubation period is highly variable but averages 6–12 weeks. Death, which rapidly follows the onset of symptoms, is inevitable without treatment and is almost certain even with treatment. Although field trials are in progress with improved vaccines, these are only helpful if administration is rapidly effected following exposure to the virus.

Rabies in southern Germany

Many transmissible diseases of man and animals occur as a series of repeating waves in time and space. The basic properties of these waves have been outlined in the preceding figure and were shown to exist in a fowlpest epizootic among poultry populations in England and Wales in 1970–1. Our second example of wave spread focuses upon the rabies epizootic which has persisted and progressed steadily across Europe for some forty years.

The epizootic started on the German–Polish border and the wave front has moved westwards at an average speed of 30–60 kilometres per year so that today it has nearly reached the English Channel coast. The main carrier is the fox which came into contact with the remainder of the wildlife population. The progress of the epizoo-

tic has assumed critical significance because foxes are increasingly found in the suburbs of the cities of Europe, so that transmission from foxes to the urban dog population is likely. In addition, certain countries like Great Britain and Sweden are presently entirely free of the disease.

The fourteen block diagrams which comprise (A) show the spread of the epizootic across part of southern Germany on a four-monthly basis from May 1963 to December 1967. A map giving the location of the 133 × 133 km study area near Stuttgart in the German Federal Republic is provided in (B). The perspective block diagrams (cf. Figure 1.5) plot the number of reported cases of rabies on the vertical axis against their location on the base formed by a 32 × 32 cell lattice which was used to partition the study area. For each of approximately 3000 animal cases in which rabies was confirmed by laboratory tests, data were collected on species, date and location of occurrence. The evidence suggested that, although the wave front generally progressed from north to south across the study area, the axis of orientation was not constant, varying between south and southeast. As the wave front of the epidemic progressed, large-

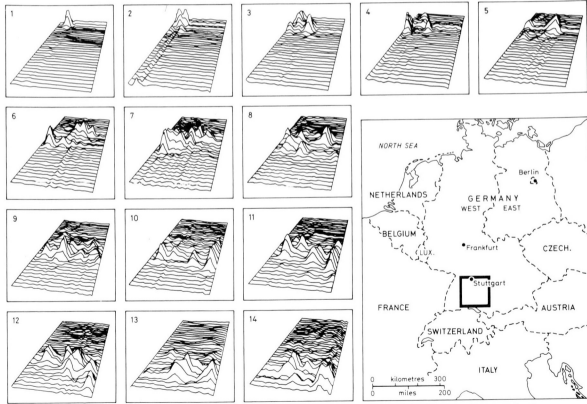

Figure 5.7 (A) North-south spread of rabies at 4-month intervals from May 1963 to December 1967 in southern Germany

Figure 5.7 (B) Location map for the area modelled in the map sequence in (A)

scale destruction of fox earths was carried out in each district until the disease disappeared. There was some evidence of separate foci for the epizootic and, after 1967, a second wave less intense than the first in some areas.

Models of rabies spread

Because of the central role of the fox in propagating the epizootic, fox ecology has been intensively studied. Detailed work by MacDonald at Oxford on the foraging range of foxes about their earths shows that the frequency distribution of distances travelled (the contact distribution) can be described by a negative exponential curve. The broad shape of such a curve is illustrated and discussed later in the first diagram of Figure 5.16(C). The shape implies that most journeys are within a short range of the earth and only a few are in excess of three miles. The theoretical properties of spread processes such as rabies epizootics, which have negative exponential contact distributions, have been investigated by Mollison who has shown that, when the negative exponential rule is obeyed, wave propagation across geographical space will be of relatively uniform velocity and the wave front will remain intact.

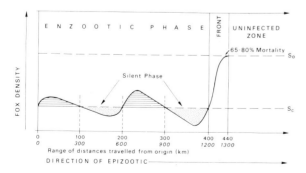

Figure 5.7 (C) Cross-section of rabies wavefronts

Developing these ideas and drawing upon the Kendall model described in Figure 5.6, Källen, Arcuri and Murray, also at Oxford, have modelled the geographical variation in rabid and non-rabid fox density as an epizootic passes [diagram (C)]. On this diagram, S_0 denotes fox population density in the absence of rabies and S_c denotes Kendall's critical susceptible population density (here for foxes) below which the epizootic will die out. The epidemic curve, as measured by rabid fox density, is shown by the heavy line. Rabies will spread (horizontally shaded areas) when the fox density lies above the threshold. The foxes will be killed off, their density will fall below the threshold and the epizootic will die out (the stippled silent phase). The fox population will then recover and the process will repeat itself, leading to recurrent waves in the enzootic area. As the frontier between the enzootic and uninfected zones is approached, fox densities will be high, leading to massive infection (Kendall type 1 waves in Figure 5.6). The authors give estimates of the speed of travel of the wave. They suggest that a wave will take between six and twelve years to travel 200–600 km so that, at a fixed location in the enzootic zone, waves of rabies cases will recur in the fox population every six to twelve years. If a cross-section in space is considered, fox density will have a 200–600 km harmonic [diagram (C)].

Forecasting rabies spread in Britain

Källen, Arcuri and Murray use their model to project the time taken for a rabies epizootic introduced into Great Britain in the vicinity of Southampton to reach different parts of the country [map (D)]. They assume that the geographical distribution of foxes is that given in MacDonald (1980). The map shows how wave

speed depends upon the susceptible fox density. Native fox density is lower in Wales, East Anglia and Scotland than elsewhere in Great Britain and it is evident that the first two stand out as relatively 'late' islands bypassed by the main wave front.

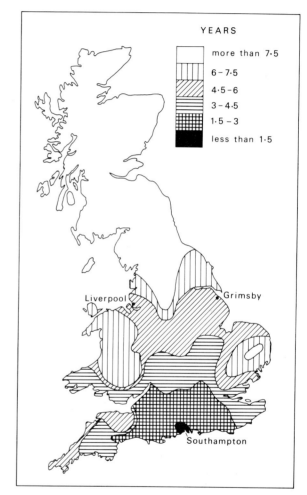

Figure 5.7 (D) Forecast map of rabies spread in Britain from hypothetical introduction at Southampton. [Subsequent models suggest a still faster rate of spread (Murray *et al.*, 1986).]

Sources and Further Reading

Map (A) is taken from B. A. McSayers, B.G. Mansourian, T.P. Tan and K. Bogel (1977), 'A pattern-analysis study of a wild-life rabies epizootic', *Medical Information*, 2, pp.11–34 and (C) and (D) from A. Källen, P. Arcuri and J.D. Murray (1985), 'A simple model for the spatial spread and control of rabies', *Journal of Theoretical Biology*, 116, pp.377–93. A subsequent, more accurate analysis and simulation can be found in J.D. Murray, E.A. Stanley and D.L. Brown (1986), 'On the spatial spread of rabies among foxes', *Proceedings of the Royal Society, London*, B229, pp.111–50. The mathematical issues in wave propagation are discussed in D. Mollison (1977), 'Spatial contact models for ecological and epidemic spread', *Journal of the Royal Statistical Society* B, 39, pp.283–326. See also F. Steck and A. Wandeler (1980), 'Epidemiology of fox rabies in Europe', *Epidemiologic Reviews*, 2, pp.71–96; D.W. MacDonald (1980), *Rabies and Wildlife: A Biologist's Perspective*, Oxford: Oxford University Press; and World Health Organization (1984), 'WHO Expert Committee on Rabies', *WHO Technical Report Series*, 709.

5.8   AVERAGE LAG MAPS

In every winter some of the common infectious diseases of man return in epidemic form to the nations of the northern latitudes. To a lesser extent, such seasonal upswings are experienced in the southern hemisphere as well (cf. Figures 4.5 and 4.6). When the onslaught of a particular disease begins in any country, a basic question which may be asked is 'how long will it be before the epidemic reaches a particular city or town?' The question is important because, in those communities for which a reasonable delay is expected, preventive action in the form of increased levels of vaccination, for example, may be taken.

Lags in measles onset

Given the recurrent nature of many epidemic diseases then, if a long enough time-series is available, it is possible to obtain an idea of which communities in a nation are generally attacked first in any epidemic, and of those which are relatively unaffected until a late stage. We call this delay the *average time-lag* to infection. Knowledge of this average or expected time to infection has implications not only for vaccination policies but, if the lag-time can be estimated for a set of places, it may provide valuable information about the way in which the disease wave moves from place to place. In this figure, we illustrate how the average lag-time to infection may be estimated by examining the recurrent

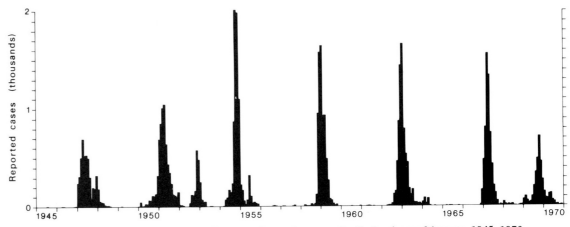

Figure 5.8 (A)   Monthly sequence of reported measles cases for Iceland over 26 years, 1945–1970

measles waves which affected Iceland between 1945 and 1970 (see box in Figure 3.3 for disease description).

The sequence of waves concerned is shown as a time-series in diagram (A). The period chosen forms part of a longer time-series covering the years since 1896 which is examined in section 6.5. As diagram (A) indicates, eight waves passed through the island between 1945 and 1970. Iceland has fifty medical districts and most were affected to some degree in each epidemic. It is from this set of eight waves that the average lag-time to infection of each of Iceland's medical districts has been calculated. The computational procedure is discussed in the technical appendix to this figure, but the results obtained are shown in the sequence of four maps comprising diagram (B). These give the average time in months from the start of all epidemics occurring between 1945 and 1970 before each medical district was reached.

Four categories have been used on the maps: less than 3 months, 3–5.9 months, 6–8.9 months, and 9 or more months. The circles are proportional to the population size of the districts in 1970. Solid circles indicate that a district was first reached in the period covered by the map; stippled circles are used to denote those districts shown as reached on an earlier map.

Sequence of spread in Iceland

The first map in (B) implies that the national capital, Reykjavík (population 73,382 in 1970), is generally the first district affected in each epidemic, on average within 1.5 months of the start. In the second time period, 3–5.9 months, two spatial processes are evident, namely (a) intensification of the epidemic in the districts immediately adjacent to Reykjavík; and (b) long distance spread to centres in the north and east. Akureyri (population 10,444) and Egilsstaðir (population 1,677) are the main shopping centres in the northern and eastern parts of the country. The third map covering the period, 6–8.9 months, sees the disease reaching almost all medical districts around the coast of Iceland.

The last medical districts to succumb are shown on the final map which covers the period, nine or more months. The districts concerned are concentrated in two areas of Iceland. In the remote northwest fjords, there are three districts with lags of 10.6, 11.0, and 16 months. In the eastern

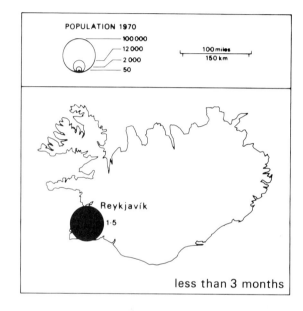

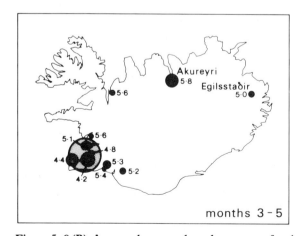

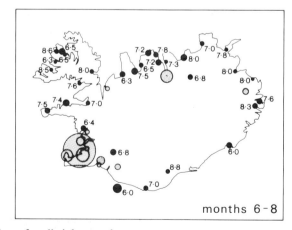

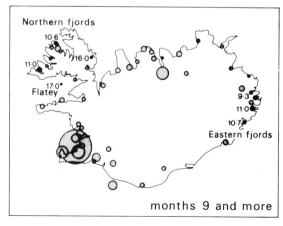

Figure 5. 8 (B) Average lag maps based on mean of arrival times for all eight measles waves

fjords there are three more districts with lags of 9.3, 10.7 and 11.0 months. The remotest medical district, the island of Flatey (population 182) off the west coast, is the last affected with an average lag of 17 months. Thus on average it is nearly 16 months after a measles epidemic commences in the capital, Reykjavík, before the same epidemic reaches Flatey.

Hierarchic effects

The patterns described support the idea of a spread model for measles epidemics which proceeds from large places to small (that is, down the urban size hierarchy), associated with contagious spread out from the initial centres of introduction into their hinterlands. The average population size of the communities on the second map of (B), which have an average lag-time to infection of 3–5.9 months, is 3,949; on the third map, where the average lag-time to infection is 6–8.9 months, the average population size is 1,399; on the fourth map, where the average lag-time is 9 or more months, the average population size is 874.

Size and distance effects

This interpretation is unfortunately complicated by the fact that the population size of settlements in Iceland generally decreases with distance from Reykjavík and from regional centres like Akureyri, Egilsstaðir and Ísafjörður (in the northwest fjords). In order to disentangle the size and distance effects stepwise regression analysis can be employed. As shown in the technical appendix, the average lag time to infection in a given medical district is expressed as a function of its population size and distance from Reykjavík.

The results of the analysis confirm that average time to infection increases as population size decreases and that it also increases as distance from Reykjavík increases. Thus, as implied by the map sequence in diagram (B), when medical districts become smaller and more remote, so they are reached later and later in the history of any epidemic. Population size also appears to be a more important determinant of time to infection than distance.

Sources and Further Reading

The analysis is discussed in detail in A.D. Cliff, P. Haggett, J.K. Ord and G.R. Versey (1981), *Spatial Diffusion: an Historical Geography of Epidemics in an Island Community*, Cambridge: Cambridge University Press, pp.95–6.

Technical appendix

For epidemic l, code the month in which the disease was first reported anywhere in Iceland as month 1, and for medical district i note the month in which the disease was first reported in the medical district as month 2, or 3, or 4, etc. Denote this month as t_{il}. The average lag time to infection over all epidemics in the i-th district, $\bar{t}_i$ is given by

$$\bar{t}_i = (1/n) \sum_{l=1}^{n} t_{il}, i = 1, 2, \ldots, 50, \quad (5.8.1)$$

where n is the number of epidemics. The $\{\bar{t}_i\}$ are plotted in (B).

If the regression model

$$\bar{t}_i = b_0 + b_1 P_i + b_2 d_i + e_i \quad (5.8.2)$$

is fitted using ordinary least squares in a stepwise regression then, at the second step, we obtain $\hat{b}_0 = 6.87$, $\hat{b}_1 = -6.56$, $\hat{b}_2 = 7.74$ and $R^2 = 0.26$. Here, P_i is the population (in thousands) of medical district i in 1970, and d_i is the distance (in tens of miles) of the principal town in the district from the capital Reykjavík. Despite the relatively low percentage of variance explained, the standard error for $\hat{b}_1$ is 2.36 and for $\hat{b}_2$ is 4.04, so that both coefficients are significant at the 95 percent significance level in a one-tailed test. Thus average time to infection is negatively related to population size and positively related to distance from Reykjavík. That is, as suggested by Figure 5.8, the smaller the place the longer the average time to infection; and the further away a place is from Reykjavík, the longer it will be before infection reaches it. The population variable was entered first in the stepwise procedure which suggests that population size is more important than distance from Reykjavík in determining time to infection.

5.9 VELOCITY MAPS

Spread within areas

When dealing with a transmissible disease, it is important to be able to determine the speed with which the disease spreads. Most geographically located medical data are collected for areal units such as countries, states, hospital areas and the like, rather than for point locations. In these circumstances, there will be two velocity components to be isolated, namely the speed with which the disease moves from area to area and, second, the speed with which the disease builds up within any geographical unit. The emphasis so far in this chapter has been upon measuring spread between areas. In this figure, we examine one way of determining rapidity of spread within an area. The methodology is illustrated by re-using the data mapped in Figure 1.3(A) which give the deaths from cholera in the registration districts of London in the cholera epidemic of 1849 (for disease description see box in section 1.1).

The speed of the London cholera epidemics

The method is summarized in the two graphs shown in (A) and (B). The registrars in each of the 34 registration districts returned data on levels of mortality from cholera on a weekly basis so that a time-series of deaths is available for each district. Instead of plotting the time-series as number of deaths (on the vertical axis) against time (on the horizontal axis), it is the *cumulative* number of deaths which is plotted against time in the two graphs. The left-hand graph (A) plots the cumulative number of deaths for the metropolis as a whole. The first cases were reported early in May and continued to trickle in until late June. The level of mortality then began to build up and, as the graph shows, rose steeply from the second week in July without respite until September 8. Thereafter the epidemic collapsed and only isolated cases were reported from the second half of September until finally ceasing in late November.

The cumulative epidemic curve has a very characteristic sigmoidal shape and the two turning points separate the growth process into three phases: (a) the slow build-up as the epidemic became established between 5 May and late June, (b) the main growth phase from July to early September occupying the segment of curve between the two turning points and finally, (c) the decay phase after 8 September. It is the relative duration of each of these phases which enables us to quantify the idea of speed of spread within any area. As graph (B) shows, the epidemic curve for rapidly moving waves will have a steep gradient between the turning points and the turning points will be well defined; slow-moving waves will grade more gently between the three stages and produce a curve with a flatter profile.

Logistic growth curves

We can therefore think of the average rate of growth or average gradient of the cumulative epidemic curve as providing one means of distinguishing areas with rapid disease spread from those in which spread is slow. Epidemic curves of the shape shown on the graphs may be readily approximated by the so-called *logistic* or *Pearl-Verhulst* distribution. Mathematical details are given in the technical appendix but, in the model, the average rate of growth or curve-gradient parameter may be identified and we denote its estimated value here by $\hat{b}$.

The logistic distribution was fitted to the time-series of deaths from cholera in each of the 34 London registration districts and the values of the parameter, $\hat{b}$ have been plotted as the four-category choropleth map (cf. Figure 1.6) shown. The areas of London served by the various metropolitan water companies are delimited by heavy lines.

Contrasts within London

The districts in the top two velocity categories are concentrated along the margins of the River Thames, and almost half are served by the Southwark and Vauxhall and Lambeth Companies. As discussed in Chapter 1, the growth of cholera in these districts may be readily related to the fact that these water companies drew their supplies from the Thames, into which the sewers containing the evacuations of the cholera patients were flushed. The situation was aggravated by the poor gradient of the sewers in the low-lying and flat areas adjacent to the Thames.

On the north side of the Thames, the area served by the East London Company also displays rapid growth. The valley of the River Lea formed the eastern border of the Company's service area, and these customers were also supplied with water drawn from the Lea within the tidal reach of the Thames. As shown in Figure 1.1(G), the Hampstead, West Middlesex and New River Companies, which served most of the area north of the Thames, drew their water from wells or surface reservoirs and so escaped the contaminated supplies piped to the populace of London south of the Thames.

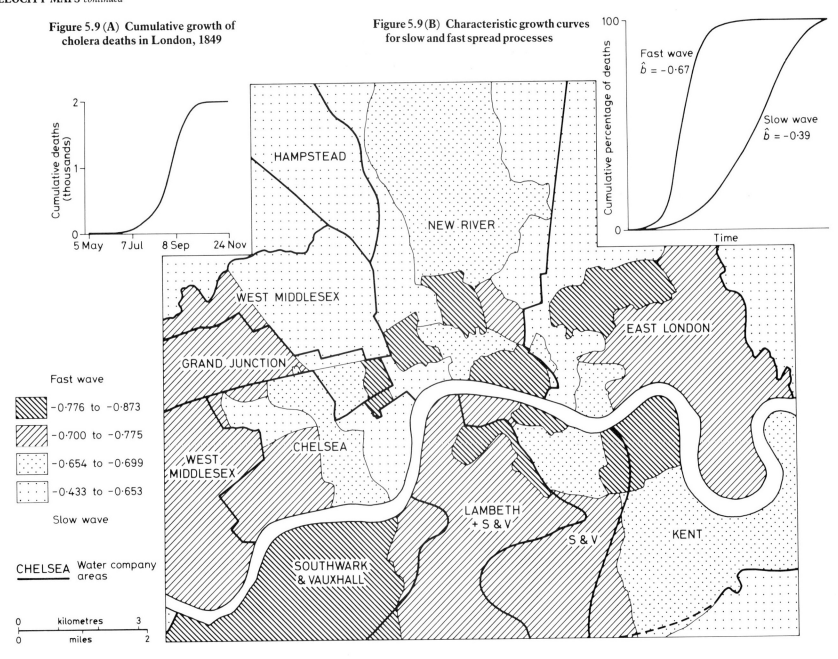

Figure 5.9 (A) Cumulative growth of cholera deaths in London, 1849

Figure 5.9 (B) Characteristic growth curves for slow and fast spread processes

Figure 5.9 (C) Velocity of cholera epidemic within each registration district, London, 1849

Sources and Further Reading

The sources of the London cholera maps are described in Figure 1.3 and the nature of cholera in Figure 1.1 of this Atlas.

The analysis here is based on methods discussed by R.M. May (1976), 'Models for single populations', in *Theoretical Ecology: Principles and Applications*, edited by R.M. May, Oxford: Basil Blackwell, pp.4–25.

Technical appendix

The logistic or Pearl-Verhulst curve has been widely used to model the growth of biological populations. Let N_t denote the cumulative number of individuals (deaths from cholera in the present context) at time t. Then the logistic curve is given by

$$N_t = K/[1 + \exp(a - bt)], \qquad (5.9.1)$$

where K, a and b are parameters. K denotes the maximum possible number (the saturation level) as t increases without limit, a determines the starting point of the curve at $t = 0$ in the sense that

$$N_0 = K/[1 + \exp(a)], \qquad (5.9.2)$$

and b is the slope coefficient which describes the average rate of growth of the process. It is the value of b which has been mapped in (C).

An alternative but equivalent form of equation (5.9.1) is

$$N_t = K/[1 + \exp(-b(t - t_{50}))], \qquad (5.9.3)$$

where t_{50} is the time at which $N_t = 0.5K$. Thus $a = bt_{50}$. When K is known, perhaps retrospectively when an epidemic is over, we may use the cumulative proportion, rather than the cumulative number, of individuals as the dependent variable; that is,

$$p_t = N_t/K. \qquad (5.9.4)$$

The structure of equation (5.9.1) becomes more apparent when we look at the first derivative, or rate of change, R_t, in p_t with respect to time. This yields

$$R_t = (dp_t/d_t) = bp_t(1 - p_t). \qquad (5.9.5)$$

Since p_t is the proportion of cases which have occurred by time t, $(1 - p_t)$ is the proportion still to come. The quantity, $2p_t(1 - p_t)$, then represents the probability that a random meeting of two individuals is between an infective and a susceptible, so that the parameter, $0.5b$, represents the rate at which meetings take place (or the rate of mixing).

There are a variety of ways in which the logistic curve may be converted into a regression equation for estimation purposes:

(a) K known or unknown; add an error term to equation (5.9.1) and fit the model by non-linear least squares. The estimation is iterative and the successive errors for the cumulative series will be strongly serially correlated so that ordinary least squares will be inefficient;

(b) K known; use the linear model

$$y_t = \ln[p_t/(1-p_t)] = -a + bt + e, \qquad (5.9.6)$$

where e is an error term;

(c) K known; from equation (5.9.5) consider the linear scheme

$$(p_{t+1} - p_t) = R_t = bp_t(1 - p_t) + e. \qquad (5.9.7)$$

When fitting the logistic model to case levels of a disease rather than to deaths, we may find that the curve grows too rapidly compared with reported case levels because the model does not allows for removals (by death or recovery) from the stock of infectives. We should then replace equation (5.9.5) with

$$(p_{t+1} - p_t) = b(1 - p_t)p_t^\star + e, \qquad (5.9.8)$$

where

$$p_t^\star = \sum_{\tau=1}^{t} (p_\tau - p_{\tau-1})g(\tau), \quad p_0 = 0, \qquad (5.9.9)$$

and $g(\tau)$ denotes the proportion of cases still infectious τ days after the onset of the disease.

5.10 CENTROID TRAJECTORIES

One way of summarizing the dynamics of a geographical spread process is to plot the trajectory followed by the centre of gravity of reported disease incidence as its location on the map changes from one time period to the next. The spatial mean is one of the simplest measures of the geographical centre of a distribution, and an application for a single time period has already been given in Figure 1.15. Locating the mean centre not only enables salient features of the spread process to be established but, by recording the distance travelled by the spatial mean between time periods, it also permits the velocity with which the disease is moving across the map to be determined.

Movements in spatial means

The equations required to calculate the spatial mean are given in the technical appendix to this figure. Their application is illustrated for a simple hypothetical example in (A). The values in the cells might represent the number of reported cases in a disease outbreak. In the bottom row of diagrams of (A), a solid circle is used to mark the centre of gravity of the cell values in each of the 2 × 2 lattices. Thus in time period 1 the geographical weight of the values is in the two left-hand cells and this is reflected in the location of the mean centre. By time period 4, the weight has shifted to the right-hand pair of cells. Time periods 2 and 3 represent intermediate positions. Diagram (B) illustrates, at a larger geographical scale, the left to right trajectory followed by the spatial mean over the four time periods.

An alternative to the spatial mean as a measure of the location of the centroid of a geographical distribution, and which has proved extremely useful in practice, has been proposed by Kuhn and Kuenne (1962). Under their approach, case levels of a disease are weighted by the distance they occur from all other locations with recorded cases. The three maps which appear in (C) apply the Kuhn–Kuenne technique to the spread of measles in the first, second and fifth of eight epidemics which affected Iceland between 1945 and 1970 (for disease description see box in Figure 3.3). The time-series of reported cases is

shown in Figure 5.8(A). The centre has been computed for the successive months of each epidemic and linked in sequence to capture the general direction of spread. Sample months have been picked out by solid circles. The numbers by some circles indicate the month in which the Kuhn–Kuenne centroid was at that location.

Icelandic epidemic trajectories

The map for Wave 1 (1 = November 1946, 19 = May 1948) plots the track followed by the

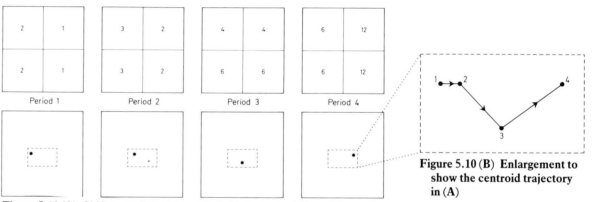

Figure 5.10 (B) Enlargement to show the centroid trajectory in (A)

Figure 5.10 (A) Shifts over four time periods in the centroid (spatial mean) of a mapped distribution

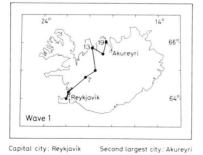
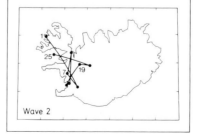
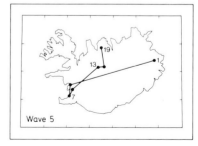

Figure 5.10 (C) Monthly shifts in the Kuhn-Kuenne centroid for four measles epidemics in Iceland

'typical' measles epidemic in Iceland in the twentieth century. It started in the Reykjavík region in month 1 (November 1946) and moved steadily northeast to finish in month 19 near the (then) second largest city in Iceland, Akureyri, located on the north coast. Wave 2 is very atypical with no clear spatial structure to it. The epidemic started, unusually, in the remote fjord region of northwest Iceland in month 1 (January 1950) before moving rapidly to the capital city, Reykjavík, in month 3. It then oscillated aimlessly in the western part of Iceland before finally involving the remote offshore island of Flatey in its decaying phase (month 25) early in 1952. The fifth wave incorporated some of the features of the first two. The epidemic started in eastern Iceland in month 1 (March 1958), well away from the capital city, Reykjavík, but soon spread to that city. It then resumed the conventional track picked out in Wave 1 and drifted steadily northeast to expire on the north coast near Akureyri.

Despite the differences between the three maps, they illustrate two repeating features of the geographical spread of measles epidemics in Iceland in this century, namely:

(a) the tendency of epidemics either to start in Reykjavík or to involve it at an early stage and

(b) the fact that most epidemics finally disappear from the island in the remoter medical districts of the north or northwest.

In interpreting the maps we should note that the location of each centroid describes an average location only. In the case of Iceland the population is distributed around the coast and therefore inland locations for the centroids do not correspond with actual settlements.

Sources and Further Reading

Centrographic methods were discussed in Figure 1.15 of this Atlas and the reader is referred to that section for further reading. The algorithm used here is that of H.W. Kuhn and R.E. Kuenne (1962), 'An efficient algorithm for the numerical solution of the generalized Weber problem in spatial economics', *Journal of Regional Science*, 4, pp.21–33, and the implications are discussed in detail in A.D. Cliff, P. Haggett, J.K. Ord and G.R. Versey (1981), *Spatial Diffusion: An Historical Geography of Epidemics in an Island Community*, Cambridge: Cambridge University Press, pp.96–9.

Technical appendix

Let the location of the jth geographical unit for which the incidence of some disease has been measured be given a horizontal cartesian coordinate u_j and a vertical cartesian coordinate v_j. Let the reported number of cases of the disease in j be denoted by I_j. The geographical mean centre of the reported number of cases in the set of $j = 1$, $2 \ldots n$ units is located at $\overline{U}, \overline{V}$ where

$$\overline{U} = \sum_{j=1}^{n} I_i u_j \bigg/ \sum_{j=1}^{n} I_j. \qquad (5.10.1)$$

and

$$\overline{V} = \sum_{j=1}^{n} I_i v_j \bigg/ \sum_{j=1}^{n} I_j. \qquad (5.10.2)$$

A more general measure of the geographical centre of a distribution has been proposed by Kuhn and Kuenne (1962); the mean centre is a special case of the Kuhn–Kuenne centroid. The Kuhn–Kuenne centroid is computed by choosing an initial starting position for the centre at the location $\hat{U}, \hat{V}$ and then employing an interactive search procedure based upon the repeated solution of the equations

$$\hat{U}_{k+1} = \sum_{j=1}^{n} I_j u_j d_{j(k)} \bigg/ \sum_{j=1}^{n} I_j d_{j(k)} \qquad (5.10.3)$$

and

$$\hat{V}_{k+1} = \sum_{j=1}^{n} I_j v_j d_{j(k)} \bigg/ \sum_{j=1}^{n} I_j d_{j(k)} \qquad (5.10.4)$$

until $\hat{U}_{(k+1)} - \hat{U}_{(k)}$ and $\hat{V}_{(k+1)} - \hat{V}_{(k)}$ are zero within some acceptable margin of error. In these equations, d_j is the distance between the latest centroid and the jth unit. The new centroid is denoted by the subscript $(k + 1)$.

5.11 STATISTICAL COMPARISON OF TIME-SERIES I: DATA DOMAIN METHODS

In most practical examples of space–time analysis, disease data will be available for a set of geographical areas over many time periods. We will then want to compare the time-series behaviour of different areas and, if we wish to understand how disease is transmitted from one geographical unit to another, to decide which areas either *lead*, or *lag* behind, others in experiencing the impact of, say, an epidemic. Understanding how regions mesh together is vital if the spread of disease is to be controlled. If we can identify any areas which tend to give early warning of the onset of disease in other areas, then medical care can be alerted to much greater effect.

Fiji and French Polynesia compared

The comparison of time-series for different geographical units can be achieved through natural extensions of the methods of autocorrelation and spectral analysis described in Figure 4.3. The methodology involved is outlined in this and the next figure by examining the monthly number of measles cases per thousand population, as reported to the World Health Organization, in two south Pacific island groups, Fiji and French Polynesia, between 1964 and 1981. A description of measles as a disease is given in the box accompanying Figure 3.3 while the locations of Fiji and French Polynesia are marked as 3 and 4 in Figure 7.2 later.

The time-series for each of these island groups

is shown in diagram (A). To reduce the impact of local variations in reporting practices, each series has been standardized by its own median and interquartile range as described in Figure 2.10. Over the 216-month study period, Fiji experienced a regular sequence of epidemics about every three or four years. *In toto*, 25,726 measles cases were reported at an average of 119.1 per month. French Polynesia displayed the same kind of epidemic regularity as Fiji at the beginning and the end of the period, but much more

erratic behaviour in the early 1970s; 13,412 measles cases were recorded at an average of 62.1 per month.

Autocorrelation and partial autocorrelation functions (ACFs and PACFs)

The internal characteristics of each series can be determined by computing their autocorrelation (ACF) and partial autocorrelation (PACF) func-

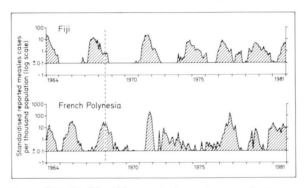

Figure 5.11 (A) Monthly reported measles cases for two Pacific countries, 1964–1981, on a standardized basis

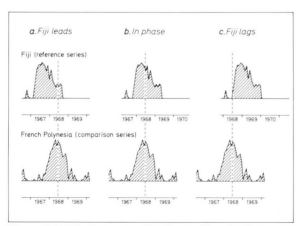

Figure 5.11 (C) Concepts of leading and lagging from a three-year section of the series in (A)

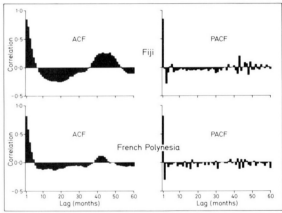

Figure 5.11 (B) Autocorrelation and partial autocorrelation functions (ACFs, PACFs) for the series in (A)

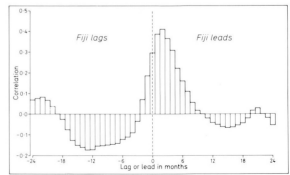

Figure 5.11 (D) Cross-correlation function (CCF) between the two series in (A)

tions. Recall from Figure 4.3 that the ACF is a plot of the degree of correlation (on the vertical axis) between all pairs of observations which are 1, 2, 3 . . . time periods (here months, on the horizontal axis) apart in the time-series. The greater the degree of association between all such pairs of observations, the bigger will be the correlation. The PACF is a similar plot which allows for the effect of any time-periods which intervene between observations which are a specified lag apart.

The ACFs and PACFs for both Fiji and French Polynesia are plotted in diagram (B). The ACF for Fiji falls off rapidly over lags 1–6, and this corresponds with the smooth build-up and fade-out of epidemics over time. The ACF becomes positive again between lags 36–53, with a flat peak between lags 41–47 which reflects the 3–4 year cycle of epidemics shown in diagram (A). The PACF plot reinforces these points. It displays high correlation at lag 1. This implies that reported case levels in adjacent months of the series are very similar. The maximum positive value of the PACF after lag 1 occurs at lag 43, suggesting a 3.5 year cycle of recurrent epidemics. The results for French Polynesia may be interpreted in the same way as those for Fiji. The evidence for cyclical recurrence is less striking because of the disappearance of the regular return interval for epidemics in the 1970s. Nevertheless, the ACF displays a smaller and slightly earlier cyclical peak than Fiji, this time between lags 41–43, which is indicative of the shorter recurrence interval in the 1960s.

Cross-correlation functions (CCFs)

To establish whether two time-series are moving together (in phase), or whether one series either leads or lags behind the other, *cross-correlation analysis* is used. Computational formulae are given in the technical appendix, but the principle involved is illustrated in diagram (C) which abstracts from diagram (A) the period from 1967–9 for Fiji (the reference series) and French Polynesia (the comparison series). If the epidemic peaks in the two series occur in the same month, the series are said to be *in phase*. However, if an event (the epidemic peak) occurs at time t in the reference series but at time $t - k$ in the comparison series, the event in the reference series is said to *lag* that in the comparison series; the extent of the lag is $-k$ $(k > 0)$ time periods. If an event occurs at time t in the reference series, but not until time $t + k$ in the comparison series, then the reference series is said to *lead* the comparison series by k $(k > 0)$ time periods. Obviously the definitions are relative; $-k$ equally implies that the comparison series leads the reference series by k time units, and $+k$ that the comparison series lags the reference series by k time units. In diagram (C), part (a) shows the actual relationship between the reference and comparison series, and it is evident that Fiji leads French Polynesia by a few months with respect to the single epidemic illustrated. Parts (b) and (c) are hypothetical and show the relative positions of the epidemics when the series are in phase (b) and when the reference series lags the comparison series (c).

Cross-correlation analysis proceeds by computing the correlation coefficient, r_k, between any pair of time-series to determine the value of k at which the maximum correlation occurs. This value of k is conventionally taken as the lead or lag of the reference series with respect to the comparison series. Diagram (D) plots the *cross-correlation function* (CCF) computed in this way between the entire series for Fiji and French Polynesia illustrated in diagram (A). The correlations reach a maximum at $1 \leq k \leq 3$, implying that measles epidemics in Fiji lead (occur before) those in French Polynesia by about 1–3 months.

Visual comparison of the two series plotted in (A) reveals that, for corresponding epidemics, those in Fiji do usually peak slightly before those in French Polynesia. The public health implications are obvious. If an island-to-island spread process had been operating, medical personnel on French Polynesia would have had some 1–3 months warning of the approach of an epidemic which, if vaccine is available, would enable preventive medicine to be practised.

Sources and Further Reading

The measles data used for the two series are taken from A.D. Cliff and P. Haggett (1985), *The Spread of Measles in Fiji and the Pacific: Spatial Components in the Transmission of Epidemic Waves through Island Communities*, Publication HG18, Canberra: Australian National University, Research School of Pacific Studies, Department of Human Geography.

Technical appendix

Let x_{it} denote the number of reported cases of some disease in time period t in region i and x_{jt} denote the corresponding value in region j. Then the cross-correlation at lag k, r_k, is given by

$$r_k = \text{corr}[x_{it}, x_{j,t+k}] =$$
$$\sum[(x_{it} - \bar{x}_i)(x_{j,t+k} - \bar{x}_j)/[\sum(x_i - \bar{x}_i)^2 \sum(x_j - \bar{x}_j)^2]^{1/2}$$
(5.11.1)

where $\bar{x}_i$ *and* $\bar{x}_j$ are the means of the series.

A basic assumption of the methods described is that the series are stationary in time. If trend or seasonal (as opposed to epidemic cycle) effects exist, these may confound the interpretation of the ACF, PACF and CCF. Trend and seasonality may be removed, as described in Figure 4.2. Since the series shown in diagram (A) appear to be free of trend, this has not been undertaken here. As discussed in Figure 4.6, seasonal effects on the Pacific islands are complex but, given the way the data have been standardized in this example, are swamped by the epidemic cycles and so have not been removed.

5.12 STATISTICAL COMPARISON OF TIME-SERIES II: FREQUENCY DOMAIN METHODS

Cross-spectral comparisons

As discussed in the preceding figure, when disease data are recorded for a set of geographical units over several time periods, then we may need to compare the time-series behaviour of the different areas. Two objectives are normally in mind when this is done. First, we wish to identify those units which *lead*, or experience the impact of a particular disease first, and those which *lag*, or are affected later. The set of units is regarded as an interacting system where events in one may produce a response in others. As we have already seen, cross-correlation analysis (Figure 5.11) provides one way of identifying leading and lagging areas.

A second objective is to identify similar components in pairs of time-series because, if we can do that, we may gain some insight into the common processes which are affecting the set of geographical units. Here, cross-spectral analysis is useful and the method is considered in this figure. The technique also permits the identification of leading and lagging areas.

To give consistency with Figure 5.11, the approach is illustrated by an application to the number of cases of measles per thousand population reported in each month between 1964 and 1981 in the Pacific island groups of Fiji and French Polynesia. A description of measles as a disease appears in the box accompanying Figure 3.3 while the locations of Fiji and French Polynesia are marked as 3 and 4 in Figure 7.2 later. The time-series are shown in diagram (A)

and the data have been standardized by their own median and interquartile ranges to reduce the impact upon the data of different reporting practices in each island group (cf. Figure 2.10).

Spectral analysis of the time-series for a single region has been sketched in Figure 4.3 and we now provide a more detailed explanation. The technique involves fitting to the data a set of cosine curves, each with its own distinctive *wavelength*, *amplitude* and offset between zero and the first peak of the curve (called the *phase-*

shift), and then calculating the percentage of the total variance in the data which is accounted for by each curve. The definitions of wavelength, amplitude and phase shift are illustrated in part (*a*) of diagram (B). The height, *y* of the curve at any point is given by the equation shown as a function of the three parameters. Part (*b*) of the diagram (B) demonstrates that a time-series with a quite complex shape can be decomposed into a sum of two simple cosine curves, and the principle can be extended.

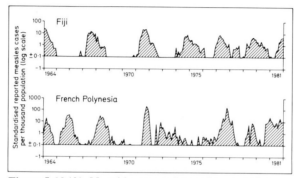

Figure 5.12 (A) Monthly reported measles cases for two Pacific countries, 1964–1981, on a standardized basis

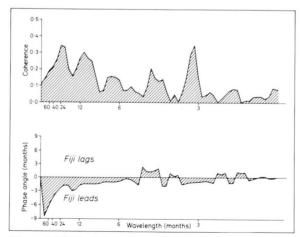

Figure 5.12 (C) Coherence and phase diagrams from the cross-spectrum between the series plotted in (A)

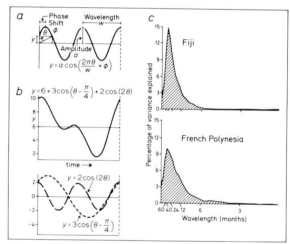

Figure 5.12 (B) (a) Concepts in spectral analysis; (b) cosine curve components; (c) spectral densities for Fiji and French Polynesia series

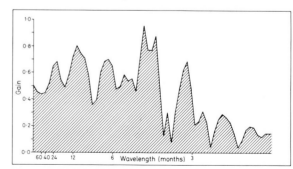

Figure 5.12 (D) Gain diagram from the cross-spectrum between the series plotted in (A)

The plot of variance explained (on the vertical axis) against wavelength (on the horizontal axis) is called the *spectral density*. The wavelength is expressed as the number of complete cycles of the given cosine curve per unit time. This is called the *cyclical frequency* and its reciprocal gives the wavelength or periodicity of the curve. The consequence of this definition of wavelength is that, on the spectral density plot, cosine curves with long wavelengths appear at the left-hand end of the horizontal axis, while the short wavelengths appear at the right-hand end.

The spectral densities of the time-series for Fiji and French Polynesia are plotted in part (*c*) of diagram (B). In the case of Fiji, peak explanation occurs with a wavelength of 40 months. This harmonic fits almost exactly the recurrence interval of the epidemics characteristic of the Fijian series in diagram (A). The spectral density for French Polynesia is less sharply peaked and, although reaching a maximum at a 40-month wavelength, a high proportion of the total variance in the time-series is explained by curves with a wavelengths between 30–39 months. Such waves have a period which mirrors closely the 2–4 year spacing between epidemics which, except for a few years in the early 1970s, is a feature of the Polynesian series.

Coherence, phase and gain

To determine the relationship between the time-series for any two areas using cross-spectral analysis, the *cross-spectrum* is calculated. This is a Fourier transformation of the cross-covariance function; the cross-covariance is the numerator of the cross-correlation defined in the appendix to Figure 5.11. Unlike the spectrum of a single series, the cross-spectrum is a complex function with real and imaginary parts; these are called the co-spectrum and the quadrature spectrum respectively.

Several functions derived from the cross-spectrum may be helpful in interpreting the cross-spectrum and we consider three here. One useful measure is the *coherence*. The coherence is the square of the correlation coefficient between the two series at a given wavelength. A plot of coherence (on the vertical axis) against frequency or period (on the horizontal axis) yields a coherence diagram. This gives the strength of the relationship (0 = no relation, 1 = perfect correlation) between the two series at corresponding frequencies. The coherence diagram is generally considered alongside the *phase spectrum*. The phase angle at a given frequency is defined as the difference between the phase shifts of the two series at that frequency. A phase diagram is a plot of the phase angle (on the vertical axis) against frequency or period on the horizontal axis. If the reference series (here Fiji) leads the comparison (French Polynesia) at a given frequency the phase angle will be negative because the phase shift of the reference series will be less than that of the comparison series. Finally, we will consider the *gain spectrum*. The gain at a given frequency is the regression coefficient of one series on the other at that frequency.

Results for the Pacific

Diagram (C) shows the coherence and phase diagrams computed from the cross-spectrum of the series for Fiji and French Polynesia. The gain is plotted in diagram (D). The greatest coherence occurs at a period of 24 months, but there is also strong association at the twelve and three-month harmonics of this fundamental periodicity. The phase diagram indicates that Fiji led French Polynesia at all wavelengths greater than five months, thus confirming the results of the cross-correlation analysis given in Figure 5.11. Gain, like coherence, also rises sharply at the 24-month period, as well as at the arithmetic harmonics of 24. Diagram (A) shows the recurrence interval of epidemics in the series for French Polynesia to be around two years in the 1960s, while that for Fiji is about four years; in the latter part of the period, both have an approximately two-year epidemic cycle. The coherence and gain diagrams reflect these features.

Thus, while cross-correlation analysis and cross-spectral analysis may both be used to explore the relationships between pairs of series, they provide slightly different information. The cross-correlations enable the leads and lags in any system to be established and we know from Figure 5.11 that epidemics in Fiji peak on average about two months before those in French Polynesia. Cross-spectral analysis, however, has enabled us to decide not only the lead-lag relationship but also that there is a 2–4 year harmonic affecting both series simultaneously; the two series are most closely associated at the two-year harmonic. The demographic factors which determine the spacing between epidemics are considered in section 6.5.

A basic assumption of the methods described is that the series are stationary in time. If trend or seasonal (as opposed to epidemic cycle) effects exist, these may confound the interpretation of the individual spectra and the cross-spectrum. Trend and seasonality may be removed as described in Figure 4.2. Since the series shown in diagram (A) appear to be free of trend, this has not been undertaken here. As discussed in Figure 4.6, seasonal effects on the Pacific islands are complex but, given the way the data have been standardized in this example, are swamped by the epidemic cycles and so have not been removed.

Sources and Further Reading

The source for the measles data is given in the preceding plate (Figure 5.11) of this Atlas. The basis of spectral decomposition of time-series is discussed in P. Haggett, A.D. Cliff and A.E. Frey (1977), *Locational Analysis in Human Geography*, second edition, London: Edward Arnold, pp.390–413. More advanced accounts are given in C. Chatfield (1980), *The Analysis of Time Series: An Introduction*, second edition, London: Chapman and Hall, pp.127–69; C.W.J. Granger (1969), 'Spatial data and time-series analysis', *London Papers in Regional Science*, 1: *Studies in Regional Science*, edited by A.J. Scott, London: Pion, pp.1–24; and G.M. Jenkins and D.G. Watts (1968), *Spectral Analysis and its Applications*, San Francisco: Holden Day.

5.13 AUTOCORRELATION ON GRAPHS I: MEASLES IN CORNWALL

Disease spread in a set of settlements

Sometimes, the spread of a disease from place to place in a country forms a continuous wave moving over space. Diffusion takes place from the initial centre of introduction to its physically nearest neighbouring centres. These, in their turn, transmit the disease to their geographically nearest neighbours and so on. The disease progresses from place to place at the leading edge of the wave and spatially divorced outbreaks ahead of the wave front are missing (cf. Figures 5.6 and 5.7).

However, such a geographically highly ordered process is rarely found in practice. The spread of a disease more often appears to be spatially erratic, with considerable distances unaffected by disease interposed between outbreaks. One of the commonest instances of such seemingly erratic geographical behaviour arises when transmission occurs through a system of cities, towns, villages and hamlets. The varying population sizes of the settlements result in spread being directed through the urban hierarchy from larger places to smaller. Typically the initial point of introduction of a disease in a region is its largest city. Then urban centres next in size follow and so on. In these circumstances, the transmission process is spatially discrete and fragmented rather than continuous because settlements such as cities and towns at high levels of the population size hierarchy will generally be some distance apart.

Often the diffusion process displays both hierarchical and contagious elements. For example,

superimposed on the downwards percolation from large settlements to small characteristic of hierarchical diffusion, simultaneous spread frequently also occurs out from each centre to its geographically nearest neighbours. Such a mixed process was examined in Figure 5.8 where the geographical spread of some measles epidemics in Iceland was considered.

In this and the next two figures, we explore ways in which spread processes can be analysed and modelled by applying the technique of spatial autocorrelation to time-series of graphs. At this point the reader may wish to refer back to Figure 1.9 where the concepts of both spatial autocorrelation and graphs are defined.

Hierarchic and contagious spread compared

The sequence of illustrations given here shows the varying efficiency with which disease is disseminated across a hypothetical geographical landscape. Suppose that, as shown in diagram (A), the landscape consists of settlements of four different sizes. Centre i is the largest and l is the smallest. Let us assume that the largest settlement, i consists of 27 population units, the second largest settlements, j of 9 population units each, the k level settlements of 3 population units each, and the l level settlements of one population unit each. Thus the total population of the region shown in diagram (A) is 81 units [that is, $(1 \times 27) + (2 \times 9) + (6 \times 3) + (18 \times 1)$]. Settlements are assumed to dominate areas of countryside in direct proportion to their population sizes to define the spheres of influence shown in diagram (B). A disease is introduced into centre i and it is allowed to spread to other places by purely contagious spread [diagram (C)], purely hierarchical spread [diagram (D)], and by a process which combines both elements [diagram (E)]. The corridors of movement are

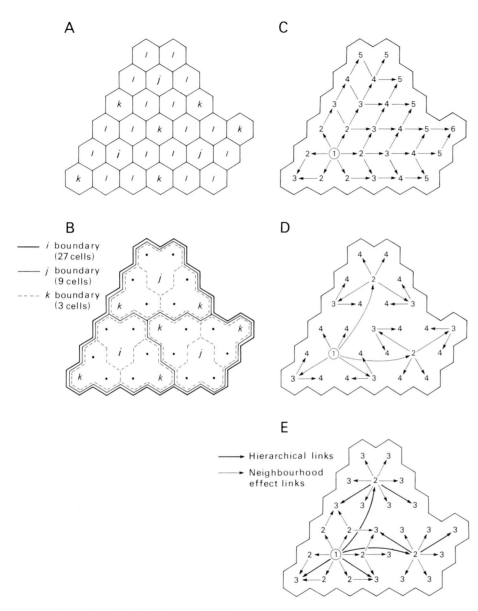

Figure 5.13 (A)–(E) Disease diffusion processes operating in hypothetical arrangements of settlements

shown by vectors in the manner of Figures 5.1, 5.4 and 5.5, while the numbers indicate the time period in which the disease reached the various settlements (1 = earliest).

Using the population sizes of the different settlements given above, we can then determine the proportion of the total population in the region infected by the end of each time period. This yields Table 5.13.1. It is evident from this table that the efficiency of different spread processes varies quite markedly. The purely contagious process shown in diagram (C) is the least efficient and it takes the longest time for all centres to be reached. The hierarchical process shown in diagram (D) is next most efficient with all centres infected by the end of the fourth time period. Not surprisingly, the process which combines the elements of both hierarchical and neighbourhood diffusion [diagram (E)] is the most efficient with all centres contacted by the third time period.

Table 5.13.1 *Comparison of speed of spread for the different diffusion processes shown in Figure 5.13 (A) – (E)*

Time Period	Number of settlements affected by each period*		
	Neighbourhood (C)	Hierarchical (D)	Mixed (E)
1	1 (33 percent)	1 (33 percent)	1 (33 percent)
2	7 (41 percent)	3 (56 percent)	9 (63 percent)
3	13 (58 percent)	9 (78 percent)	27 (100 percent)
4	19 (85 percent)	27 (100 percent)	
5	26 (98 percent)		
6	27 (100 percent)		

*Figures in brackets indicate the proportion of the total population of 81 units contacted by each time period.

Cornwall as a test area

A specific application of this approach is given in diagrams (F) – (H) and is taken from Haggett (1976). This shows the county of Cornwall in southwest England. The nodes on the graph are the General Register Office (GRO) areas which comprise one of the basic geographical frameworks for the collection of medical data in the United Kingdom. The size of each node has been drawn proportional to its population in 1970. The links in the graph represent the contacts based on adjacency. The spread of measles through this graph was examined for a 222-week period extending from the autumn of 1966 to the end of 1970 (see box in Figure 3.3 for a description of measles as a disease). Maps of Cornwall were constructed for every week of the study period, with each of the 27 nodes coded to show presence (black) and absence (white) of the disease. Diagram (F) shows one of the maps in the sequence in which the disease was strongly concentrated in west Cornwall.

Six other graphs were constructed linking the nodes in the graph of Cornwall in different ways. Each network defined corresponded with a hypothesized spread pattern for the disease. Diagrams (G) and (H) present a generalized picture of the results obtained. The advance phase of a measles epidemic in Cornwall is marked by a rapid increase in both the number of cases and, as judged by the number of GRO areas affected, the geographical extent of the disease; see diagram (G). During the subsequent retreat phase after the peak case load has passed, the number of cases falls off rapidly. This is not associated with a corresponding reduction in the geographical extent of the disease; the number of areas still affected falls off much more slowly, so that the epidemic appears to decay spatially *in situ* rather than retreating in a spatially organized manner.

Identification of spatial processes

The onset and decay phases are characterized by marked differences in the relative importance of the seven graphs. A graph was said to be important if, at the 95 percent significance level, it displayed significant positive spatial autocorrelation (clustering) of the GROs coloured black; the *BW* join-count statistic was used and technical definitions are given in Figure 1.9. As shown in diagram (H), the diagram (D) graph, spread down the urban population size hierarchy, is important at the onset of an epidemic. It becomes progressively less important as wave contagion in the shape of either mixed [diagram (E)] or purely contagious [diagram (C)] spread takes over. At the epidemic peak, local contagion effects dominate, setting up strong regional contrasts between the compact clusters of infected and uninfected GRO areas. In the decay phase, the general level of autocorrelation falls steadily on almost all graphs. The one exception is the spatial interaction graph. This graph takes into account travel between urban areas and the homes of people living within their spheres of influence, and has somewhat greater sustained importance just after epidemic peaks.

Whether the patterns found in Cornwall are general remains to be seen. The Icelandic evidence presented in Figure 5.8 is consistent with the results reported here. Nevertheless, it must be remembered that the Cornish results are for a restricted geographical area and a limited number (2) of epidemic waves. More complex examples are considered in Figures 5.14 and 5.15.

Sources and Further Reading

Maps (B) and (C) are based on P. Haggett (1976), 'Hybridizing alternative models of an epidemic diffusion process', *Economic Geography*, 52, pp.136–46, and P. Haggett (1978), 'Regional and local components in elementary space–time models of contagious processes', in *Spacing Time*, vol. 3, edited by T. Carlstein, D. Parkes and N.J. Thrift, London: Edward Arnold.

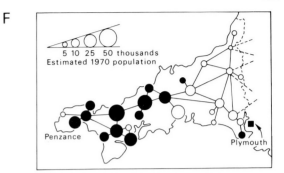

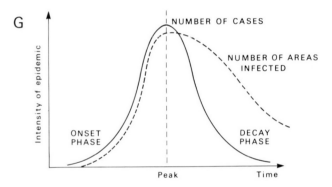

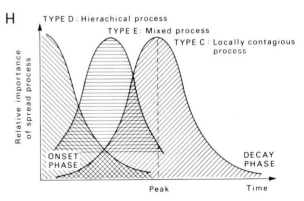

Figure 5.13 (F) – (H) Tests of disease diffusion processes operating in an actual arrangement of settlements (Cornwall)

5.14 AUTOCORRELATION ON GRAPHS II: MEASLES IN SOUTHWEST ENGLAND

Southwest England as graph

The geographical spread of common transmissible diseases like measles in urbanized societies frequently exhibits two components. Relatively long-distance diffusion occurs by spread from city to city and from town to town, often leapfrogging the intervening countryside between urban areas. The second component consists of the in-filling of the space between towns by localized spread outwards from each infected urban centre into the surrounding countryside which falls within its sphere of influence (cf. Figure 5.13). In less urbanized regions, the component of spread between urban areas is often reduced so that diffusion is much more wave-like from the initial points of introduction of the disease.

The way of assessing the relative importance of these spread components is to map geographical space onto a graph, as defined in Figure 1.9, and to examine the temporal evolution of the disease on the graph defined. The approach is illustrated in diagrams (A) and (B) by considering the spread of two measles epidemics which affected southwest England between October 1966 and December 1970. A description of measles as a disease appears in the box accompanying Figure 3.3.

The main units used by the General Register Office (GRO) for gathering disease data in the United Kingdom are the local authority administrative areas of county boroughs, municipal boroughs, urban districts and rural districts. The six counties of southwest England, namely Corn-

wall, Devon, Somerset, Gloucester, Dorset and Wiltshire, are divided into 179 such areas. If we ignore the Scilly Isles, the remaining 178 areas comprise a contiguous network that may be represented as a graph. Each GRO area forms a *vertex* on the graph while the existence of a common boundary between any pair of areas is indicated by a *link*. The number of links in the shortest route between any pair of GRO areas is referred to as the *spatial lag* between the two areas. The process of translation of the GROs onto a graph is shown for Cornwall in diagram (B).

For the 151 vertices relating to GROs not located at the junction of the Southwest with adjacent regions of England, the average number of links with other vertices is 3.22. This is slightly less than the 5.79 expected for a random set of contiguous areas and reflects the strongly peninsular and linear form of the graph in Devon and Cornwall. The linear nature of the graph also produces 22 links in the shortest route through the graph from the extreme southwest to the extreme northeast. Table 5.14.1 gives the relative location of the three main diffusion centres for measles in the southwest in relation to the rest of the graph. The greater connectedness of the largest centre, Bristol, is evident.

Space-time correlograms

The 179 GRO areas permit a large number (15,842) of pairwise comparisons to be made between their time-series. The data analysed consist of the reported number of cases of measles in each GRO area in each week of the time-series from 1966 (week 40) to 1970 (week 52). If the average correlation on reported cases between all pairs of time-series which are 1, 2 . . . spatial lags apart on the graph is computed for each of the 222 weeks of the study period, the complex time-space correlogram shown in diagram (A) can be constructed. The average correlation is plotted on the vertical axis, while spatial lag and time form the axes of the base of the block diagram. Only the positive correlations are shown. The upper part of diagram (A) is based upon the calculated values of the correlation coefficients. In the lower part of the diagram, the average correlations have been smoothed using a running mean to bring out the broad space-time patterns more clearly. On the backplane of the lower block, the number of areas reporting cases in each week is plotted in the diagonally shaded histogram.

The first of the major measles epidemics which occurred in the time period studied

Table 5.14.1 *Relative location of the three major measles centres in the southwest on the graph of the region*

GRO area:	Bristol CB	Plymouth CB	Penzance UD
Total link distance	1,090	1,141	2,576
Mean link distance	6.12	8.02	14.47
Maximum link distance	16	15	22
Percent of GRO areas within three links	24	11	6

Note: CB denotes country borough; UD denotes urban district

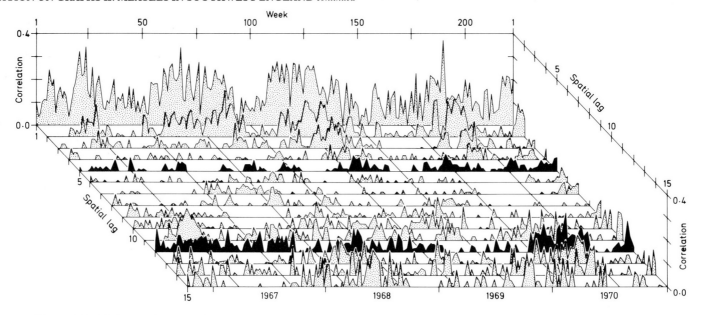

Figure 5.14 (A) Space–time correlogram for areas at spatial lags up to 15 for weekly measles records in southwest England, late 1966–1970

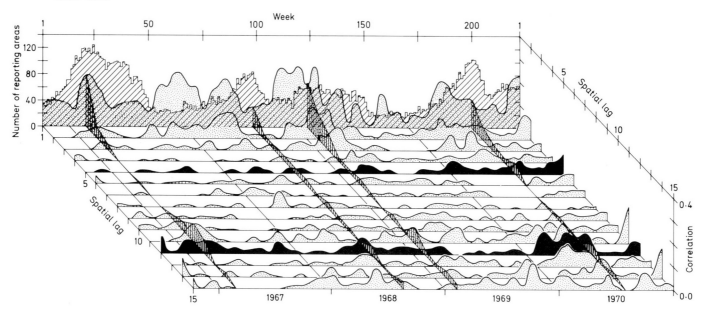

Figure 5.14 (B) Smoothed version of diagram (A) with cross-sectional slices at the peaks of measles epidemics

peaked in the southwest in February 1967 (week 20). It was characterized by a strengthening of the correlation bonds at some spatial lags (for example at one, two and eleven). The second major epidemic peaked in the summer of 1970 (weeks 186–204) and produced marked positive average correlations at spatial lags from one to four and at eleven and twelve. Other peaks appear in an irregular fashion on the correlogram in the inter-epidemic periods and reflect a scatter of small, localized outbreaks throughout the study period.

The four vertically shaded cross-sectional slices parallel to the spatial lag axis on the lower block diagram show clearly how the average correlation falls exponentially with increasing spatial lag [cf. Figure 5.6(B)]. This implies that, at any time, similar case levels are found in GRO areas which are close together on the graph of the southwest (cf. Figure 5.2) and is produced by the spread of disease from urban areas into their spheres of influence.

Local maxima on the correlation profiles

Special interest attaches to the two local maxima in the correlation profiles, shown in black, at around spatial lags five and twelve. These maxima imply greater than expected correlation (since the correlation should continue to fall exponentially with increasing spatial lag) between places at these lags on the graph. As Table 5.14.1 demonstrates, the average separation between all GROs and Bristol on this graph is six links and this is the main endemic reservoir for measles in the southwest. The separation between Bristol and Plymouth is twelve links. These centres, with their adjacent urbanized areas, had populations of one half and one quarter of a million respectively in 1970, when they made up about one fifth of the total population of the study area.

The two cities were persistent centres of measles infection and recorded a continuous trace of cases over the entire study period. The local maximum at lag five is related to the fairly persistent pockets of infection in the smaller urban centres. Apart from Bristol and Plymouth, there were four urban areas with populations in excess of 100,000 namely Gloucester–Cheltenham (200,000), Poole (120,000), Swindon (120,000), and Torbay (100,000). There were two towns (Exeter and Bath) between 50,000 and 100,000 and a further nine with populations between 20,000 and 50,000. These seventeen population clusters together made up one half of the southwest region's estimated civil population of 3.7 millions in 1970. The average distance between GROs and these centres on the graph of the southwest is approximately five.

Thus the spread of measles in the southwest appears to show both the diffusion components mentioned initially namely, spread between urban areas and spread from urban areas into their hinterland regions.

Sources and Further Reading

The correlograms are based on A.D. Cliff, P. Haggett, J.K. Ord, K.A. Bassett and R.B. Davies (1975), *Elements of Spatial Structure*, Cambridge: Cambridge University Press, pp.100–1. See also P. Haggett (1972), 'Contagious processes in a planar graph: an epidemiological application', in *Medical Geography: Techniques and Field Studies*, edited by N.D. McGlashan, London: Methuen, pp.307–24.

For an ecological application of spatial correlograms see R.R. Sokal (1979), 'Ecological parameters inferred from spatial correlograms', in *Contemporary Quantitative Ecology and Related Econometrics*, edited by G.P. Patil and M.L. Rosenzweig, Fairland, Md: International Cooperative Publishing House. One interesting epidemiological application to one-dimensional cross-sections of the United States is B.J. Glick (1982), 'The spatial organization of cancer mortality', *Annals of the Association of American Geographers*, 82, pp.471–81.

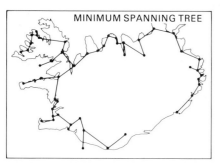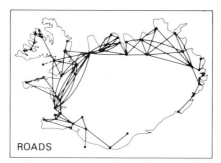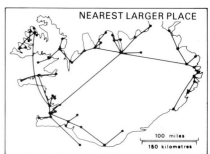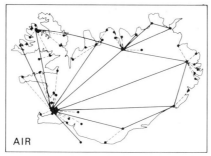

Figure 5.15 (A) Alternate graphs linking Iceland's fifty medical districts

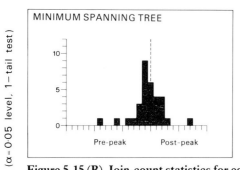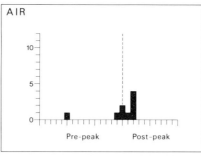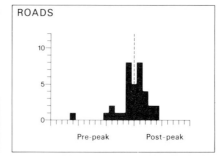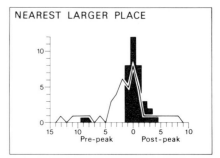

Figure 5.15 (B) Join-count statistics for estimating paths followed by influenza epidemics, 1945–1970

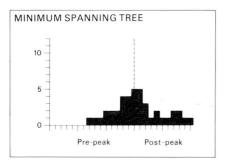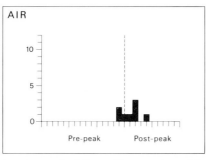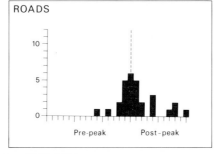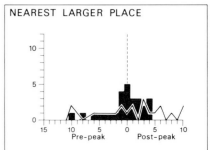

Figure 5.15 (C) Join-count statistics for estimating paths followed by measles epidemics, 1945–1970

Number of significant deviates (α = 0·05 level, 1−tail test)

5.15 AUTOCORRELATION ON GRAPHS III: MEASLES IN ICELAND

Iceland as a graph

As we have seen in the two preceding figures, one way of studying the spatial spread of diseases is to treat the area over which spread is occurring as a graph. The nodes on the graph consist of the settlements through which the disease is moving, while the links between the settlements may be chosen to reflect the potential transmission corridors. A small-scale example showing how the link structure may be varied to reflect the spread process has been given in Figure 5.13 (F) – (H). In the present figure, the methodology is developed more fully in a comparative study of the diffusion corridors followed by epidemics of measles and influenza in Iceland between 1945 and 1970. Disease descriptions for measles and influenza appear in the boxes in Figure 3.3 and section 6.4 respectively.

As discussed in Figure 2.11, the basic geographical unit for the collection of epidemiological data in Iceland is the medical district, of which there were 50 in the period from 1945–70. We can thus view Iceland as a graph consisting of a set of nodes (the medical districts) and the links between them. Since measles and influenza rely primarily upon person-to-person transmission for their spread, the geographical patterns of diffusion may be expected to reflect the movements of the Icelandic population for work, schooling, holidays and so on. We can conveniently call someone who is infectious at a particular moment with either measles or influenza an index case. In theory, an *index case* could travel from any one of the 50 districts to any of the others to pass on the disease to someone else. So with 50 nodes we could draw a graph with each medical district linked to every other medical district, yielding 2450 links in all. In practice, we can limit the number of links to give a graph which corresponds as closely as possible to the probable paths for the diffusion of the diseases being studied.

Four alternate graphs

The four maps in (A) show the medical districts of Iceland connected as graphs which reflect different aspects of the likely movements of index cases. The first illustrates Iceland as a minimum spanning tree (MST), which is the simplest network configuration in which all nodes are linked to their nearest neighbouring medical districts. Given 50 medical districts (n), the number of such links is 49 (or $n - 1$). This network of links implies a highly localized spread process round the coast, with each centre open to infection only from its two physically adjacent medical districts. Such a spread model reflects short distance travel by the index cases, mainly by local roads, possibly for work or schooling. Obviously longer distance trips are made and the remaining three graphs take these into account.

Because of the difficult terrain in Iceland, the relatively poor roads away from towns and the long distances between major settlements Iceland possesses the most heavily used internal airline network, per head of population, of any country in the world. The second map therefore gives the graph obtained from the network of domestic airline links. Medical districts without an airport have been joined with a pecked line to the nearest node on the airline graph. The third map shows a road graph giving connections based on the road network in the 1970s. Although most roads in Iceland are simply dirt-graded and many become impassable in winter, car ownership is high and an extensive round-the-island bus service is available in the summer months. The last map is based on the population size of settlements. Each district is linked to the medical district which is as geographically close to it as possible, and yet is also larger than it in population size. Such a nearest larger place (NLP) graph reflects the commonly observed fact that people tend to make regular trips to nearby settlements larger than their own for specialized shopping and other services not available in the local village or community.

We now consider which of the four networks gives the closest approximation to the channels actually followed by an infectious disease as it spreads through the Icelandic population. To do this, we consider the post-war epidemics of influenza and measles. For each of the 312 months between 1945–70 in which cases were reported, a graph was drawn on which nodes were coded black (B = cases reported) or white (W = no cases reported) and the BW join count statistic defined in Figure 1.9 evaluated. The histograms presented in diagrams (B) and (C) show the results of this analysis for influenza and measles respectively. On each histogram the vertical axis plots the number of occasions on which the BW statistic, and therefore the graph or network, was statistically significant at the 95 percent level in a one-tailed test for positive spatial autocorrelation. The horizontal axis shows time in months ranging from 15 months before epidemic peaks (marked by the vertical pecked lines) to 10 months after. This allowed all 17 influenza and all 8 measles epidemics to be plotted on a common basis using the maximum number of monthly cases as a crude indicator of epidemic peak.

Pathways for influenza epidemics

In the case of influenza the following points may be noted from diagram (B). The MST and road network graphs, which represent spatially contagious spread, are important from one month before epidemic peaks until two to four months after. The NLP graph, which represents spatially constrained hierarchical spread, is important from one month before until two to three months after epidemic peaks. If we relax the requirement of contiguity in the NLP graph and repeat the analysis for a hierarchical spread process which moves from larger to smaller places in a strict population size succession (irrespective of location), then the line trace on the NLP diagram shows the results obtained for the *BW* statistic. This revised graph is important from four months before until one month after epidemic peaks. Taken together the findings suggest a disease transmission process which starts through the urban hierarchy (pure population size graph) in the build-up phase of an epidemic. This is taken over by spatially contagious diffusion (MST, road and NLP graphs) around the epidemic peak and geographically *in situ* decay during the fade-out phase.

Pathways for measles epidemics

The results for measles are shown in diagram (C) and tell a slightly different tale. Purely hierarchical spread, which appears as the line trace on the NLP histogram, is insignificant at all stages in the history of the epidemics. Contagious spread, as exemplified by the MST graph, dominates the build-up phase of measles epidemics and is also important at epidemic peaks; it is also at the time of peak case-load that the road network graph becomes important. In the fade-out stage of epidemics after the month of peak case-load, the NLP graph appears to dominate, implying that measles epidemics tend to fade out partly through the urban system and partly locally.

Comparison of results for influenza and measles

A striking feature for both measles and influenza is the lack of importance of the airline network as a diffusing agent. This graph and the pure population size graph, which is important for influenza but not measles, are the two aspatial spread processes considered. In contrast, all the spatially constrained graphs are significant in varying degrees and their importance appears to wax and wane with the growth and decay of the epidemics. This changing importance of spatial proximity with the stage of the epidemic was also noted in Figure 5.14 where the spread of measles in southwest England was considered. Perhaps we may account for the dominance of geographical proximity over aspatial spread in the transmission of these diseases by remembering the relatively short infectious periods of both before isolation of patients is likely, thus restricting the distances over which travel and therefore contact with those at risk is possible.

Sources and Further Reading

The results mapped here are taken from A.D. Cliff, P. Haggett, J.K. Ord and G.R. Versey (1981), *Spatial Diffusion: an Historical Geography of Epidemics in an Island Community*, Cambridge: Cambridge University Press, pp.99–102. Parallel results for influenza are described in A.D. Cliff, P. Haggett and J.K. Ord (1986), *Spatial Aspects of Influenza Epidemics*, London: Pion, pp.182–5.

5.16 SPACE–TIME CLUSTERS: BURKITT'S LYMPHOMA

BURKITT'S LYMPHOMA (BL) falls in class 202 of the ICD list. See Figure 2.1. It is a malignant lymphoma of children occurring with highest frequency in hot, wet lowland parts of Africa and New Guinea where malaria (cf. Figure 3.5) is hyperepidemic. It is found with low frequency throughout the world and in non-malarious areas. One of the early maps of the distribution of the tumour produced by Burkitt in 1962 [diagram (A), left] shows, using solid circles to represent BL cases, a belt of incidence across Africa. This highly structured geographical distribution led Burkitt to hypothesize that the causal agent might be a vectored virus related to malaria transmission. Later work on BL has focused upon identifying a role for the Epstein-Barr virus (EBV) in the development of the tumour (cf. Figure 3.7). Although there has never been any direct epidemiological evidence that BL is caused by the EBV, there seems to be some association. For example, the tumour itself usually contains the EBV genome and certain antigens, while EBV producing cell lines can be derived from the tumours.

The possibility that BL might have a viral origin has spawned several studies which have attempted to determine whether clusters of BL exist in time and space that can be related either to the geographical distribution of an arthropod-borne agent or to some geographically or time-varying trigger mechanism which provokes the oncogenic potential of the globally ubiquitous EBV. Some of the evidence is reviewed in this figure.

Burkitt's lymphoma in central Africa

The maps illustrate the geographical distribution of BL cases in two areas of Africa, West Nile district [diagram (B)] and North Mara district [diagram (C)]. The locations of the two districts are shown in diagram (A), right. Diagram (B) gives the geographical location of 14 histologically confirmed BL cases found among some 42,000 children studied in the West Nile district between February 1972 and September 1974 (Thé *et al.*, 1978). Diagram (C) shows the location of histologically confirmed BL cases in North Mara district in each year from 1971 to 1977 (Siemiatycki *et al.*, 1980). Forty cases in all are mapped. The position of each new crop of cases in relation to those diagnosed in the previous year is portrayed using solid and open circles.

Detecting space–time clusters

The space-time clustering technique seeks to determine whether the number of pairs of cases of the disease which are 'close' in space and 'close' in time is so great that there is a only a very low probability that the pairs could have arisen by chance, as opposed to being linked by some mechanism. Application of the method depends critically upon the definition of 'close'. Although statistical details are given in the technical appendix, the earliest development of the method, by Knox (1964), signalled pairs which were 'close' by 1 and those which were 'not close' by 0.

Subsequent generalizations by Mantel (1967) and Hubert *et al.* (1981) permitted pairs to be given general weights according to their closeness in time and space. For example, pairs might be weighted according to a negative exponential series in time and space. This gives great emphasis to pairs occurring in adjacent time and space locations, but falls off rapidly as the time and/or space gap between observations increases. General weighting is important if there is space–time clustering due to a communicable agent. Then, in areas of even population density (cf. Figure 5.13), one would expect the probability of two cases being related to be highest if they occurred at the same place and to decline gradually as geographical distance increased. The same might be true of temporal distance.

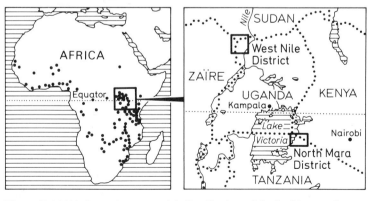

Figure 5.16 (A) Location map with distribution of the incidence of Burkitt's lymphoma across central Africa

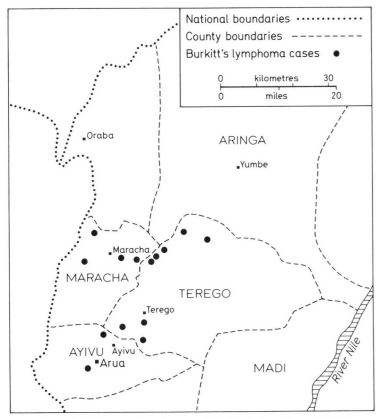

Figure 5.16 (B) Distribution of cases of Burkitt's lymphoma in West Nile district

West Nile and North Mara results

The space–time clustering method has been applied by Siemiatycki *et al.* to both the West Nile and North Mara data using a variety of functions to define closeness or proximity; some are illustrated in the first block of diagram (C). In the spatial domain, two Knox-type functions were tried, one defining proximity as within 5 km of an existing case and a second with a threshold of 20 km. The Mantel-type functions were all negative exponential in form. The

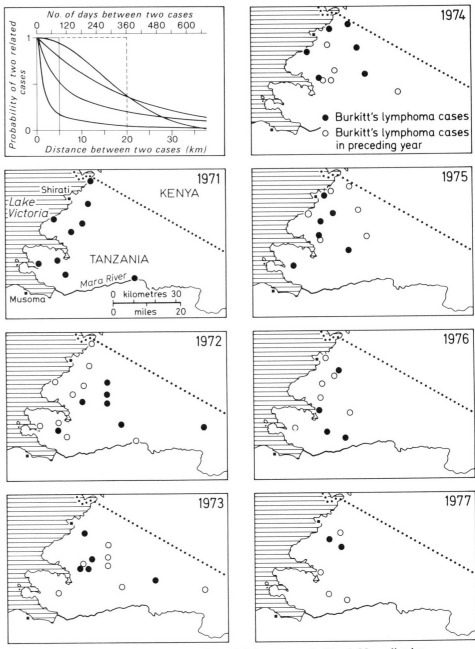

Figure 5.16 (C) Distribution of cases of Burkitt's lymphoma in North Mara district

gradients were chosen to decay, with various degrees of rapidity, the probability of contact over increasing distances. Similar functions were used in the time domain. The equation and a test of significance for the Knox and Mantel space–time clustering index (STI) are given in the technical appendix.

The results obtained were highly variable. Using West Nile data for the period 1961–65, very significant space–time clustering was found with every proximity function. For data relating to 1966–70, only the Knox and very rapid exponential decay functions were statistically significant. However, the standard Normal deviates were positive for all the space–time proximity functions, providing weak evidence of clustering. For the data illustrated in diagram (B), the degree of clustering increased, compared with 1966–70, for most of the proximity functions, with all the Mantel-type yielding positive standard Normal deviates. In North Mara district, every proximity function yielded STI values close to random expectation; many of the standard Normal deviates were negative.

The results of the analyses are conflicting. The general message from West Nile is of some space–time clustering but often very weakly developed, while in North Mara there is no support for clustering. The aetiological implication is that BL does not result from a single agent operating evenly in space and time, otherwise clustering would not be found on some occasions but not on others. Nor is the latent period fairly constant; if that were so, again space–time clustering would be expected as cases of BL 'batched' through in time and space.

Sources and Further Reading

The maps are taken from the West Nile study described in G. de Thé (1978), 'Epidemiological evidence for causal relationship between Epstein-Barr virus and Burkitt's lymphoma from Ugandan prospective study', *Nature*, 274, pp.756–61, and from the re-examination of the North Mara data by J. Siemiatycki, G. Brubaker and A. Geser (1980), 'Space–time clustering of Burkitt's lymphomas in East Africa: analysis of recent data and a new look at old data', *International Journal of Cancer*, 25, pp.197–203.

Burkitt's original ideas are discussed in D. Burkitt (1962), 'Determining the climatic limitations of a children's cancer common in Africa', *British Medical Journal*, 2, pp.1019–23, and in P. Cook and D. Burkitt (1970), *An Epidemiological Study of Seven Malignant Tumours in East Africa*, London: Medical Research Council. See also S.A. Hall and B.W. Langlands (1975), *Atlas of Disease Distribution in Uganda*, Nairobi: East Africa Publishers. An up-to-date collection of papers on BL and its epidemiology has been edited by G.M. Lenoir, G.T. O'Connor and C.L.M. Olweny (1985), *Burkitt's Lymphoma: A Human Cancer Model*, International Agency for Research on Cancer (IARC), Scientific Publication No. 60, Oxford: Oxford University Press.

The STI index is summarized in A.D. Cliff and J.K. Ord (1981), *Spatial Processes: Models and Applications*, London: Pion, pp.22–4. More detailed accounts are those of E.G. Knox (1964), 'The detection of space–time interactions', *Applied Statistics*, 13, pp.25–9; N. Mantel (1967), 'The detection of disease clustering and a generalised regression approach', *Cancer Research*, 27, pp.209–20; and L.J. Hubert, R.G. Golledge, C.M. Constanzo and G.D. Richardson (1981), 'Assessing homogeneity in cross-classified proximity data', *Geographical Analysis*, 13, pp.38–50.

Technical appendix

Let STI denote an index of space–time clustering where

$$\text{STI} = \sum\nolimits_{(2)} w_{ij} y_{ij}, \qquad (5.16.1)$$

and $\sum_{(2)} = \sum\limits_{i} \sum\limits_{j}.$

Here the $\{w_{ij}\}$ are weights used to define closeness in space, while the $\{y_{ij}\}$ measure closeness in time. For example, if the ith event occurred at time t_i, we may define

$$y_{ij} \begin{cases} = 1 \; if \; |t_i - t_j| \leqslant u \\ = 0, \text{otherwise}, \end{cases}$$

for a suitable choice of u. We always take $y_{ii} = 0$ for all i.

As summarized in Cliff and Ord (1981), under the null hypothesis of no association we may regard all the assignments of the $\{w_{ij}\}$ as fixed and then consider every possible permutation of rows (and corresponding permutations of columns) of $n \times n$ matrix, $\mathbf{Y} = \{y_{ij}\}$. Using this approach, the expected value of STI is

$$\text{E(STI)} = S_0 T_0 / [n(n - 1)], \qquad (5.16.2)$$

where $S_0 = \sum_{(2)} w_{ij} \; and \; T_0 = \sum_{(2)} y_{ij}.$

To specify the variance we set

$$T_1 = \tfrac{1}{2} \sum\nolimits_{(2)} (y_{ij} + y_{ji})^2, \quad T_2 = \sum_i (y_{i.} + y_{.i})^2,$$

where $y_{i.} = \sum\limits_{j} y_{ij}$ and $y_{.i} = \sum\limits_{j} y_{ji}.$

Similar definitions may be given for S_1 and S_2 in terms of the $\{w_{ij}\}$. For convenience we assume that $y_{ij} = y_{ji}$ for all i and j, so that

$$\text{var(STI)} = S_1 T_1 / (2n^{(2)}) + [(S_2 - 2S_1)(T_2 - 2T_1)] / (4n^{(3)})$$
$$+ [(S_0^2 + S_1 - S_2)(T_0^2 + T_1 - T_2)] / n^{(4)}$$
$$- [\text{E(STI)}]^2. \qquad (5.16.3)$$

Here $n^{(k)} = n(n - 1) \ldots (n - k + 1)$. For large n and general weights, appeals to asymptotic Normality are made, but with limited justification without some structure being imposed upon the $\{y_{ij}\}$. Under Normality, equations (5.16.2) and (5.16.3) provide a test of significance using a standard Normal deviate (cf. Figure 1.7).

5.17 BIPROPORTIONATE MATRICES

Comparing changes over time

When disease data have been collected for a series of areas over several time periods, the conventional way of studying changing temporal incidence is to plot the values on a graph as in the main part of diagram (A). Here some hypothetical values are shown for two areas, A and B, at five different points in time. Incidence starts at a very much higher level in A than in B, but falls more rapidly so that, by time period five, both display similar levels of infection.

In making this interpretation we must remember that the data for each area have been plotted independently of the data for the other and so absolute changes are being compared. However, there will be many occasions on which we will want to assess relative rather than absolute change. Thus when studying a set of areas, we may wish to comment upon the degree of temporal change which has taken place in any one, compared with the amount of change experienced in the others. Alternatively, we may want to establish which of the time periods in the time-space matrix exhibits the most change over the set of areas.

Matrix standardization

A variety of methods exist for standardizing a matrix so that relative change may be assessed. One of the most common is to use row and column totals to generate expected values in each area in each time period and then to examine the departures of the actual values from these

expectations (cf. Figures 1.8, 3.10, 3.13, 3.14 and 3.15). A particularly powerful alternative method is to use *biproportionate scores* and we illustrate the computational procedures involved by examining the data plotted in the main part of diagram (A). The raw data appear in part (A) of Table 5.17.1.

Suppose a matrix of observations is available in which the areas form the rows (denoted by i) and the time periods form the columns (denoted by j). The quantity in any cell of the matrix gives the value of the variable of interest (disease incidence, say) in a particular area in a selected time period. In step one of the standardization procedure, the values are scaled so that each row sum is equal to the number of columns in the matrix, here five. This is achieved by calculating the row sums in the original data (for example 1550 in the case of area 1) and then dividing these totals by five to give a scaling factor for each row of the data matrix. For the first row,

Table 5.17.1 *Hypothetical data for two regions and five time periods*

Areas	Time periods					
	1	2	3	4	5	Total
	PART (A) ORIGINAL DATA					
1	800	400	200	100	50	1500
2	80	40	20	10	5	155
Total	880	440	220	110	55	
	PART (B) FIRST ITERATION SCORES					
1	258	129	65	32	16	500
2	258	129	65	32	16	500
Total	516	258	130	64	32	
	PART (C) SECOND ITERATION SCORES					
1	100	100	100	100	100	500
2	100	100	100	100	100	500
Total	200	200	200	200	200	

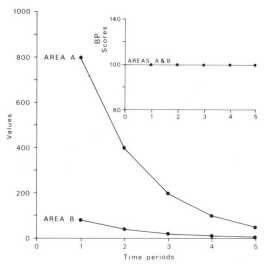

Figure 5.17 (A) Biproportionate scores for two exceptionally declining trends in two areas

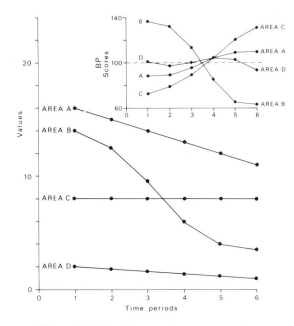

Figure 5.17 (B) Biproportionate scores for contrasting time trends in four areas

this procedure yields 1550/5 = 310, and for the second row, 155/5 = 31. The adjusted scores are then obtained by taking the values in each row of the original data matrix and dividing them by their corresponding scaling factor. This step produces the matrix given in Table 5.17.1(B) where, to eliminate decimal points, all values have been multiplied by 100.

The standardization process then continues by scaling the columns of the matrix given in part (B) so that each column sum is equal to the number of rows in the matrix, here two. This yields the matrix given in Table 5.17.1(C) where again all values have been multiplied by 100. The process of adjustment is continued, operating alternately on rows and columns until the adjusted matrix converges; that is, the values in the matrix cease, within some margin of error set by the researcher, to change. In the simple example given here convergence has already occurred by the end of the second cycle, but in large matrices with irregular relationships between the areas, a substantial number of iterations may be required.

In the matrix recorded in part (C) of Table 5.17.1, reading down the columns gives the relative change in each area over time, while reading across the rows gives the relative change in each time period over the set of areas. If the time-series for both areas change exponentially (either both upwards or both downwards) over time, as in the example used here, then the adjusted or standardized values will be unity (100). These standardized values have been plotted on the inset graph of diagram (A). A value of unity (100) in the biproportionate matrix is the expected value if an area is changing exponentially over time, so that cells with values greater than unity have experienced relatively greater change; cells with values less than unity have experienced relatively less change. In diagram (A), the line graphs for the raw data show that disease incidence in both areas has declined exponentially over time, while the biproportionate scores confirm that their relative behaviour is the same.

A more complex example appears in diagram (B) involving four areas and six time periods. The time trends for the raw data in each of the four areas have been plotted on the main graph, along with the biproportionate scores on the inset graph. Thus in terms of the original data, where each area is being examined in isolation and independently of every other area, we see that A starts at a high initial level in the first time period and exhibits a steady decline in disease intensity. Area B shows a rapid decline from high levels of intensity. Area C appears to have been steady throughout the period at an intermediate level of intensity. Area D is always at a low level of intensity but with a slight decline over time. In terms of the biproportionate scores, however, which enable us to look at the comparative performance of each area we see that A and D are relatively stable over time, but that the changes in areas B and C are dramatic.

Area B has, relatively speaking, experienced a marked decline in intensity over time whereas area C has increased equally clearly.

Biproportionate maps of Icelandic measles waves

Diagram (C) applies the method to fifteen measles epidemics which affected Iceland between 1900 and 1970 (for disease description see box in Figure 3.3). A six-region division of Iceland has been taken, namely the Reykjavík area, the Southwest (SW), the Northwest (NW), the North (N), the East (E) and the South (S). These divisions are shown on the diagram and regions with biproportionate scores in excess of 100 have been shaded black; as before, all scores have been multiplied by 100 for convenience in plotting. The size (thousands of reported cases), the geographical spread (number of medical districts affected) and intensity (cases per thousand population) of each epidemic is shown using bar

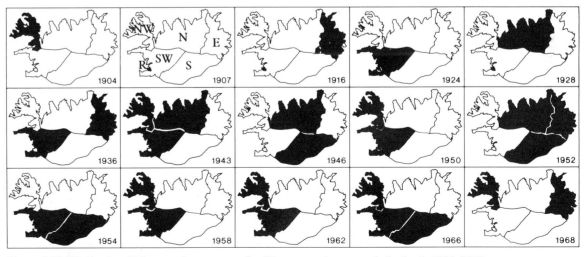

Figure 5.17 (C) Regional biproportionate maps for fifteen measles waves in Iceland, 1904–1968

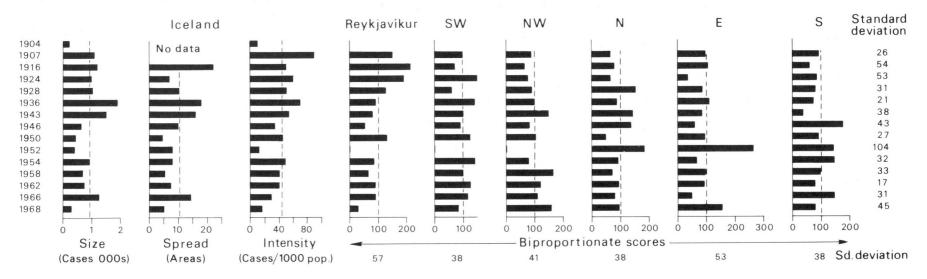

Figure 5.17 (D) Biproportionate scores for fifteen measles waves in Iceland, 1904–1968

graphs in diagram (D) above. Averages are marked by the vertical pecked lines. The biproportionate scores, along with the row and column standard deviations, are also given in diagram (D). Geographically, the maps and graphs indicate that the eastern region played an important role in the epidemics of 1916, 1936, 1952 and 1968 but, with negative residuals in the other ten epidemics, suffered relatively slightly compared with other regions. Overall, it was the Reykjavík region and the East which displayed the greatest relative variability in the extent to which they were affected in epidemics, with standard deviations of 57 and 53 respectively. When time slices are compared, it is noticeable that there were intense regional contrasts in the 1952 epidemic (standard deviation of 104) and relatively low regional contrasts in the 1962 epidemic (standard deviation of 17).

Sources and Further Reading

The biproportionate maps of Iceland shown in (C) are taken from A.D. Cliff, P. Haggett, J.K. Ord and G.R. Versey (1981), *Spatial Diffusion: An Historical Geography of Epidemics in an Island Community*, Cambridge: Cambridge University Press, pp.113–15. The methods are discussed at length in M. Bacharach (1970), *Biproportionate Matrices and Input–Output Change*, Cambridge: Cambridge University Press.

5.18 REGRESSION MODELS

Structure of regression models

The format of regression models has been illustrated earlier in Figure 1.14. Adapted into a framework which handles space–time interactions by Box and Jenkins (1970), the number of cases of a disease in the typical geographical area i at time t (called the effect or dependent variable and denoted by x_{it}) is expressed as a function of x in previous time periods, $(t - 1)$, $(t - 2)$ . . . ; these are called the cause or explanatory variables. The model may relate x both to its past history in the reference area i and to the history of x in other areas, so building up the cone of dependencies projecting back through time shown historical part of Figure 3.1(C).

The approach relies heavily on identifying leading and lagging areas and so the methods of *cross-correlation analysis* and *cross-spectral analysis* discussed in Figures 5.11 and 5.12 are important elements in the methodology. Because the model regresses x upon past values of itself, it is called an *autoregression*. It is usually given the shorthand nomenclature of an AR(k) model where k is an integer denoting the number of time periods in the past upon which x_{it} is regressed.

Formulation of local and neighbourhood terms

To illustrate the structure of AR models in more detail we return to the 1849 cholera epidemic considered in Chapter 1. Suppose we wish to model the number of cases of cholera per 10,000 population occurring in each of the 34 registration districts of London in each week of the epidemic, using the case rate in the preceding week as the explanatory variable. The raw

cholera and population data are mapped in Figure 1.8. Taking Bethnal Green [see diagram (A)] as an example, diagram (B) shows how the death rate from cholera in Bethnal Green in week 12 may be viewed as a function both of the death rate in Bethnal Green (a local effect) and of the death rate in registration districts contiguous to Bethnal Green (a neighbourhood effect) in week 11. Thus the rate in Bethnal Green in week 12 may be viewed as a weighted sum of the rates in Bethnal Green and its neighbours in week 11.

The same argument holds for all the other registration districts. The average contribution to the dependent variable of the local effect is summarized through the coefficient b_1, and of the neighbourhood effect through the coefficient b_2. The statistical formulation is given in the technical appendix.

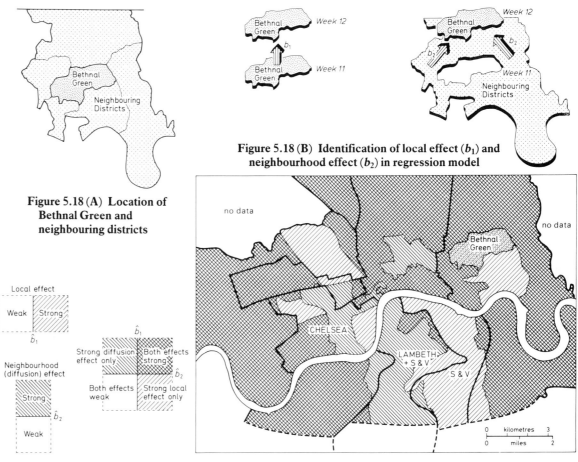

Figure 5.18 (A) Location of Bethnal Green and neighbouring districts

Figure 5.18 (B) Identification of local effect (b_1) and neighbourhood effect (b_2) in regression model

Figure 5.18 (C) Cross-classification of regression terms and their application to modelling cholera spread in London, 1849

Application to the London cholera epidemic, 1849

As discussed in Chapter 1, cholera is a water-borne disease and the 1849 epidemic had its seat in the sewerage-contaminated water supplied to dwellings by the Southwark and Vauxhall (S & V) and Lambeth Companies. The water company areas are marked with heavy lines in diagram (C). A qualitative model of the process whereby the epidemic spread across London would be to regard the registration districts served by these companies as diffusion poles so that, for example, people working in districts supplied by these companies but living elsewhere might move the disease across the city before being stricken. Once cholera became established within a district, we might also expect substantial within-registration district growth of cases to occur. In terms of the AR model already outlined, the stronger the within-district growth, the larger will be the b_1 coefficient; the greater the diffusion component (spread from one district to another), the larger will be the b_2 coefficient.

These ideas have been tested by fitting equation (5.18.1) using ordinary least squares to the time-series of weekly death rates from cholera in each registration district from May 12 ($t = 1$) to November 24 ($t = 29$), 1849. Diagram (C) uses choropleth techniques (cf. Figure 1.6) to summarize the results. An effect (local or diffusion) was judged as strong if the corresponding regression coefficient (b_1 or b_2) was statistically significant at the 95 percent level in a one-tailed test. Otherwise it was coded as weak.

In diagram (C) the diffusion or neighbourhood effect is significant in the areas served by the S & V, Lambeth and Chelsea Companies. As discussed in Figures 1.1 and 1.13, the Chelsea, along with the S & V and Lambeth, all drew

their supply water from the Thames which was used for the discharge of sewerage. There is also one unexplained diffusion pole north of the Thames. Most other parts of London are significant on both effects.

Taken together, these results suggest that transfer of the disease took place at an early date from the source areas to other districts. Once established in other areas, these experienced both continued local growth and simultaneously acted as diffusion poles in their own right to promote the disease in neighbouring districts.

Sources and Further Reading

The data sources for the London cholera maps are described in Figure 1.3, and the nature of cholera in Figure 1.1 of this Atlas.

The concept of regression was introduced in Figure 1.14, and the reader is referred to this plate for basic references. The use of regression models in analysing space–time series is discussed in P. Haggett, A.D. Cliff and A.E. Frey (1977), *Locational Analysis in Human Geography*, second edition, London: Edward Arnold, pp.390–413, and applied to epidemiological data in A.D. Cliff, P. Haggett, J.K. Ord and G.R. Versey (1981), *Spatial Diffusion: An Historical Geography of Epidemics in an Island Community*, Cambridge: Cambridge University Press, pp.132–58. See also G.E.P. Box and G.M. Jenkins (1976), *Time Series Analysis: Forecasting and Control*, San Francisco: Holden-Day.

Technical appendix

Using the notation already given we may write

$$x_{it} = b_0 + b_1 x_{i,t-1} + b_2 \sum_{j \in \mathcal{J}} w_{ij} x_{j,t-1} + e_{it}, \qquad (5.18.1)$$

where the summation is over the j registration districts believed to affect i, and e_{it} is a stochastic error term. The $\{w_{ij}\}$ are structural weights proportional to the influence registration district j exerts on i. A simple choice would be $w_{ij} = 0$ if j is not contiguous to i and $w_{ij} = 1$ otherwise. The term in b_1 summarizes the local effect shown in (B) and b_2 the neighbourhood effect.

Other terms may be added to the basic model given in (5.18.1). For example, a moving average (MA) component is possible, yielding an ARMA structure. In the same way non-autogressive explanatory variables (for example, supplying water company, height above the Thames) may also be added to the right-hand side. The justification for these variables is given in Figures 1.13 and 1.14

While the example described here has used historical data, so that the form of equation (5.18.1) covers the present and historical components of Figure 3.1 (C), the model can be readily extended to the forecasting domain by changing the subscripting in t; that is

$$x_{i,t+1} = b_0 + b_1 x_{it} + b_2 \sum_{j \in \mathcal{J}} w_{ij} x_{jt} + e_{i,t+1}. \qquad (5.18.2)$$

With this structure, it could be used to forecast future maps (see Chapter 7).

CHAPTER SIX

SPATIAL DYNAMICS
OF EPIDEMICS

Figure over   Scanning electron microscopy of HIV-1 infected H9 cells. (a) Overview of a virus-producing cell at magnification × 11,000.
(b) The same cell, at magnification × 22,000, clearly shows abundant virus particles on the cell surface. Numerous cell blebs are visible,
indicative of the virus-induced cytopathic effect
Source   Specimen and micrograph by courtesy of Dr Muhsin Özel of the Robert Koch Institut, Berlin

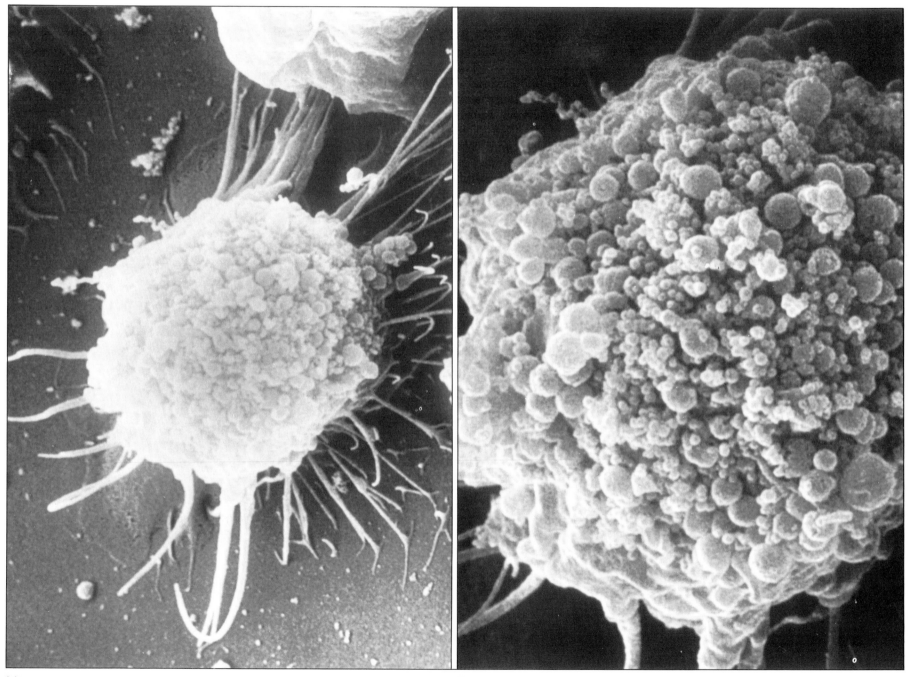

(a)   (b)

SPATIAL DYNAMICS OF EPIDEMICS

6.1   FOUR CONTRASTING EPIDEMIC DISEASES

Introduction

In this chapter we examine some spatial aspects of four communicable diseases, drawing upon the full range of methods outlined in the previous five chapters. We begin with a consideration of the geography of **ACQUIRED IMMUNE DEFICIENCY SYNDROME** or **AIDS** (ICD 279.1). One of the quarantine diseases, **SMALLPOX** (ICD 050), is examined next, before we turn our attention to spatial aspects of **INFLUENZA** epidemics (ICD 487). The chapter is concluded with an analysis of the space–time patterns woven by **MEASLES** (ICD 055).

Although this list appears eclectic, there is a rationale behind it. AIDS is included because of its projected critical importance in the remainder of this century. The long incubation period of the disease, the current lack of a cure, high virulence, and spread encouraged by one of the most basic urges of the human race have combined to create a crisis mentality which was characteristic of the nineteenth-century cholera epidemics in Victorian cities (see Chapter 1 of this Atlas). Our narrative thus comes full circle, with projections of deaths from AIDS, although speculative, engendering fear in the same way as cholera and other plagues of history.

The geography of smallpox in the 1960s and 1970s is one of the best examples of the achievements of medical science at an international level. Articulated through the World Health Organization, it is a story of the gradual elimination of the disease from its remaining strongholds in Latin America, Africa and Asia until the last recorded case, outside laboratory accidents, occurred in Somalia in October 1977. The methods by which this was achieved involved not only mass vaccination but also meticulous fieldwork on a large scale to identify patients and their contacts.

Influenza has been described by Professor Sir Charles Stuart-Harris as 'the last of the Great Plagues . . . one of the few communicable diseases we are still unable to control.' While Stuart-Harris's remarks were made before the current AIDS epidemic, it is still nevertheless true that influenza remains, through mortality, reduced quality of life and absence from work, one of the most important sources of economic loss in the developed nations. Loss of working days from influenza far exceeds loss from strikes.

With the elimination of smallpox, international attention has switched to other virus diseases which might yield to the same methods. Measles has been identified as a possible candidate. Apart from its complications, it is not now a life-threatening disease in the context of the developed world but, in the less developed nations of Africa, it frequently carries 30–40 percent mortality. It is also the disease which provides a natural bridge between the methods of the physician, the virologist and the mathematician for, as we shall see, the classic epidemiological work on mathematical models of the spread of disease in human populations nearly always took the well-understood and predictable measles virus as its test-bed. This section therefore forms a bridge to the concluding chapter of the Atlas where models to forecast future maps of disease are studied.

6.2 AIDS: THE START OF A NEW PANDEMIC

The causative virus of AIDS is the lymphadenopathy-associated virus/human T-cell lymphotropic virus type III (LAV/HTLV-III). It is classified under ICD 279. In May 1986, the International Committee on the Taxonomy of Viruses agreed to give the virus the generic name, the **HUMAN IMMUNO-DEFICIENCY VIRUS** (HIV), covering all strains. The virus's host cells in the human body are a type of white blood cell or lymphocyte known as T4 cells. The reproductive mechanism of the virus kills these cells which are a crucial part of the human immune system, laying the body open to a wide range of chance infections which would normally be dealt with by the body's defences. The range of manifestations accordingly range from none, through non-specific illnesses and opportunistic infections, to autoimmune and neurological disorders and several types of malignancy, especially Kaposi's sarcoma.

Two main transmission corridors exist between individuals. The first is through contact with infected blood and blood products. Given the screening and treatment of such products before use in the hospital services of the western nations which has followed the emergence of AIDS, the most common way that infected blood transfers occur in these countries is via the habit of sharing syringes among intravenous drug abusers. The use of unscreened and untreated blood and blood products remains a problem in the developing nations. The second corridor is through sexual contact with an infected person. In the developed countries, the homosexual community where promiscuity is common is most at risk on frequency grounds, but it is important to recognize that spread occurs through conventional heterosexual contact.

---

[1] Analysis of deep-frozen tissue from a 16-year old boy who died with mysterious symptoms, including Kaposi's sarcoma, in St Louis, Missouri, in 1969 has fuelled speculation about earlier existence in the United States of the AIDS virus in minority communities than the first official diagnosis of the disease in

Introduction

Many of the diseases mapped in this Atlas have been scourges of man over the centuries and their origins lie beyond scientific investigation. AIDS had its apparent genesis in more recent years. For the western world, the ostensible start came in the summer of 1980 when, after a long illness, a patient died in a New York City hospital from infections that the human body can normally fight without undue difficulty (Koch, 1987, p.46).[1] Cross checks with other United States hospitals and with other countries revealed not only an alarming number of parallel cases but a very steep rise in hospital admissions of individuals suffering from illnesses which pointed to collapse of the immune system. Because the condition was a result of the breakdown of the immune system, it was called acquired immune deficiency syndrome, or AIDS. The world was on the edge of another of its great pandemics.

Nature of AIDS

The HIV virus is a retrovirus, a group of viruses which can convert their genetic material, RNA, into the genetic material, DNA, which is found in human cells. The virus does its damage by impairing the body's immune system. It has surface proteins which bind to the protein receptors on the surface of a type of white blood cells or lymphocytes known as T4 cells. It then enters the cells and eventually the cytoplasm. Here the viral structure disintegrates, releasing

---

1979. The tissue and blood samples examined by Dr M. Witte of the University of Arizona and Dr R. Garry of Tule University reacted positively to standard tests for HIV.
(Report in *The Daily Telegraph*, November, 1987.)

from its core its genetic RNA and copies of the reverse transcriptase enzyme which the virus uses to multiply itself. The reverse transcriptase first copies the viral RNA into DNA. The DNA then enters the nucleus of the cell, where it becomes incorporated into the cell's own DNA. This makes the virus a permanent part of an infected person's own cells. The original infective virus has given rise to a latent 'provirus' which sits in the cell's DNA to await chemical signals to start it multiplying. The T4 cells are 'helper' cells in fighting infection and, as such, form a crucial part of the human immune system. The reactivating signal thus occurs with

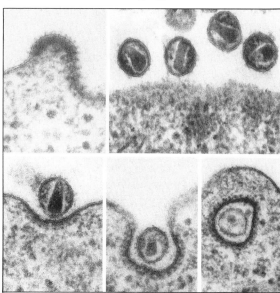

Figure 6.2 (A) Electron micrographs of ultrathin sections of human immunodeficiency virus.
Upper row (left), virus assembly takes place at the cell surface as a budding process; (right), cell-released HIV after maturation show tubulo-prismatic cores containing the ribonucleoprotein portion of the virion.
Lower row, sequential stages in the up-take of HIV by a receptor-mediated process.
Magnification × 120,000.

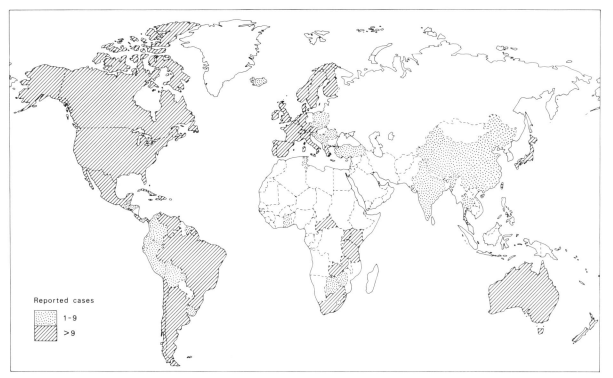

Figure 6.2 (B) Countries reporting AIDS cases to the World Health Organization, 1986

Reported cases
1-9
>9

the arrival in the body of some other infection. This activates the infected T4 cell and with it the latent viral genes. The cell begins to make copies of the viral genes and eventually a new generation of viruses buds from the T4 cell to repeat the process elsewhere in the body. Diagram (A) shows the virus budding from a cell (top) and invading a cell (below). While the virus may spread to other types of cells throughout the body including the brain, the most crucial effect of HIV infection is that it kills the T4 cells in the budding process. It thus selectively damages immune defences, leaving the body vulnerable to other diseases.

There is debate as to the origins of HIV. It is often suggested (Koch, 1987, p.49) that the virus has a common ancestor with a virus found in several African monkeys which it resembles, and that it jumped the species barrier somewhere in Central Africa, probably near the west coast of Lake Victoria where the AIDS epidemic is at its worst. The evidence is, however, speculative.

___

AIDS: the global picture

International information on the AIDS pandemic is available through the World Health Organization's *Weekly Epidemiological Record*. The published data are obtained through regional surveillance systems, national committees or other task forces for the containment of AIDS, epidemiological newsletters and other official sources of information in member countries. As a result, the reporting fabric is very patchy both in time and space. Diagram (B) shows the countries reporting AIDS cases to WHO at the end of 1986 at two levels of intensity. What is more significant is the large number of countries which do not report. These include parts of the globe worst affected by the pandemic, such as Africa and the East Indies, as well as countries, like the USSR, which traditionally have a low WHO reporting record.

There are two causes for the non-reporting of the disease. First, as we have seen in Figures 2.2, 2.3 and 2.5, variable levels of medical care between developed and developing countries and different reporting conventions from country to country result in missing data for even the simplest of diseases. Second, in the case of AIDS there are frequently political and social reasons for the non-reporting of a sexually transmissible disease. However, the data which are assembled by WHO include information on reported cases of AIDS in member countries, along with periodic analyses of its age, sex and risk group distribution.

Diagram (C) shows the cumulative number of reported cases of AIDS in the WHO major world regions on an annual basis from 1979–86. Because of the small number of cases involved and the great variability in accuracy both of the AIDS data and estimates of population from one part of the world to another, the data have been plotted as totals rather than as rates. Note that a logarithmic scale has been used on the vertical axis of each graph to enable widely different case levels to be plotted. Nevertheless, the approximately straight-line growth evident on all the graphs implies, in terms of the original data, exponential growth over the time period considered. Over a longer time period, we would expect logistic rather than continued exponential

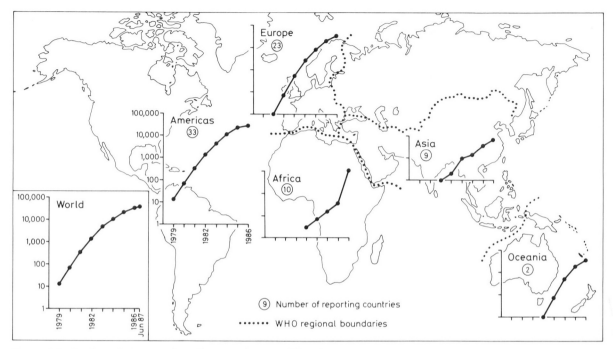

Figure 6.2 (C) Cumulative number of reported cases of AIDS in world regions as defined by the World Health Organization on an annual basis, from 1979 to June 1987

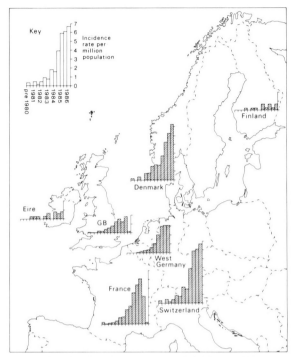

Figure 6.2 (D) Incidence rates for AIDS per million population on a six-monthly basis for 7 European countries, 1979–1986

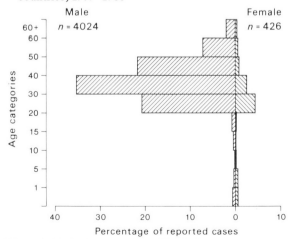

Figure 6.2 (E) Age–sex pyramid of AIDS cases reported for 27 European countries up to the end of 1986

growth [cf. diagram (G), below, for the United States]. As Figure 5.9 shows, the logistic is exponential in its initial stages.

Because of detailed surveillance programmes which exist both in North America and in Europe, data from these regions are among the most reliable returned to WHO. Diagram (D) therefore plots the (non-cumulative) incidence rates for AIDS per million population on a six-monthly basis from 1980–86 for a selection of contrasting European countries. As on the global scale, the initial exponential growth in cases is evident in those countries, like Denmark and Switzerland, with high incidence rates. The German Federal Republic (West Germany) has already assumed the classic logistic shape, while in Finland and Eire an epidemic curve has not yet become established.

The age–sex distribution of AIDS cases is highly characteristic in the countries of the northern hemisphere. Diagram (E) plots the percentage of cases reported in 27 countries of the WHO European region up to 1986 which fell in different age cohorts; an age–sex pyramid has been used (cf. Figure 2.6). Two features merit comment. First, up to the age of 4 years, males and females have the disease in equal proportions. After the age of 15, a concentration of the disease in the male population is found which reflects the transmission routes produced by sexual promiscuity and intravenous drug abuse. The focusing of the disease upon the male population is spectacular between the ages of 20 and 50. The excess in this age group is reinforced if the pyramid is compared with the usual demographic pyramid for the developed nations;

that for Iceland, which is representative, is plotted in Figure 2.6(A).

AIDS in the third world: central Africa

Central Africa displays the impact of AIDS in its most extreme form. It appears, on presently available evidence, to be the most severely affected part of the world, with over two millions probably infected by HIV out of the WHO's estimated world total of 5–10 millions (Mann, 1987, p.43). A substantial amount of research effort has attempted to trace the origins of the disease in the continent and, although medical records have been scoured, the hard evidence suggests that the epidemic started there in the late 1970s and early 1980s concurrent with the epidemics in the United States and Haiti.

The epidemic is worst in central, eastern and parts of southern Africa [map (F), shaded area]. It threatens the economic and social development of the continent; as in Europe, the virus is found primarily among those aged between 20 and 30 years, but it is the urban middle classes (teachers, administrators, doctors, engineers,

traders, mechanics and military officers) whose skills are essential for the future of African countries who are primarily involved. These are the people who travel and have more opportunity for promiscuity than the urban and rural poor.

In Africa there is one fundamental difference in the pattern of the disease compared with the rest of the world. From the outset, a large number of cases have appeared both among women and in the heterosexual community. Roughly half of the African cases are women compared with fewer than 10 percent in the United States and Europe. Spread through sexual contact has therefore been much more rapid.

AIDS in the western world: the United States

Diagram (G) shows both the number and the cumulative number of AIDS cases reported in the United States on a quarterly basis from 1979 to mid-1987. Also shown is the estimated doubling time for cases, in months, calculated from the data at various dates. In an exponential growth process, these doubling times should be

constant when plotted against time. Instead the graph shows that, although constant doubling times are a feature of the start of the epidemic, from mid-1983 the estimated doubling time has increased steadily. This implies that epidemic growth has now slowed and that transfer to the conventional logistic model may be expected to occur [compare the quarterly totals curve in diagram (G) with that for West Germany in diagram (D)]. Using this growth curve approach, the Centers for Disease Control's *Morbidity and Mortality Weekly Report* (MMWR) as of January 1987 projected a cumulative case total in the United States of 270,000 by 1991.

Illustration (H) shows the geographical patterns formed when the initial 10,000 AIDS cases reported (upper map) and the cumulative number recorded per 100,000 population between 1979 and mid-1987 (lower map) are plotted on a state-by-state basis. The distribution of initial cases broadly reflects the distribution of the population, with the interesting anomaly of the state of Colorado. Extremely high concentrations are to be found in California (San Francisco and Los Angeles) and New York (New York City).

By the middle of 1987, the cumulative number of AIDS cases in the United States had reached 38,000. The distribution by states is very skewed, with only Washington DC, New York, New Jersey and California reporting a cumulative rate exceeding the United States average of 16.14 per 100,000 population. Nevertheless, the states in which the initial cases were concentrated [upper map (H)] have continued to record the highest rates throughout the epidemic [lower map (H)]. While most reports of women with AIDS come from the states of Florida, New Jersey and New York, the patterns shown in (H) are dominated by the incidence of the disease in male homosexuals and drug abusers in the major cities.

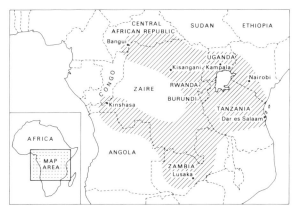

Figure 6.2 (F) Principal areas of Africa affected by AIDS , shown by diagonal shading

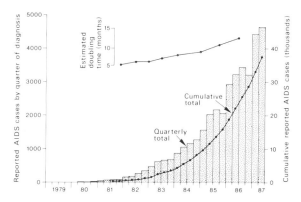

Figure 6.2 (G) Quarterly and cumulative totals of AIDS cases reported for the United States, from 1979 to June 1987

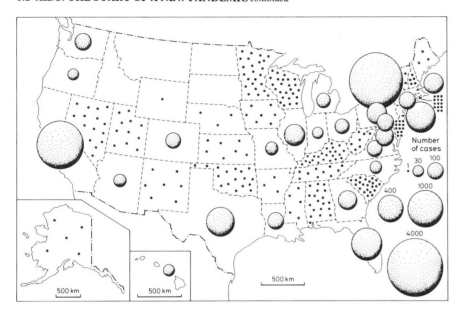

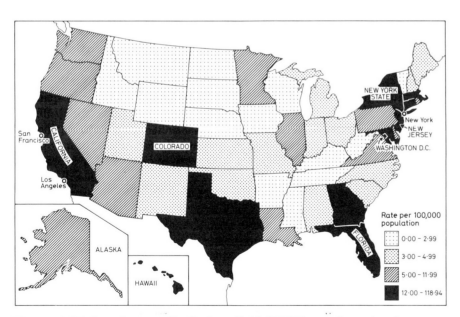

Figure 6.2 (H) State-by-state distribution of initial 10,000 cases (upper), and cumulative number of AIDS cases, per 100,000 population (lower), in the United States, 1979 to mid-1987

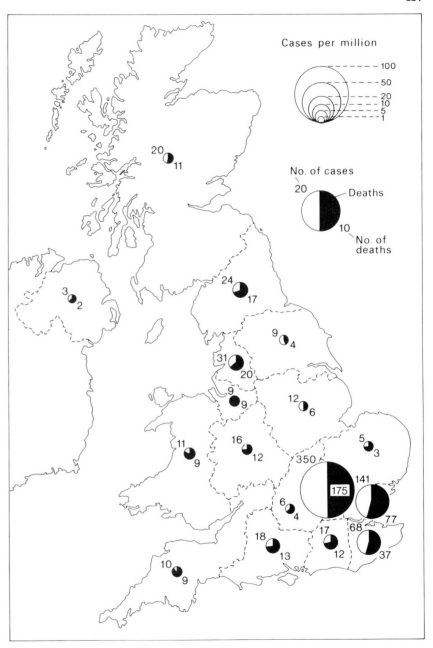

Figure 6.2 (I) Cumulative number of AIDS cases and known deaths for United Kingdom area health authorities to April 1987

AIDS in the western world: England and Wales

In the United Kingdom HIV and AIDS data are published by the Public Health Laboratory Service. Diagram (I) uses proportional circles to show the cumulative number of AIDS cases per million population reported by the end of April 1987 in Wales, Scotland, Northern Ireland and in each of the 14 area health authority areas of England. The segments of the circles which have been shaded black give the cumulative number of deaths, also as a rate per million population. The numbers associated with each circle and slice give the cumulative totals of cases and deaths to set against the rates illustrated by the pie-charts.

The data are interesting for two reasons. First, whether mapped as rates or case levels, diagram (I) shows a clear concentration of the disease in the London area. Second, as we shall see below, although the number of individuals known to be infected with the virus is large, the number who have developed full-blown AIDS or who have died from the disease is small in statistical terms.

If we recognize that most biological growth processes conform to a logistic curve of the type illustrated in Figure 5.9, critical questions are the likely ultimate size of the epidemic and when it will be reached. Given the long incubation period of the disease, relatively imprecise estimates can be obtained of the number of HIV positive patients who will eventually develop full-blown AIDS. As a result, any forecasts of ultimate size are likely to be extremely speculative, with large margins of error.

Diagram (J) shows the cumulative number of HIV positive patients, as a rate per million population, reported on a monthly basis in Wales, Northern Ireland and in each of the regional health authority areas of England since the end of 1984. We use y_{it} to denote the value of

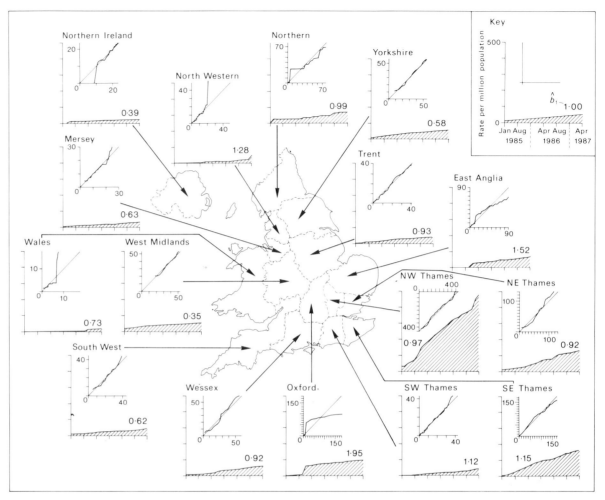

Figure 6.2 (J) Cumulative number of HIV positive patients per million population in Northern Ireland, Wales and the area health authorities of England, by months, from 1985 to April 1987

this variable in area i at time t, and it is plotted on each of the main graphs using diagonal shading below a heavy line. The country divides into two parts. The Northwest Thames, Northeast Thames, Southeast Thames and Oxford health authority areas have experienced much more rapid growth than others and may be regarded as diffusion poles leading the epidemic.

Bearing in mind the exponential growth experienced in other countries in the early stages of the AIDS pandemic, a naive way of generating short-term forecasts is to fit the log regression model,

$$\log y_{i,t+1} = b_0 + b_1 \log t + e_{it}, \qquad (6.2.1)$$

where the $\{e_{it}\}$ are stochastic error terms. The inset graphs on each of the main charts use a heavy line to plot, on the horizontal axis, the rates predicted by the model against, on the vertical axis, the corresponding observed values. Underestimation by the model occurs where points lie above the 45° line; overestimation of rates produces points which lie below the 45° line. With the exception of the Oxford health authority area, good fits are obtained in the core areas of the epidemic, and the fit of the model generally deteriorates as distance from the south-east epicentre increases. The estimated value of b_1, denoted by $\hat{b}_1$, in equation (6.2.1) is shown on each graph.

An alternative to this curve-fitting approach to forecasting is to build a process model based upon likely probabilities of contact between risk groups. Diagram (K) plots by transmission characteristics the percentage of AIDS cases recorded in the United Kingdom up to the end of April 1987. The disease is overwhelmingly concentrated in the male homosexual community, although it is important to stress that the disease has entered the population at large. Knox (1986) has proposed a mixing model based upon this kind of information to examine rates of spread in the population of the United Kingdom. A simplified version is shown in diagram (L) where the risk groups are identified by the ellipses and the vectors give the transmission paths. The numbers indicate the maximum transmission risk as a probability and reflect the known concentration of the disease and level of contact between members of the homosexual community.

Knox's model predicts:

(a) the infection will be self sustaining in the heterosexual as well as in the homosexual community.

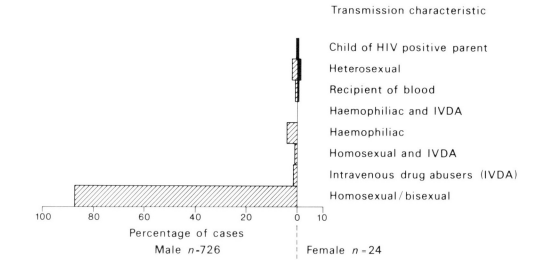

Figure 6.2 (K) Transmission characteristics of all AIDS cases in the United Kingdom to April 1987

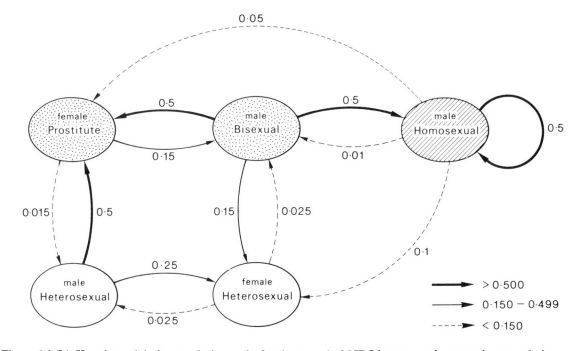

Figure 6.2 (L) Knox's model of transmission paths for the spread of AIDS between sub-groups in a population

(b) the equilibrium prevalence of HIV infection may attain 500–800 per thousand among promiscuous male homosexuals and female prostitutes; 1 to 5 per thousand among non-promiscuous heterosexual males and females; and 8 to 15 per thousand overall.

(c) these equilbria will be reached in about 10 years among the promiscuous classes but not for 40 years among the less promiscuous.

(d) this implies 20,000 to 40,000 deaths per year from AIDS in the United Kingdom; this is about the levels occurring from tuberculosis at the turn of the century, or lung cancer in the 1980s.

Obviously these estimates will be modified by behaviour changes in the population in response to education and fear of infection, but Knox believes that substantial control will depend upon the production of a suitable vaccine. So far, there is no real sign of this occurring.

Conclusion

While it is clear that the AIDS epidemic is a major public health problem, there is some evidence to suggest that in the developed countries a conventional logistic growth process is beginning to assert itself. However, the gradient of the curve is steep and so the equilibrium case totals are likely to be large. For example, Knox's estimated annual death toll of 20–40,000 in the United Kingdom implies, on a pro rata basis, an annual mortality of the order of three millions on a global scale. There is some hard American evidence that public education is having an effect. The WHO *Weekly Epidemiological Record* for 15 November 1985 reports (p.354–55) a survey conducted in August 1984 and April 1985 among homosexual and bisexual males living in San Francisco on the impact of a campaign to encourage them to avoid unsafe sexual practices. As a result of the campaign, the proportion who reported that they were monogamous, celibate or performed unsafe practices only with their steady partner increased from 69 to 81 percent. A fall was also reported in the number having more than one sexual partner in a 30-day period.

One of the great difficulties facing researchers trying to establish the extent of the public health problem is the lack of accurate data on a space-time framework. While confidentiality of the individual is essential, it should be possible, without infringing those rights, to provide fuller information on a finer space–time mesh than is presently available. Only in this way can researchers hope to develop the conceptually elegant, but data demanding, models like that of Knox into a space–time forecasting format.

Sources and Further Reading

Specimen and micrograph for diagram (A) was supplied by Dr Hans Gelderblom of the Robert Koch Institut, Berlin. International data on AIDS cases from the WHO's, *Weekly Epidemiological Record* form the basis of diagrams (B), (C), (D) and (E). Map (F) of AIDS in Africa is redrawn from *The Daily Telegraph*, 6 October 1987. United States data from the Centers for Disease Control's *Morbidity and Mortality Weekly Report* have been used in diagrams (G) and (H, *lower*). The map of the initial 10,000 US cases (H, *upper*) is redrawn from T.A. Peterman, D.P. Drotman and J.W. Curran (1985), 'Epidemiology of the Acquired Immune Deficiency Syndrome (AIDS)', *Epidemiologic Reviews*, 7, pp.1–21, Figure 1, p.7. See also A.K. Dutt, C.B. Munroe, H.M. Dutta and B. Prince (1987), 'Geographical patterns of AIDS in the United States', *Geographical Review*, 77, pp.456–71. The United Kingdom data illustrated in (I), (J) and (K) are taken from the weekly *Communicable Disease Report* of the Public Health Laboratory Service Disease Surveillance Centre, London. The transmission pathways in (L) are drawn from data in E.G. Knox (1986), 'A transmission model for AIDS', *European Journal of Epidemiology*, 2, pp.165–77. See also R. May and R.M. Anderson (1987), 'Transmission dynamics of HIV infection', *Nature*, 326, pp.137–42.

The epidemiological literature on AIDS is growing explosively and any figures are soon outdated. New journals such as *AIDS Research* are being founded to provide new channels for the flood of research papers. A special issue of the *Journal of the Royal Statistical Society*, A151, Part 1 (1988) is devoted to the mathematical modelling and epidemiology of AIDS transmission. A useful review is given in National Academy of Sciences (1986), *Mobilization Against Aids: The Unfinished Story of a Virus*, Cambridge, Mass.: Harvard University Press.

6.3 SMALLPOX: THE END OF AN OLD PANDEMIC

Introduction

So far in this book, we have been concerned primarily with techniques for understanding how diseases spread from place to place. In these circumstances, the area affected becomes steadily larger over time. But it is the objective of both medicine and public health agencies to reverse this process; to interrupt the spread of disease and to push back its geographical extent so that the area affected becomes smaller and smaller.

The outstanding example of such 'diffusion in reverse' is the eradication of smallpox. The story of smallpox is a dramatic tale of a disease with such potential epidemic violence that it has shaped the past, certainly in the New World, but which has now been globally eradicated. Historically, it devastated whole populations; its disappearance was the result of a remarkably persistent and organized effort.

The nature of smallpox

SMALLPOX or **VARIOLA** (ICD 050) was an acute infectious disease caused by an *Orthopoxvirus*, a genus that also includes cowpox, monkeypox and vaccinia viruses. It was caused by a large brick-shaped virus measuring about 250–300 nm × 200–250 nm, with genome consisting of a single molecule of double-stranded deoxyribonucleic acid. In individuals not protected by vaccination, the case fatality of variola major was 15–25 percent overall, rising to 40–50 percent in the very young and the very old. There was a characteristic pustular rash, which left facial pockmarks on most survivors. It was transmitted through oropharyngeal secretions, by direct face-to-face contact between a susceptible person and a patient with a rash. Occasionally airborne spread occurred over longer distances, and infection could also occur via inanimate objects, such as patient's bedding.

Seasonality The virus does better in conditions of relatively low temperature and humidity. As a result, the disease is seasonal (Sarkar, Ray and Manji, 1970). In Bangladesh the seasonality is so marked that the Bengali word for the spring of the year, *bashunto*, is the word for smallpox. In the Punjab there was a distinct winter peak (November to February), with very few cases between June and September (Benenson, 1976). Henderson (1974) gives data on 27 introductions of smallpox into Europe between 1961 and 1973. Twenty in the period from December to May spawned 483 subsequent cases (an average of 4.025 per introduction per month); seven between June and November produced 11 subsequent cases (0.262 per introduction per month).

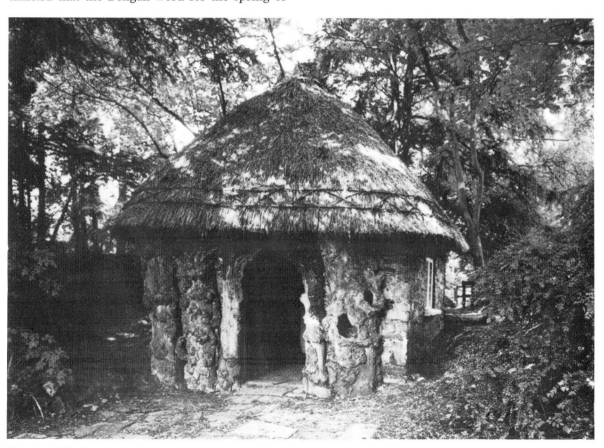

Figure 6.3(A) A current photograph of Jenner's 'Temple of Vaccinia' at Berkeley near Gloucester, England, built *c.* 1800

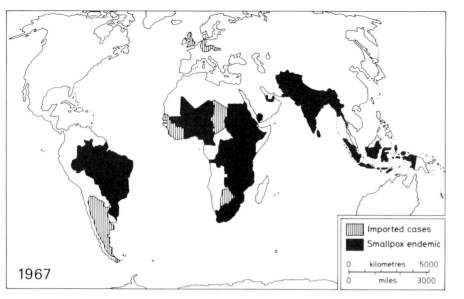

1967

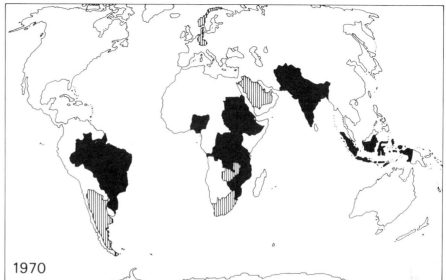

1970

Imported cases

Smallpox endemic

| 0 | kilometres | 5000 |
| 0 | miles | 3000 |

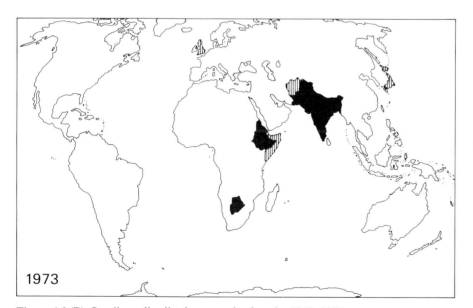

1973

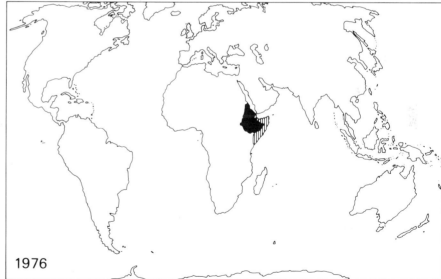

1976

Figure 6.3 (B) Smallpox distribution over the decade, 1967–1976

Historical extent

There are reasons to believe that smallpox as a human disease is of great antiquity. Lesions on the mummified face of Rameses V, dated 1160 BC, suggest that he died of smallpox (Dixon, 1962) and the disease is first clearly described by the Persian physician, Rhazes, in about 900 AD (Kahn, 1963). It was spread through Europe by the Saracen invaders and by the returning Crusaders. The Spaniards took smallpox with them to the West Indies in 1507 and to Mexico in 1520, decimating the Indian population.

In the seventeenth and eighteenth centuries it was the most devastating disease of the Western and in endemic areas generally contracted the disease before the age of ten. In 1707 some 18,000 of the total population of 50,000 of Iceland died from the disease in a single year. In the New World, Boston experienced eight epidemics during the eighteenth century with attack rates as high as 52 percent of the population (Downie, 1970).

The coming of vaccination

Such was the fear of smallpox that experiments in inoculation of smallpox were practised in both the New and the Old Worlds throughout the eighteenth century, often with disastrous consequences. The great advance in the smallpox story was the experiment carried out by the English physician, Edward Jenner, to test the old wives' tale that those who had had cowpox were not susceptible to smallpox. On 14 May 1796 he vaccinated one James Phipps with material obtained from a pustule on the hand of a milkmaid. Six weeks later he attempted, without success, to infect Phipps with pus from a smallpox patient. After several more successful vaccinations, he submitted a report which was rejected but which he later published privately (Jenner, 1798). Photograph (A) shows the hut near his home at Berkeley in Gloucestershire, England, in which Jenner vaccinated many of the poor of the neighbourhood in which he lived.

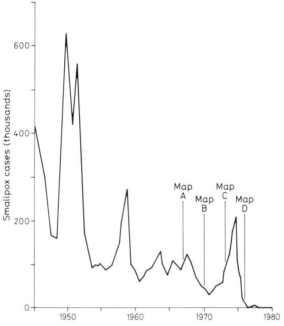

Figure 6.3 (C) Graph of recorded smallpox cases, world scale, 1945–1980

Despite the availability of vaccine, smallpox continued to be endemic over large tracts of the globe. As international travel grew, checks on movement as well as vaccination became routine by the middle of the nineteenth century in western Europe in order to break the chains of infection between individuals. The Atlantic was no barrier to the adoption of similar procedures in North America. As a result the disease was effectively eliminated in the developed nations by the mid-1950s, although sporadic restricted outbreaks still occurred as a result of interna-

tional travel. Map (B) and graph (C) illustrate the last years of this retreat by showing the parts of the globe affected by the disease and the number of reported cases at four dates spaced at three-year intervals (1967, 1970, 1973 and 1976). The final places in which endemic smallpox survived were, as the maps show, located in the Tropics; as late as 1949–51, a massive and uncontrolled epidemic swept through Indonesia and India.

The WHO control programme

Until the mid-1960s control of smallpox was based primarily upon mass vaccination to break the chain of transmission between infected and susceptible individuals by eliminating susceptible hosts. Although, as already shown, this approach had driven the disease from the developed world, the less developed world remained a reservoir area. Thus between 1962 and 1966 some 500 million people in India were vaccinated, but the disease continued to spread. Between 5–10 percent of the population always escaped the vaccination drives, concentrated especially in the vulnerable under-15 age group. The main reason for the missed vaccinations was the great difficulty in vaccinating even 80 percent of a highly mobile population in a poor but very populous country. School children were vaccinated often; pre-school children (particularly in villages) were much harder to trace and vaccinate. Nevertheless, the susceptibility of the virus to concerted action had been demonstrated, and led to critical decisions at the Nineteenth World Health Assembly in 1966.

Nineteenth World Health Assembly This Assembly embarked upon a ten-year Intensified Smallpox Eradication Programme which was launched in 1967. The programme was based upon a series of facts about the disease. Smallpox is transmitted from man to man; infection is manifest and silent carriers are of no epidemiological importance; the infectious period is relatively brief (2–4 days); the incubation period is relatively long (two weeks) allowing intervention to occur; individuals who recover from the disease are resistant to reinfection; vaccination confers long-lasting immunity.

The World Health Organization (WHO) Intensified Smallpox Eradication Programme started with mass vaccination, but rapidly recognized the importance of selective control. Contacts of smallpox cases were traced and vaccinated, as well as the other individuals in those locations where the cases occurred.

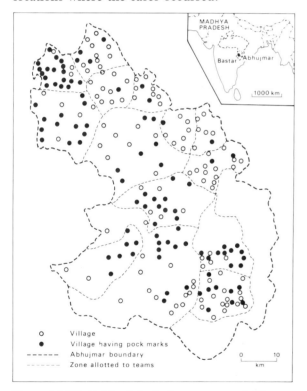

Figure 6.3 (D) Epidemiological assessment of villages in an Indian district, Abhujmar, in the preparatory phase of the WHO Intensified Smallpox Eradication Programme

The Programme had four main phases in each area targeted. In the *preparatory phase*, before active eradication was started, time was allowed for the epidemiological assessment of the distribution of smallpox and immunity in the local population. Map (D) shows how epidemiological assessment was organized in Abhujmar, Bastar District, Madhya Pradesh, India. The area was divided up into some 14 zones, into which small teams of health workers were put. Their task was to record the location of each village in their zone, and whether or not evidence of smallpox was to be found in the village population. During the preparatory phase, health-care personnel were also recruited and trained. Education programmes were established to ensure acceptance of vaccination.

The *attack phase* (while the incidence of smallpox in the targeted community was five or more cases per 100,000 population per annum, and less than 80 percent of the population was vaccinated) consisted of systematic mass vaccination and the establishment of a surveillance programme with follow-up vaccination of contacts and individuals in local areas where cases occurred.

The *consolidation phase* was reached when smallpox incidence fell below 5 cases per 100,000 population per annum and primary vaccination had extended to over 80 percent of the population. This phase consisted of a 'maintenance vaccination programme' for new-borns and those, such as immigrants, missed in the attack phase. The surveillance network now became critical, with every suspected case followed up by field investigation and action where necessary.

The *maintenance phase* was reached when there was no endemic smallpox in the targeted area for more than two years while the disease still persisted on the continent concerned. Maintenance vaccination was continued and intense surveillance continued. Each report of a sus-

pected case was treated as an emergency until final elimination occurred.

The success of this four-phase programme after 1966, following upon the efforts of individual nations in the post-war period, may be judged from map (B) and graph (C). By 1970, retreat was in progress in Africa. By 1973 the disease had been eliminated in Latin America and the Philippines; a few strongholds remained in Africa, but most of the Indian subcontinent

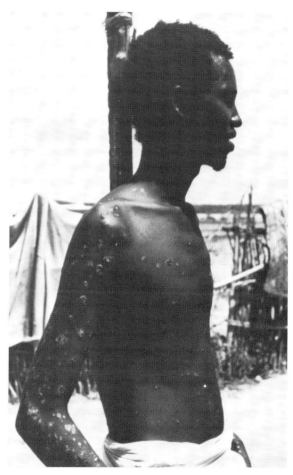

Figure 6.3 (E) The world's last naturally-occurring smallpox case, a 23-year-old Somalian

remained infected. Despite a major flare-up of the disease in 1973 and 1974, the hunt by WHO for cases and case contacts continued. By 1976 the disease had been eradicated in southeast Asia and only a part of East Africa remained to be cleared. The world's last recorded smallpox case (except for a laboratory accident in an English hospital) is shown in photograph (E), 23-years-old Ali Maow Maalin of Merka town, Somalia, who succumbed with the disease on 26 October 1977. After a two-year period during which no other cases (other than the laboratory accident) were recorded, WHO formally announced in December 1979 that the global eradication of smallpox was complete.

The eradication campaign in India

The Indian subcontinent was, as shown in map (B), one of the last strongholds of the disease. Although mass vaccination was practised from 1962, India demonstrated the limitations of such a strategy alone. The large population of the country (543 millions in 1971) and the dense level of settlement in many areas meant that, although primary vaccination was performed on a very large scale, there always remained a large pool of unvaccinated persons which was constantly added to by the high birth rate. Even when vaccination coverage reached 85–90 percent, which was difficult enough in itself to achieve, there remained in many Indian states where smallpox was endemic, a population numbering tens of millions among whom smallpox transmission readily occurred.

In general WHO found that the number of smallpox foci in the country was greater than expected. In some districts the findings showed that up to five percent of the villages were still affected even at the low point of the transmission season. It is a measure of the earlier levels of

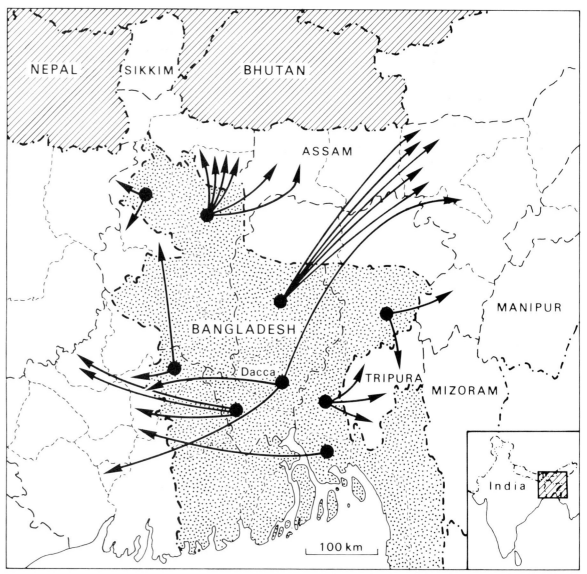

Figure 6.3 (F) Smallpox cases in India in 1975 which originated from movements across the international border with Bangladesh

under-reporting that previous observations suggested smallpox outbreaks did not reach such high levels even during the peak incidence months.

Not only did smallpox remain circulating within India itself but, as map (F) shows for Bangladesh, continual leakage of cases occurred across India's international frontiers until the neighbouring countries were also effectively purged. On map (F), the vectors plot, for 1975, the destination of smallpox cases within India which originated Bangladesh. It was, of course, a two-way process, since India also exported small-pox cases to countries sharing its international frontiers. The dates of the last reported cases in the subcontinent were 16 October 1974 in Pakistan, 6 April 1975 in Nepal, 24 May 1975 in India and 16 October 1975 in Bangladesh.

Once the active surveillance and containment programmes of the later attack and consolidation phases of the WHO campaign were fully implemented, India, with its large number of trained health personnel, was able to complete eradication within a relatively brief period. As graph (G) shows, the intensified smallpox campaign using surveillance methods began in the autumn of 1973. Regular active search was instituted. This inevitably led to a large number of previously unreported cases being discovered and their contacts traced, so that over the next nine months case levels rose sharply. The maps in diagram (H) give, as a point pattern, the geographical locations of cases in four of the north-central states (Madhya Pradesh, Uttar Pradesh, Bihar and West Bengal) discovered by the active searches undertaken in October, November and December of 1973.

Once the first flush of cases discovered by active search throughout India had been dealt with, new cases began to decline in frequency from the middle of 1974 [see graph (G)]. Operation 'Smallpox Zero' began in December 1974, and India was freed of the disease by June 1975. It is important to note, however, that each of the peaks of cases in (G) between October 1973 and October 1974 correspond with the work in the field of the active search teams. For example, in Madhya Pradesh in the week before the first search only nine cases in two of the state's 45 districts were reported, but during the

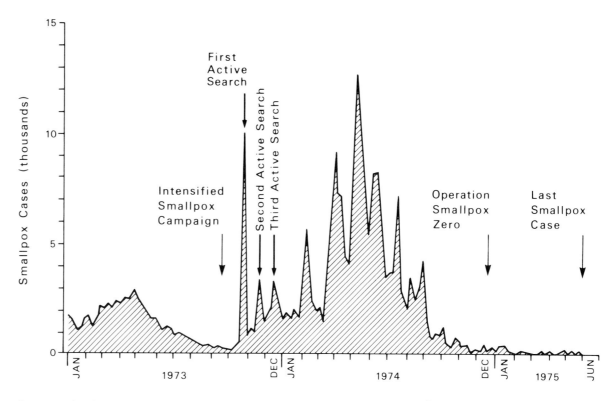

Figure 6.3 (G) Graph of weekly smallpox cases in India from January 1973 to June 1975

first search 1216 smallpox cases were discovered in 164 villages and six municipalities in 16 districts. As shown on the inset graphs of diagram (H), a similar pattern emerged in other states.

The sheer magnitude of the task of freeing a country the size of India of disease like smallpox is staggering. From September 1974 until 1977, a total of 611,495 villages and 1276 towns in 397 districts of the country were searched periodically during each search operation. All endemic states were searched, on average, three times during the last quarter of 1973, eleven times in 1974, nine times in 1975 and three times in 1976. An average of nine searches was conducted in each of these states after they achieved zero incidence status, followed by a further seven after India achieved zero status.

Conclusion

The elimination of smallpox occurred as a result of intense international effort over a substantial period of time. It demonstrated the ability of organized vaccination programmes to break the diffusion links between infectives and contacts, initiating geographical contraction and, ulti-mately, extinction of the disease. The methods employed raise the critical question of whether the same approach might work for other virus-borne diseases and this issue is considered in the next two sections.

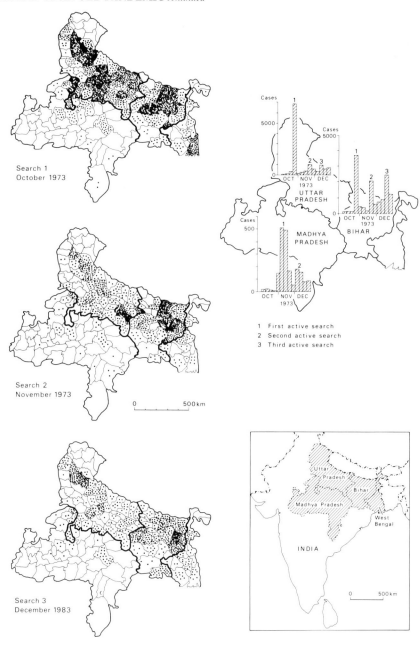

Figure 6.3 (H) Geographical local of smallpox cases found in four Indian states in active searches in October, November and December 1973

Sources and Further Reading

The diagrams in (B) to (G) are based on a series of World Health Organization reports, *The Global Eradication of Smallpox* (1980), *Eradication of Smallpox from India* (Basu *et al.*, 1979) and *Eradication of Smallpox from Bangladesh* (Joarder *et al.*, (1980). The photograph in (A) is by the authors, and (E) from WHO/J. Wickett, and published on p.1067 in F. Fenner *et al.* (1988); see below.

Jenner's classic account of vaccination against smallpox is given in E. Jenner (1798), *An Inquiry into the Causes and Effects of the Variolae Vacciniae, a Disease Discovered in Some of the Western Counties of England, Particularly Gloucestershire, and Known by the Name of Cowpox*, London: Sampson Low. Subsequent steps in the battle against smallpox are traced in C. Kahn (1963), 'History of smallpox and its prevention', *American Journal of Diseases of Children*, 106, pp.597–609. The best recent account of the history of smallpox is D.R. Hopkins (1983), *Princes and Peasants: Smallpox in History*, Chicago: Chicago University Press.

The classic and definitive account of the WHO campaign for the global eradication of smallpox is F. Fenner, D.A. Henderson, I. Arita, Z. Jesek and I.D. Ladnyi (1988), *Smallpox and Its Eradication*, Geneva: World Health Organization. See also F. Fenner (1977), 'The eradication of smallpox', *Progress in Medical Virology*, 23, pp.1–21. An early study of eradication possibilities is given in E.H. Hinman (1966), *World Eradication of Infectious Diseases*, Springfield, Ill.: Thomas.

The basic epidemiology of smallpox is reviewed in A.B. Benenson (1984), 'Smallpox', in *Viral Infections of Humans: Epidemiology and Control*, second edition, edited by A.S. Evans, New York: Plenum, pp.541–68. See also C.W. Dixon (1962), *Smallpox*, London: Churchill Livingstone; A.W. Downie (1970), 'Smallpox', in *Infectious Agents and Host Reactions*, edited by S. Mudd, Philadelphia, Penn.: Saunders, pp.487–518; D.A. Henderson (1974), 'Importation of smallpox into Europe', *WHO Chronicle*, 28, pp.428–30; and J.K. Sarkar, S. Ray and P. Manji (1970), 'Epidemiological and virological studies in the off-season smallpox cases in Calcutta', *Indian Journal of Medical Research*, 58, pp.829–39.

6.4 INFLUENZA: A CHANGING VIRUS WITH UNIQUE EPIDEMIC WAVES

INFLUENZA (ICD 487; see Figure 2.1) is the clinical illness caused by some members of the myxoviruses. Influenza viruses occur as one of three main types, A, B or C. It is influenza A which generally causes the great pandemics and regular epidemics of the disease. The A virus has the ability to change its surface antigen structure to a degree which gives it the means of bypassing population immunity acquired from exposure to a strain of the virus with a different surface antigen structure. Major changes in the surface antigens are termed shifts and produce the great pandemics like that of 1957 considered in this section. Minor changes are called drifts and lead to regular epidemic cycles of the disease witnessed in most winters.

The clinical onset of influenza is marked by shivering, sweating, coughing and aching pains in the muscles of the back and limbs. The total course of an attack from initial virus receipt to recovery may be up to ten days.

Introduction

Influenza has been described by Stuart-Harris and Schild (1976, p.96) as 'an unchanging disease due to a changing virus', and it is the continually changing character of the virus which makes its epidemiology so fascinating to study.

In this section, we explore some of the space–time patterns of influenza at several spatial scales in an attempt to improve our understanding of the geographical characteristics of the disease. Prior to the main discussion, we outline some of the difficulties involved in estimating influenza prevalence. Then the 1957 pandemic is used to illustrate the important relationships between the size and rapidity of spread of the global pandemics and the normal years of influenza epidemics which both precede and follow them. These ideas are tested first at the global scale (population about 3.5 to 4 billions in 1957), then at the regional scale and finally at the local scale in a single country doctor's practice of about 3,500 to 4,000 patients in Cirencester, England. The regional settings selected are Iceland (population about 180,000 in 1957) and England and Wales (population about 45 millions in 1957).

Measuring influenza prevalence

So that a proper assessment can be made of the geographical patterns to be presented, it is important to be aware of the difficulties involved in estimating influenza prevalence. Reporting practices for influenza vary greatly from country to country. Globally in 1957 some 110 countries reported influenza morbidity and about 90 influenza mortality [cf. Figure 2.3]. Iceland records both morbidity and mortality while in the United Kingdom only mortality is reported. To estimate morbidity in the United Kingdom, two indirect measures are generally used (see Figure 2.4 for details). In the first, a panel of general practitioners in different geographical regions of England and Wales notify the occurrence of cases of acute respiratory illness in their practice to the Epidemiological Research Unit of the Royal College of General Practitioners. These returns provide a sensitive index of influenza prevalence when suitably scaled up; the data are further refined by tests on throat swabs. For the second measure use is made of the weekly data on new claims for sickness benefit in the working population recorded in National Insurance returns.

Even using influenza mortality returns to assess prevalence is not straightforward. In the United Kingdom, for example, the disease may be recorded on death certificates as a primary or secondary (associated) cause of death. The complications of influenza can affect the cardiovascular and nervous systems as well as the lower respiratory tract. Increases in influenza incidence can therefore show up in increased deaths from heart disease as well as in deaths from influenza and pneumonia (cf. Figure 3.13).

The implication of the above discussion is that reported levels of influenza prevalence greatly underestimate the actual cases occurring, especially at the global level. Cliff, Haggett and Ord (1986, pp.90–93) have estimated that the 'real' total of influenza cases may be anywhere between three and 15 times greater. This recording gap means that caution must be exercised in studying influenza patterns. On the other hand, the data are not so far out that they are beyond analysis. For example, the use of changes in levels is an effective way of tackling the data. In addition, the selection of Iceland is deliberate because, as discussed later in section 6.5.2, the Icelandic data are known to be highly reliable. In the same way, the particular doctor's practice in Cirencester was selected because the great majority of clinical cases of influenza reported there were confirmed in the laboratory as being either sero- or virus-positive.

The Kilbourne model

Influenza follows the typical seasonal pattern of many respiratory virus diseases in having, at all spatial scales, a low summer and a high winter incidence. Over a longer time scale, the regular annual cycles of influenza epidemics are interrupted by major pandemics at intervals of ten to forty years associated with fundamental changes,

called *shifts*, in the haemagglutinin (H) and
neuraminidase (N) surface antigens of the virus
(Stuart-Harris, Schild and Oxford, 1985). The
conventional argument is that the antigenic shifts
produce a virus which has not been met before
by most members of the population (and certainly not by most children) and to which they
have little or no antibody protection. The shifted
virus produces pandemics which result in the
infection of a large proportion of the world's
population, perhaps between one and two thirds,
and they are followed by smaller annual
epidemics involving variants which have *drifted*
from the current pandemic strain.

Diagram (A) shows a schematic model, proposed by Kilbourne (1973), of the relationship
between the number of cases produced by the
original pandemic and later epidemics. Once the
new strain, A2, is introduced into the population
and individuals become infected, so antibody
levels to the strain build up in the population
over time (pecked line). This process leads to a
diminishing population stock susceptible to the
strain and so to successively smaller epidemics
with a greater time interval between them (solid
line). Kilbourne argued that the natural selection
pressures forced upon the virus trigger antigenic
drift, eventually causing a new strain [A3 in
diagram (A)] to emerge which would not have
been previously encountered by individuals in
the population and to which antibody levels
would be low [chain pecked line in diagram (A)].
This new virus causes the next pandemic and the
process is repeated.

Despite the conceptual elegance and
seemingly obvious nature of Kilbourne's model,
evidence for its existence is elusive whenever raw
influenza data are studied. A major difficulty is
that relatively few shifts (only some four or five)
have occurred in the last hundred years. In
addition, there is some suggestion in more recent
years of more than one A-type virus circulating

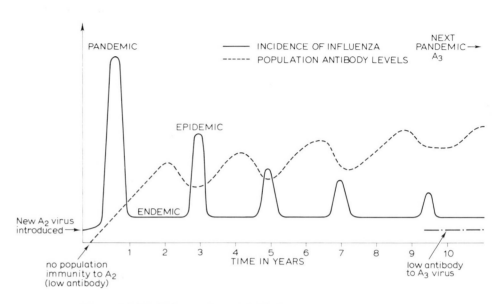

Figure 6.4 (A) Kilbourne's model of influenza waves

in the population at the same time, a possibility
which is not considered in the Kilbourne model.

Notwithstanding these difficulties we define in
the technical appendix to this section a measure
of *average epidemic intensity*, denoted by b_0,
which, when calculated for the recorded case
levels of the 1957 pandemic and epidemics in
preceding and succeeding years, points strongly
to the validity of the Kilbourne model. Although
mathematical details are given in the appendix,
we note here that large values of b_0 correspond
with high incidence rates and small values with
the lower levels of infection observed in most
winters. We should therefore expect a plot of b_0
against time to display the cycles shown in
diagram (A) if the Kilbourne model is applicable.

The Asian influenza pandemic: global patterns

In February 1957 a new strain of influenza virus
appeared for the first time in an epidemic in the
Kweichow province of China. Eventually designated A/Asian/57 (H2N2), and popularly called
Asian influenza, this virus differed fundamentally from the H1N1 strain which had
been in circulation, along with variants, certainly
since 1947 and possibly for much longer.
Because of the fundamental shift in the character
of the surface antigens, neuraminidase (N) and
haemagglutinin (H), this new strain was able to
by-pass the immunity in the world's population
to previous strains of the virus and, wherever it
was encountered, major attack rates ensued
leading to a world-wide pandemic.

From its initial hearth in China, the virus spread rapidly across the world. The corridors it followed are mapped in (B). On this diagram, the digit of the month in which infection was first reported in each country is recorded; the spread vectors are constructed from this sequence of dates. The pandemic seems to have spread from China by two pathways: westwards via the Trans-Siberian railway into European Russia, and by sea from Hong Kong to Singapore and Japan (Stuart-Harris, 1965, p.102). It had reached the Indian subcontinent by May, Africa by July, Western Europe by June, the United Kingdom by September, Australia by July and both seaboards of the United States by June. The new virus thus swept around the globe in about eight months from its time of first recognition. While still within the first season of the virus, a second wave of the disease affected Western Europe between September 1957 and January 1958; these outbreaks are denoted by squares on map (B).

The number of cases of influenza caused by the virus is recorded in the World Health Organization's (WHO) *World Health Statistics Annual*. As noted above, much care is needed in interpreting the figures. Many of the world's countries do not return influenza morbidity data to WHO, while significant levels of under-reporting occurs among those which do. Major omissions include the United States, the United Kingdom, Canada, Australia, New Zealand and the USSR. Bearing this limitation in mind, we have mapped in (C) the reported cases of influenza per thousand population in each of the WHO reference regions; the regional boundaries are shown by the heavy lines.

The world-wide nature of the pandemic is reinforced by this diagram when we bear in mind that the average incidence of influenza per thousand population reported by WHO between 1945 and 1977 was 19.2 for Europe, 2.7 for

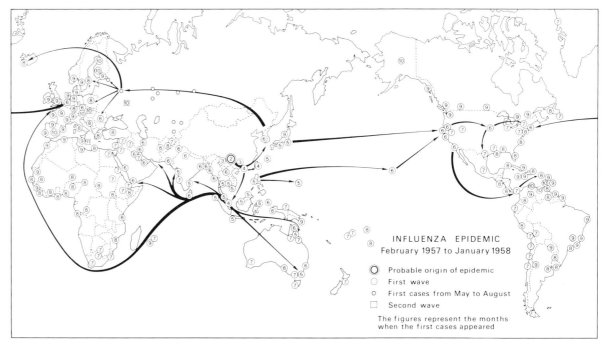

Figure 6.4 (B) Global sequence of spread of the 1957–1958 influenza pandemic

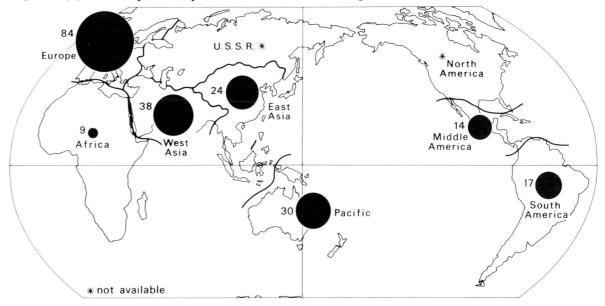

Figure 6.4 (C) Reported cases of influenza per thousand population in seven of the nine WHO regions, 1957

Africa, 7.5 for West Asia, 4.1 for East Asia, 29.5 for the Pacific, 3.8 for Middle America and 4.1 for South America. All the regional rates shown in (C) greatly exceed these figures. Nevertheless, map (C) still conceals considerable variation between individual countries. Thus the European average of 84 cases per 1000 population included Finland (150), Denmark (121), Iceland (111), and Czechoslovakia and Poland (110). In the Pacific, the place-to-place contrasts were even greater, with small islands like Niue reaching rates of 526 cases per 1000 population, while the Gilbert and Ellice group and Tonga both returned values of over two hundred cases per thousand population. Worldwide, there was a tendency for smaller territories, especially if they were also islands, to show rates which were much more extreme than those of larger countries.

In terms of the Kilbourne model, the 1957 pandemic thus displayed the rapid geographical spread and high attack rates expected of a new virus strain. In the time domain, the relationship between cases per thousand population in the pandemic and case rates reported to WHO in other influenza years is examined in diagram (D). Using annual data between 1945 and 1977 for the seven world regions shown in map (C), the upper graph in (D) plots the value of b_0 (denoted by $\hat{b}_0$), average epidemic intensity, against time as a pecked line. The solid line is a running mean of the values. Comparison of the smoothed values for $\hat{b}_0$ with the theoretical curve (A) shows the basic similarity between observation and theory. The average attack rate in the seven regions fell steadily between 1946 and 1956. An upturn occurred with the virus shift from H1N1 to H2N2 in 1957; this is much more apparent in the unsmoothed than in the smoothed values for $\hat{b}_0$. Attack rates fell again after 1957. A slight increase developed prior to the 1968 shift which may have been caused by

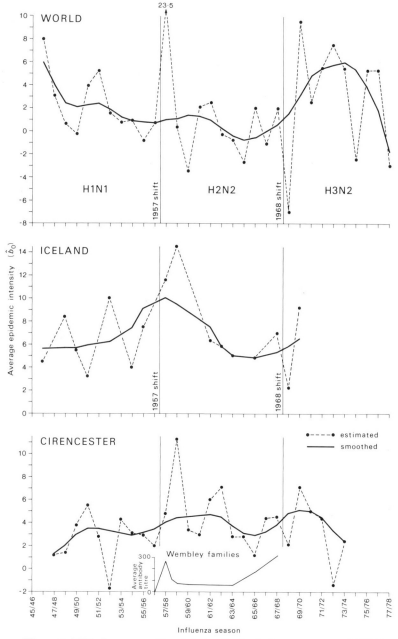

Figure 6.4 (D) Average epidemic intensity for influenza seasons 1945/6 to 1977/8 at three geographical scales

drift of the parent H2N2 virus in its later years. The first four seasons of the H3N2 virus were marked by a dramatic increase in attack rates but, as predicted by the Kilbourne model, these have declined since 1971.

The Asian influenza pandemic: national patterns

Iceland One country in which the history of the pandemic is particularly well recorded is Iceland. As described later in section 6.5.2, the basic source of data is *Heilbrigðisskýrslur* (1957, pp. 75–9 and 1958, pp.72–3). In the spring and early summer of 1957 cases of influenza from the previous season continued to be reported at a low level. However in late April the Icelandic authorities became aware of the influenza epidemic in China and other southeast Asian countries 'caused by a previously unknown strain of virus'. They noted its subsequent spread and

In July and August news then began to be brought from Europe that the disease had arrived there, in Holland, in England, and West Germany. Our first dealings with the disease . . . happened as a result of air communications [from the international airport and military airfield at Keflavík in southwest Iceland] with the military airfields at Thule in Greenland. The disease began there on 3 July, reached a peak on 12 July, and attacked sixty to seventy percent of the airfield's employees. Consequently on 15 July, four Icelandic pilots and two air hostesses were quarantined after returning from there but none of them fell ill . . . On 22 August two ships arrived from abroad, *Gullfoss* from Copenhagen and *Koöperatio* from Russia, with participants in the youth

meeting in Moscow. They brought news . . . of a disease . . . said to be Asian influenza at the Moscow meeting.

Thus despite the early summer alarms, the disease eventually arrived in Iceland via the Soviet route shown on the global map of influenza, (B).

The quotation also gives the first hint of the extremely high attack rates associated with the new virus strain which were to be experienced by Iceland in the pandemic. In this first season of Asian influenza, the reported case rate was 111 per thousand population, equalled or exceeded in this century only by the seasons of 1928–9 (111), 1936–7 (189) and 1958–9 (the second Asian influenza year, 116). The geographical distribution in the medical districts is shown in map (E) using the method of proportional circles. The frequency distributions of cases against time for both Iceland as a whole and Reykjavík appear as bar graphs, along with the values of the Pearson measures of skewness (b_1) and kurtosis (b_2). During the peak months of October and November, the level of sickness

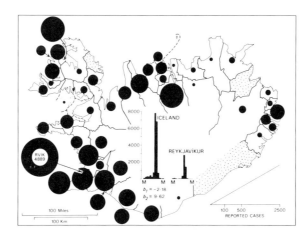

Figure 6.4 (E) Distribution of influenza cases in Iceland during the 1957–1958 pandemic

caused doctors in four districts to report closure of schools for periods of about two weeks. The disease seems to have affected the age groups of 5–10 years and 40–60 years most severely.

The new virus also brought high mortality. The Director-General of Public Health commented 'this is the fourth greatest year for influenza deaths since 1918 when the Spanish disease itself was raging. The figures for influenza deaths for these four years are 1919 : 91,   1921 : 79,   1937 : 87,   1957 : 55, 1919–57 average for all years 22.3.' In terms of the Kilbourne model, the high level of infection and mortality produced in Iceland by the new strain was thus the same as on the world stage.

To place the 1957 pandemic in an Icelandic context, we consider how it compared with the intensity of the seventeen influenza epidemics to have affected the country between 1945 and 1970. Returning to diagram (D) and using the same methodology as with the international data already analysed, the middle graph plots the average epidemic intensity ($\hat{b}_0$) estimated from the number of reported cases of influenza per thousand population in each medical district in each year, 1945–70. The smoothed intensity curve is identical in form to Kilbourne's model shown in diagram (A), with a substantial increase in influenza intensity around the virus shift year of 1957. A steady decline is evident after 1957, with a second upturn after the virus shift to Hong Kong influenza in 1968. Thus the Icelandic data, like the global, show the cycles in case levels predictable from the Kilbourne model.

England and Wales Given the absence of official notifications of influenza, the geographical distribution of the disease in the United Kingdom in any year has to be determined from the surrogate sources outlined in Figure 2.4 (Cliff, Haggett and Ord, 1986, pp. 18–24). The spread

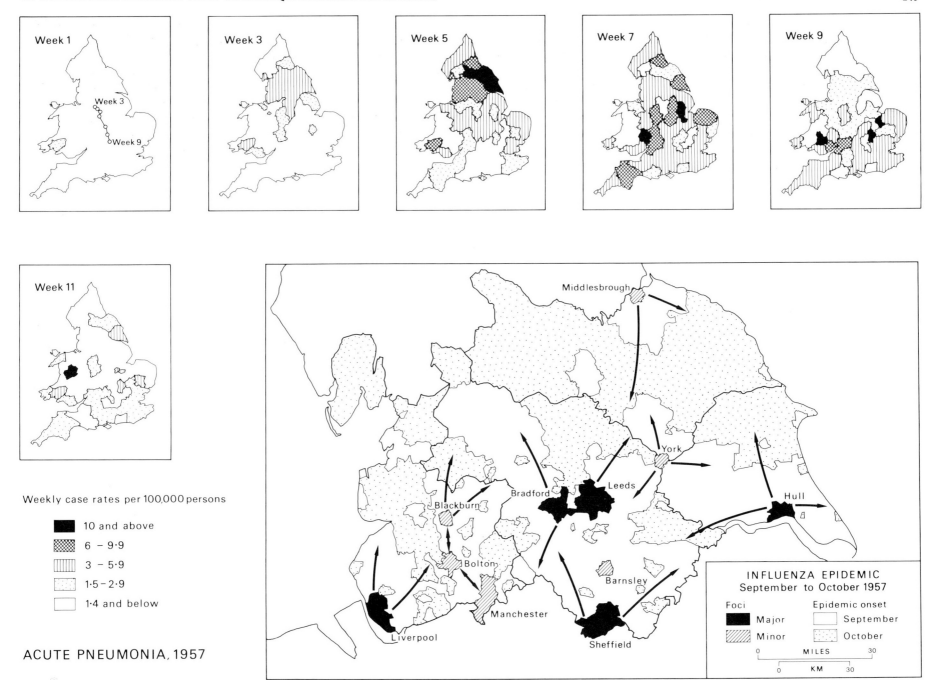

ACUTE PNEUMONIA, 1957

Figure 6.4 (F) **Geographical path of the influenza pandemic of 1957 plotted for England, Wales and northern England**

of Asian influenza in its first season in England and Wales has been so reconstructed by Hunter and Young (1971). Again the high attack rates and rapid spread postulated for a new virus strain in the Kilbourne model are evident.

The disease entered England and Wales in June and, as in Iceland, the main points of ingress appear to have been seaports rather than airports. The epidemic flowered in September and, over the next twelve weeks, about six million cases of the disease occurred, an estimated incidence of 11.5 percent. This compares, for example, with a rate of about 6.2 percent per annum in Iceland between 1945 and 1970, where notification of influenza cases is compulsory. Distinct regional variations in attack rates were evident. Roughly twenty percent of the population in the north was affected compared with only ten percent or less in the south. Still lower rates were found in the Welsh hill counties and in the more isolated parts of northwest England.

The maps of weekly spread shown in diagram (F) are based upon the notifications of acute pneumonia cases in the General Register Office (GRO) areas of England and Wales. The maps have been drawn at two-weekly intervals and the shading is proportional to the weekly case rate per 100,000 persons. As well as showing the initial outbreak of the disease in west Wales, the map for week one in diagram (F) also plots the trajectory followed by the centre of gravity of the epidemic over the full twelve-week period (cf. 5.10). Until early October, the centre was firmly located in northern England. Most counties in southern England escaped until the fourth week of the epidemic. Then as the epidemic began to wane in the north, the centre began to shift rapidly southwards and, by week six, only three counties in southern England and five in central and west Wales were uninfected. Thus the whole of southern England and Wales was invaded within a two-week period.

A more detailed view of the spread of influenza within northern England also appears in diagram (F). The map shows the eleven influenza foci of Lancashire and Yorkshire from which the disease diffused throughout northern England. Three were major seaports (Liverpool, Hull and Middlesbrough). The remaining eight were inland centres. Schematic diffusion corridors have been added the basis of an analysis of the weekly returns from each GRO area. Areas of early onset in September form rings around the initial foci. Areas in which onset of the epidemic was delayed until October have been stippled. The disease thus seems to have spread out from its core areas in a simple wave-like progression. However, once the epidemic reached any location, its subsequent history in that area seems to have been effectively independent of the starting date; acute epidemic conditions (with over 42 percent local infection) occurred in 29 GRO areas widely scattered throughout both urban and rural districts.

Although the graph of cases against time in most communities displayed a single and well-marked peak, a few GROs experienced a double wave or biphasic epidemic curve. The latter were particularly common in cities with communities which were distinct in terms of either ethnic origin, socio-cultural identification or occupational structure. In Bradford, a Yorkshire textile city whose location is shown on (F), a small wave peaked in a Pakistani community in advance of the main wave [graph (G)]. This was probably related to the early introduction of the disease into the community by an infected air passenger visiting from Pakistan. According to local general practitioners in the area, rapid spread seems to have ensued because of the custom among Pakistanis of visiting the sick in large numbers. Double peaks were also identifiable among the steel workers of Sheffield and the coal-miners of Barnsley.

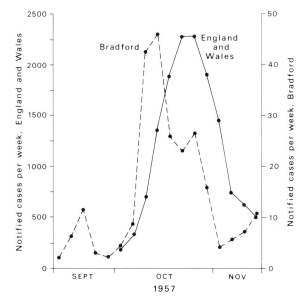

Figure 6.4 (G) Comparison of Bradford with England and Wales of the timing of the Asian influenza pandemic of 1957

The Asian influenza pandemic: local patterns

A micro-level example of impact of the pandemic is provided by the single doctor's practice of R. E. Hope-Simpson in Cirencester, England. This market town, which lies between Gloucester and Swindon in the English Cotswolds, had a population of about 12,000 in 1957. Hope-Simpson's practice covered an area of about eighty square miles, extending up to seven miles from the centrally located surgery in Cirencester. In this practice, individual patients were identified and influenza was diagnosed and studied by a single doctor and his partner over a thirty-year period following the end of the Second World War.

The panel consisted of between three and four thousand patients and Hope-Simpson kept very detailed daily records of the incidence of several infectious diseases, but especially influenza, for each patient. Working with the help of his wife and later with the support of the Medical Research Council and the Public Health Laboratory Service he set up an Epidemiological Research Unit in Cirencester. By converting cottage rooms at his surgery in Dyer Street, he established a laboratory to permit identification of the viruses isolated from his patients. As a result, this unique practice became internationally known and it provides an unrivalled window into the operation of epidemiological processes at the micro-scale. The period from about 1961 to 1973, when Higgins was in charge of the laboratory and Hope-Simpson was director of the unit as a whole, was particularly profitable, and most of the basic virological work was undertaken in these years.

Using Hope-Simpson's data, some of which are published in Cliff, Haggett and Ord (1986, pp. 45–86), the features of rapid geographical spread and high attack rates predicted by the Kilbourne model can be as readily detected in the 1957 pandemic at this local geographical scale as they have been at the regional and the global. In the first season of the disease, Hope-Simpson recorded 669 clinical cases compared with an average rate of only 351 over the other

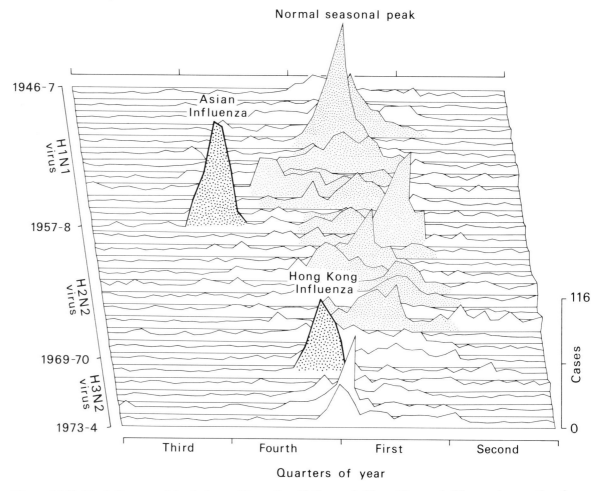

Figure 6.4 (I) Block diagram of the timing and intensity of influenza in Hope-Simpson's Cirencester practice, from 1946/7 to 1973/4

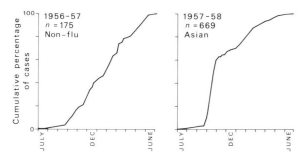

Figure 6.4 (H) Cumulative percentage of influenza cases for a non-epidemic year (left) and an epidemic year (right) for Hope-Simpson's Cirencester practice

years between 1946 and 1974. Diagram (H) gives the cumulative percentage of cases for the weekly incidence of influenza in the practice for two seasons, 1956/57 (which was a non-epidemic year for influenza in Cirencester) and for 1957/58 (the first season of Asian influenza). The striking contrast in the gradient of the two curves is apparent, with almost sixty per cent of the cases occurring between the last week in September

and the middle of October in the first season of Asian influenza; this appears as the vertical section of curve of the 1957/58 chart. Conversely, in the non-epidemic year, the 175 cases arrived as a steady trickle throughout the season.

If the 1957/58 season is looked at in the context of all influenza seasons between 1946 and 1974, it is possible to produce the block diagram shown in diagram (I). It is evident from this diagram that, in the first season of Asian influenza, like the early years of the Hong Kong virus (since 1968/69), the peak incidence of influenza occurred much earlier in the year than was usual in the practice. In the case of Asian influenza the peak month was October, compared with February and March in most other seasons. The two peaks corresponding with the major virus shifts stand out on the diagram well to the left of the main range of peaks representing the normal late winter seasonal maximum. This appearance of an early peak at times of antigenic shift in the causative virus can be related to the larger stock of susceptibles available for immediate infection on such occasions.

The test of the Kilbourne model by plotting average epidemic intensity against time appears in the last graph in diagram (D); the calculations have been based upon the number of clinically identified cases of influenza in the Hope-Simpson practice in each influenza season, 1947–74. The lower part of the diagram gives the average antibody titre (informally defined as a measure of the amount of antibody present, in this case to the H2N2 virus, as determined by titration) recorded in fifteen individuals sampled at regular intervals during the H2N2 virus period. These are the so-called 'Wembley families data' and are unpublished. They have been kindly supplied to us by M.S. Pereira, formerly of the Public Health Laboratory Service, Colindale.

The message conveyed is clear and is consistent with diagram (A). As the Wembley families data show, exposure for the first time to the H2N2 virus caused a rapid rise in antibody levels to the virus. This resistance fell steadily with time until antibody levels were sufficiently low towards the end of the H2N2 period for reinfection to be possible; then antibody levels rose again. The smoothed curve for $\hat{b}_0$ in the upper part of the diagram shows average influenza intensity in the Hope-Simpson practice rising during shift years and falling in the second half of each virus period as the susceptible population diminished.

Conclusion

Study of the rates of geographical spread and levels of cases reported in the 1957 influenza pandemic at global, regional and local scales has shown that virus drift and shift are potent methods by which influenza renews itself periodically to sweep the globe on a scale akin to the great nineteenth-century cholera pandemics discussed in Chapter 1. In addition, the method of analysis described in the technical appendix to this section has enabled the Kilbourne model to be detected in case-rate data for influenza at a variety of spatial scales. Given the continually changing nature of the influenza virus, the prospects for control are somewhat bleak. Thus Smith (1976, p.291) states:

> The attempted elimination of either pandemic or inter-pandemic influenza is, therefore, unrealistic at the present time. It is, however, entirely reasonable to attempt seriously to mitigate the impact of the disease . . . [by] annual vaccination of those at greatest risk.

In contrast, as the United States experience discussed in Figure 4.9 has shown, the global elimination of measles is much more foreseeable and we consider the geography of this disease in the next section.

Sources and Further Reading

The standard reference book on the disease is Professor Sir Charles Stuart-Harris, G.C. Schild and J.S. Oxford (1985), *Influenza: The Viruses and the Disease*, 3rd edn, London: Edward Arnold, and diagram (B) is redrawn from the first (1965) edition of this book. Maps (F) and (G) which show the spread of the 1957 Asian influenza pandemic in England and Wales, have been redrawn from J.M. Hunter and J.C. Young (1971), 'Diffusion of influenza in England and Wales', *Annals of the Association of American Geographers*, 61, pp.637–53. The source for the remaining diagrams in this section is A.D. Cliff, P. Haggett and J.K. Ord (1986), *Spatial Aspects of Influenza Epidemics*, London: Pion.

The Kilbourne model is described in E.D. Kilbourne (1973), 'The molecular epidemiology of influenza', *Journal of Infectious Diseases*, 127, pp.478–87. The economic impact of influenza upon populations is discussed in J.W.G. Smith (1976), 'Vaccination strategy', in *Influenza: Virus, Vaccines, Strategy*, edited by P. Selby, London: Academic Press, pp.271–94.

Recent Russian work on influenza modelling is described in O.V. Baroyan, L.A. Genchikov, L.A. Rvachev and V.A. Shashkov (1969), 'An attempt at large-scale influenza epidemic modelling by means of a computer', *Bulletin of the International Epidemiological Association*, 18, pp.22–31, and in O.V. Baroyan, L.A. Rvachev and Y.G. Ivannikov (1977), *Modelling and Prediction of Influenza Epidemics in the USSR*, Moscow: Gamaleia Institute of Epidemiology and Microbiology. See also L.A. Rvachev and I.M. Longini (1985), 'A mathematical model for the global spread of influenza', *Mathematical Biosciences*, 75, pp.3–22, and L.R. Elveback, J.P. Fox, E. Ackerman, A. Langworthy, M. Boyd and L. Gatewood (1976), 'An influenza simulation model for immunization studies', *American Journal of Epidemiology*, 103, pp.152–65.

An excellent critical review of influenza modelling is given in P.E.M. Fine (1982), 'Applications of mathematical models to the epidemiology: a critique', in *Influenza Models: Prospects for Development and Use*, edited by P. Selby, Lancaster, Penn.: MTP Press, pp.15–85.

Technical appendix

A regression formulation of the Kilbourne model

Let I_{it} denote the number of cases of influenza (per thousand population) reported in a given area at a time t of the T-time period influenza season i. Set

$$I_{it} = b_0 + b_1 I_{i-1,t} + e_{it}, \; t = 1,2, \ldots ,T. \qquad (6.4.1)$$

Equation (6.4.1) allows the average behaviour of influenza season i to be expressed as a linear function of that behaviour in season $i-1$. Denote the ordinary least squares estimates of b_0 and b_1 by $\hat{b}_0$ and $\hat{b}_1$ respectively. It is well known from the statistical theory of the general linear model that the relationship,

$$\hat{I}_{it} = \hat{b}_0 + \hat{b}_1 \hat{I}_{i-1,t}, \qquad (6.4.2)$$

implies

$$\bar{I}_{it} = \hat{b}_0 + \hat{b}_1 \bar{I}_{i-1,t}, \qquad (6.4.3)$$

Here the bars are used to denote the means of the variable. Taking equation (6.4.3) from equation (6.4.2) yields

$$(\hat{I}_{it} - \bar{I}_{it}) = \hat{b}_1 (I_{i-1,t} - \bar{I}_{i-1,t}). \qquad (6.4.4)$$

That is, the constant $\hat{b}_0$, absorbs the mean of the process; it may be interpreted as the level of $\hat{I}_i$ expected when $\hat{I}_{i-1}$ is zero. Plotted against time, b_0 should display the cycles shown in diagram (A) if the Kilbourne model is detectable in the data, with large values of $\hat{b}_0$ occurring around virus shift years.

6.5 MEASLES: A STABLE VIRUS WITH REPETITIVE EPIDEMIC WAVES

Introduction

With the elimination of smallpox from the World Health Organization's list of infectious diseases in 1979, attention has been focused upon other viruses to assess their potential as candidates for worldwide eradication. Among these, the measles virus (see box in Figure 3.3) deserves special attention. Already the introduction of measles vaccination programmes in many developed countries since the 1960s has produced sharp falls in incidence (cf. Figure 4.9). But a gap has opened between the attack and death rates reported there and those in less developed countries where they remain at a level typical of Europe or the United States in the nineteenth century. Mortality rates of 20–30 percent are commonly reported in African countries today, and the latest United Nations figures suggest that measles still retains the position it has held since the Second World War in the top ten causes of death in the world as a whole. In addition to deaths directly attributable to measles, there is evidence points linking measles in childhood to the subsequent development of some neurological diseases. The two most commonly cited are subacute sclerosing panencephalitis (SSPE) and multiple sclerosis (MS). See Figure 4.9.

In this section, we examine the circumstances under which measles, like smallpox, might be eradicated, and illustrate the basic principles involved by considering measles epidemics in the mid-Atlantic island of Iceland in the twentieth century.

Critical community size for virus maintenance

When considering world-wide eradication of measles as a possible goal, it is worth recalling that the virus is already periodically eliminated through natural processes in restricted geographical areas. It was the fact that measles cannot persist indefinitely in small, isolated communities that led Sir Macfarlane Burnet (1972, p. 17) to argue that 'in principle vaccination against measles could allow eradication of measles from the globe.'

A crucial question, therefore, is the size of the human population required to maintain the measles virus. This was investigated by the Oxford statistician, M. S. Bartlett (1957), who suggested from his study of British and American cities that between 4,000 and 5,000 measles cases each year in a community was just enough to sustain endemicity. Given the reporting and attack rates prevalent at the time of Bartlett's study, this implies that a city of around a quarter of a million inhabitants is the lower population size threshold for a permanent measles virus reservoir to exist.

What happens below this level is shown in diagram (A). In large cities above the size threshold, like community A, a continuous trickle of cases is reported. These provide the reservoir of infection which sparks a major epidemic when the population at risk (susceptibles, S) builds up to a critical level. Since clinical measles confers subsequent life-long immunity to the disease, this build-up occurs only as children are born, lose their mother-conferred immunity and escape vaccination or the disease. Eventually the S population will become sufficiently large for an epidemic to break out. When this happens, the S population is diminished and the stock of infectives, I increases as individuals are transferred by infection from the S to the I

population. This generates the characteristic 'D'-shaped relationship over time between the sizes of the S and I populations shown on the end plane of the block diagram.

If the total population of a community falls below the quarter of a million size threshold, as in settlements B and C of diagram (A), measles epidemics can only arise when the virus is introduced into it by the influx of infected individuals (so-called *index cases*) from reservoir areas. These movements are shown by the broad arrows in diagram (A). In such smaller communities, the S population is insufficient to maintain a continuous record of infection. The disease dies out and the S population grows in the absence of infection. Eventually the S population will become big enough to sustain an epidemic when an index case arrives. Given that the total population of the community is insufficient to renew by births the S population as rapidly as it is diminished by infection, the epidemic will eventually die out.

It is the repetition of this basic process which generates the successive epidemic waves witnessed in most communities. Of special significance is the way in which the continuous infection and characteristically regular Type I epidemic waves of endemic communities break down, as population size diminishes, into first, discrete but regular Type II waves in community B and then, second, into discrete and irregularly spaced Type III waves in community C. Since the S population continues to grow by births in the absence of infection, very large epidemics can occur in small and isolated communities if build-up takes place in the absence of vaccination and index cases over a long period of time. Note also, in communities below the population size threshold, that the base of the 'D' relationship between the S and I populations is at zero with respect to I between epidemics. This contrasts with communities like A where the non-zero

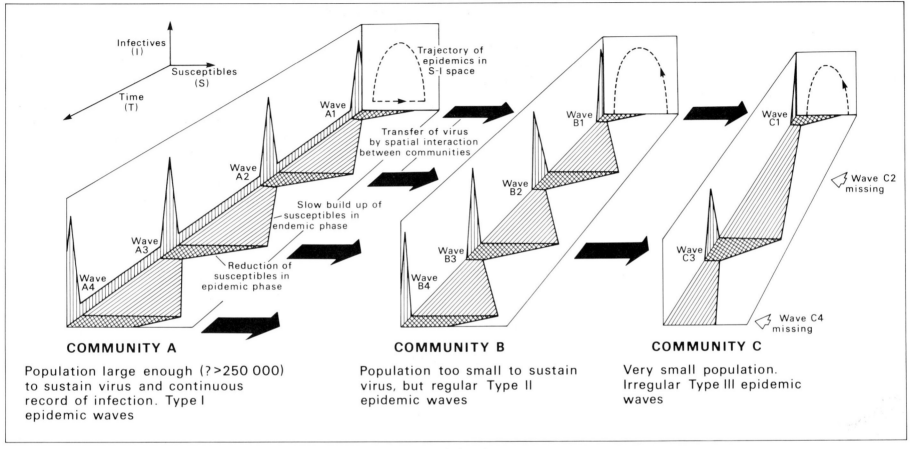

Figure 6.5 (A) Bartlett model of measles spread through communities of different population sizes

base reflects the continuous trickle of cases in the inter-epidemic phases.

Bartlett's calculations for cities were re-examined by F.L. Black (1966). This time, however, the units of observation were not cities but eighteen islands. Of these, only Hawaii with a total population of 550,000 had a continuous Type I pattern of measles infection over the sixteen-year study period considered by Black. Type II patterns were found in islands with population totals as low as 10,000. Below this population level

measles epidemics were temporally irregular and the Type III pattern predominated.

In the remainder of this section, we build upon the Bartlett–Black model by taking one of the islands in Black's sample, Iceland, and subjecting it to very detailed geographical examination. We attempt to find answers to some of the following questions. What is the population size for endemicity suggested by the Icelandic data? Since the total population of Iceland even in 1987 is still below Barlett's

endemicity threshold, how does the virus reach the island on a regular basis? How often do major epidemics occur? What is the geography of the disease transmission paths within the island? Are these stable or random? If the former is the case, then are they consistent enough to allow mathematical models to be built of the spread processes involved? And are such models sufficiently accurate to direct vaccination programmes to interrupt the chains of infection so that Burnet's hope of eradication can be fulfilled?

Iceland as a laboratory

To answer these questions Iceland, the second largest island in Black's sample, is a most appropriate laboratory area. Map (B) shows it to be a large island (about the size of southern England or the state of Indiana) located just south of the Arctic Circle. The biggest single settlement is the capital, Reykjavík, which has been growing both in absolute population size and in its relative share of the Icelandic total. In 1901 its 6,700 inhabitants accounted for less than a tenth of the island's 78,000; by the mid-1970s, Reykjavík had grown to 87,000 out of a total population of 213,000.

The geographical distribution of Iceland's population by medical districts in 1973 is shown on map (B), using the method of proportional circles. Iceland is the least densely settled country in Europe. The harsh environment of the interior plateau has restricted settlement to the peripheral lowlands [stippled in Figure 6.5 (B)]. Given a deeply indented fjord coastline around much of the island, communities tend to be rather separate and remote from each other. Until the end of the Second World War, most communication was by sea. It is therefore often more appropriate from an epidemiological point of view to think of Iceland as an archipelago of population islands rather than as a single cohesive unit.

The external isolation of Iceland's settlements from the rest of the world and their internal separation from each other has, when linked to the island's lack of measles endemicity, profound epidemiological consequences. As we shall see, measles waves arrive discretely in both time and space in the island's settlements, with each epidemic episode separated by a virus-free window. Such waves are much easier to analyse than the continuous and overlapping wave trains

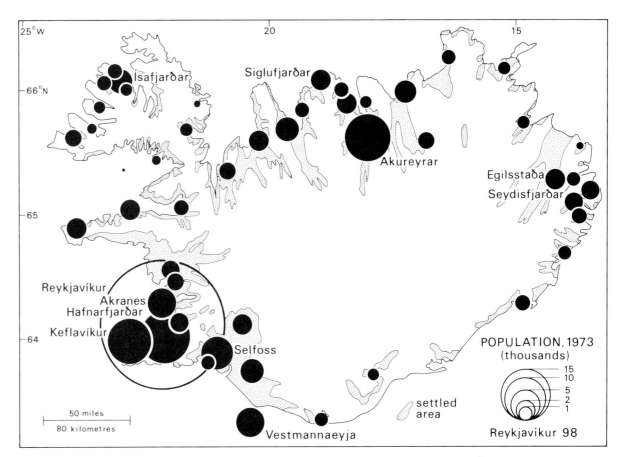

Figure 6.5 (B) Population distribution in Iceland, 1973

experienced in continental areas where the measles virus is endemic.

The data base A second reason for selecting Iceland is the quality of the country's demographic and epidemiological data. These are among the most complete in the world. Records in reasonable detail go back to 1751 and through them it is possible, as shown in diagram (C), to build up an accurate picture of Iceland's demographic and epidemiological history over the last 200 years.

Iceland has experienced a population explosion since 1900 which, as shown in the left-hand graphs of (C), reflected in the early years the declining mortality, especially among infants, common to most industrialized counties and, latterly, sustained high birth rates. As a result, Iceland has the youngest population in the industrialized world. Since Iceland has no co-ordinated measles vaccination programme, this relatively large young population has ensured a reasonable case load for analysis in epidemic

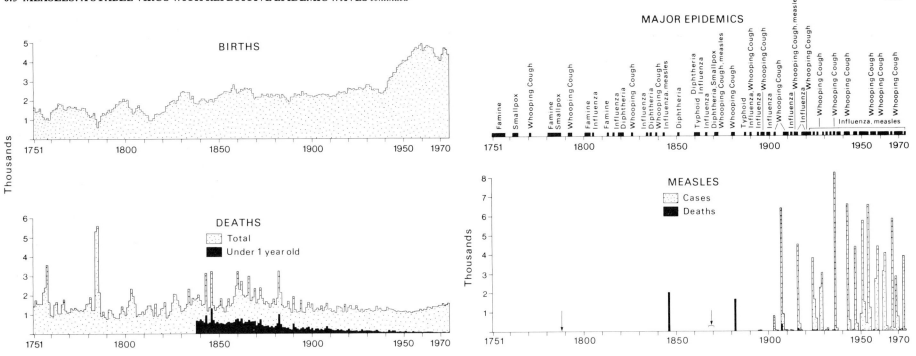

Figure 6.5 (C) Demographic and epidemiological record for Iceland over a 220-year period, 1751–1971

periods. The data are also reliable. On the basis of birthrate and serological information Black, in his work discussed earlier, considered Iceland's data on measles case levels to have an accuracy of better than 40 percent, substantially more than in other western countries.

In addition to quantitative information on the country's demographic and epidemiological past, an important feature of the Icelandic data is the availability of detailed qualitative information which may be used to supplement the numerical record. Both kinds of data are included in the one publication, *Heilbrigðisskýrslur*, the annual report of the state of public health in Iceland. First published in 1896, *Heilbrigðisskýrslur* not only provides on a monthly basis figures for measles cases reported in each of some fifty

medical districts (cf. Figure 2.11), but it also contains written accounts by local medical officers of the course of the disease in their own district. These give details of the severity and spread of the various epidemics in each community and indicate, where known, the external source of the disease and how it diffused from village to village or even from farm to farm within the district. We have already shown in Figure 5.5 how it is possible to use these accounts to construct a picture of an epidemic in a community. Not surprisingly, this information was easier to obtain when most movements were by local boats and, with the coming of the motor car, aircraft and tourism, the quality of this evidence deteriorates.

Characteristics of Iceland's measles waves

General features Focusing first upon the quantitative record, the right-hand graphs of diagram (C) show that, throughout the period since 1751, the population of Iceland has been affected by epidemics of many infectious diseases, notably the great smallpox surge of the 1780s. Among a familiar list which includes diptheria, influenza, smallpox, typhoid and whooping cough, measles has played a quantitatively important role. Until the early part of the twentieth century, measles epidemics were infrequent but were associated with severe mortality. In this century, epidemics have become more and more frequent with declining mortality levels.

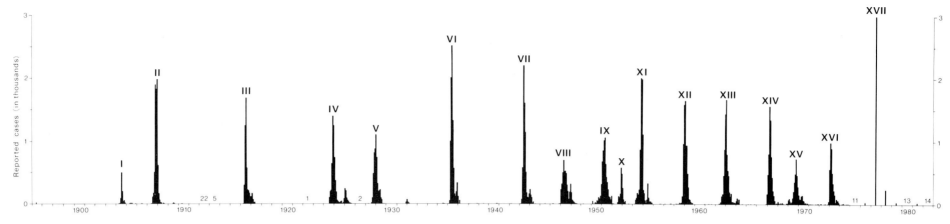

Figure 6.5 (D) Iceland's monthly record of reported measles cases, 1896–1982

The bare statistics of Iceland's measles records underline the frequency and severity of epidemic attacks. Over the period between 1896 and 1982 for which, as discussed below, very reliable morbidity data are available, 89,506 measles cases were reported with 658 directly attributable deaths.

The cases were generated in the form of seventeen distinct epidemic waves which are illustrated in graph (D). Since 1975 only annual, rather than monthly, totals are given in published sources, so that the annual figure has been plotted at mid-year in 1977. The waves ranged in size from 822 cases (Wave I, April to November 1904) to 8,408 cases (Wave VI, February 1936 to March 1937). Each lasted on average nineteen months and spread over most parts of the island. If we ignore the aberrant 1904 epidemic, then generally only five of Iceland's fifty medical districts could expect to escape infection in any one wave. Between the epidemic waves were quiet periods, averaging three years in length, when the island was free of the measles virus.

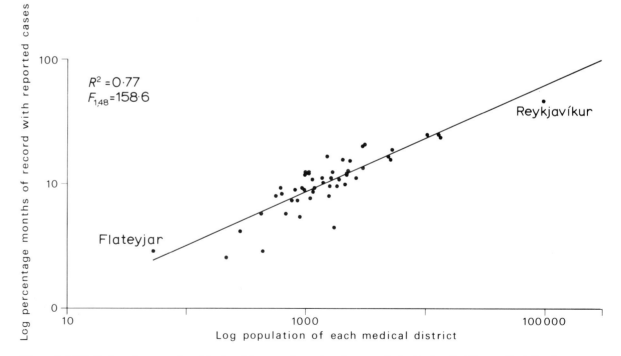

Figure 6.5 (E) Estimating an endemicity level for measles using the records for Iceland's fifty medical districts, 1945–1970

Endemicity For the period between 1945 and 1970, diagram (E) replicates Black's (1966) approach to the problem of identifying the minimum population size required to sustain a permanent measles virus reservoir. For each of the country's fifty medical districts, *i*, the percentage of the 312 months with reported measles cases, T_i has been plotted against its population, P_i. Note that both axes of the graph have been logarithmically transformed and that, to allow for population growth, the population has been estimated as the midpoint value between 1945 and 1970. The fitted linear regression equation is

$$\log T_i = -0.36 + 0.43 \log P_i, \qquad (6.5.1)$$

with an estimated threshold of around 290,000. This compares very closely with the value of 250,000 suggested by Bartlett's (1957) study (see early part of section).

Geographical spread Because Iceland is below Bartlett's population threshold for measles endemicity, for a measles attack to occur on an Icelandic farmstead, the virus has to be carried by one infected individual (or, like an Olympic torch, by a chain of infected individuals) across several hundred miles of ocean, from the seaport or the airport to the rural community, and finally to the farm itself. Temporarily foresaking the quantitative information in *Heilbrigðisskýrslur* for the qualitative, we find that Iceland's records contain evidence of just such movements. Up to the end of the Second World War, the country of origin of all of Iceland's measles epidemics is reported in *Heilbrigðisskýrslur*. Since 1945, the

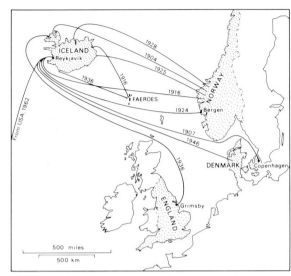

Figure 6.5 (F) External epidemic pathways: known international movements of index cases to Iceland at the start of eleven measles epidemics

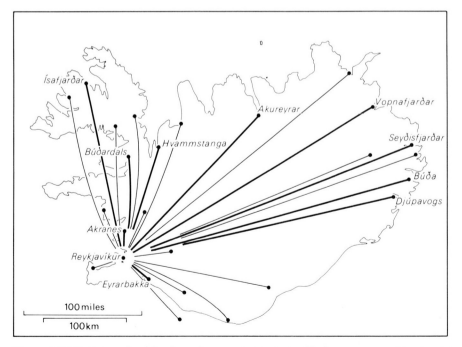
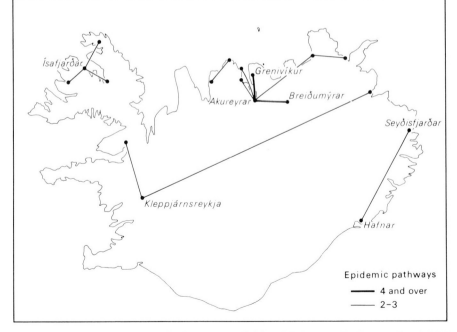

Figure 6.5 (G) Internal epidemic pathways: movements of index cases noted in physicians' records between Reykjavík and other centres (left) and between all other centres (right)

information is very incomplete. All the known international epidemic pathways by which measles reached Iceland since 1896 to start an epidemic are mapped in diagram (F). It shows that the main reservoir of infection is northwest Europe and reflects the strong bonding of Iceland to other Scandinavian countries.

Once within Iceland a multiplicity of routes may be followed. By combining all the known movements of index cases noted in the pages of *Heilbrigðisskýrslur* as being responsible for transmitting the measles virus from one settlement to another within the island, we can determine whether there is any stability in the pattern of geographical spread. Diagram (G) plots these internal epidemic pathways. The left-hand map shows those based upon the capital, Reykjavík, while the right-hand map shows those between all other pairs of settlements. On both only links

which are mentioned on two or more occasions in *Heilbrigðisskýrslur* are illustrated.

The left-hand map clearly demonstrates the importance of Reykjavík as a centre for virus spread. The large regional towns such as Ísafjörður, Akureyri and Seyðisfjörður are all strongly linked to Reykjavík in terms of epidemic movement (pathway category 4 and over). The right-hand map indicates that, superimposed upon this wave movement between the capital and the other main urban centres, are localized epidemic circulation cells, especially around Akureyri and Ísafjörður.

Taken together, (F) and (G) suggest a three-stage qualitative model by which a measles epidemic passes through Iceland. First, introduction occurs from the rest of the world, or else at a very early stage from elsewhere in Iceland, to the capital Reykjavík. Second, spread takes place

from the capital to regional centres in the northwest (Ísafjörður), north (Akureyri) and east (Seyðisfjörður) of the island. Using the ideas of Figure 5.13, this represents diffusion down the urban population size hierarchy. Simultaneously, there is also localized contagious diffusion from Reykjavík into southwest Iceland. Third, there is restricted spread out from the regional centres into their hinterlands.

Quantitative evidence for this model is given earlier in Figure 5.8. If the average time taken for measles to reach each of the Icelandic communities is computed for the eight waves to have affected the country between 1945 and 1970, the following results are obtained: capital (Reykjavík), 1.5 months; regional centres (Ísafjörður, Akureyri, Seyðisfjörður, and Egilsstaðir), 6.7 months; northwest Iceland, 9.2 months; Reykjavík region, 5 months.

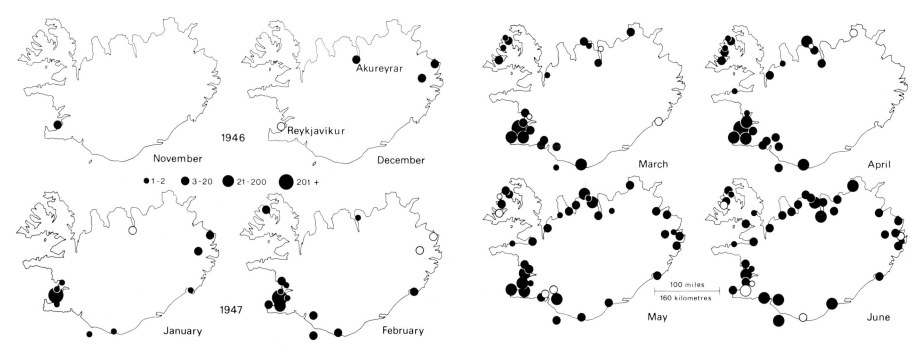

Figure 6.5 (H) Monthly sequence of measles cases from November 1946 to June 1947

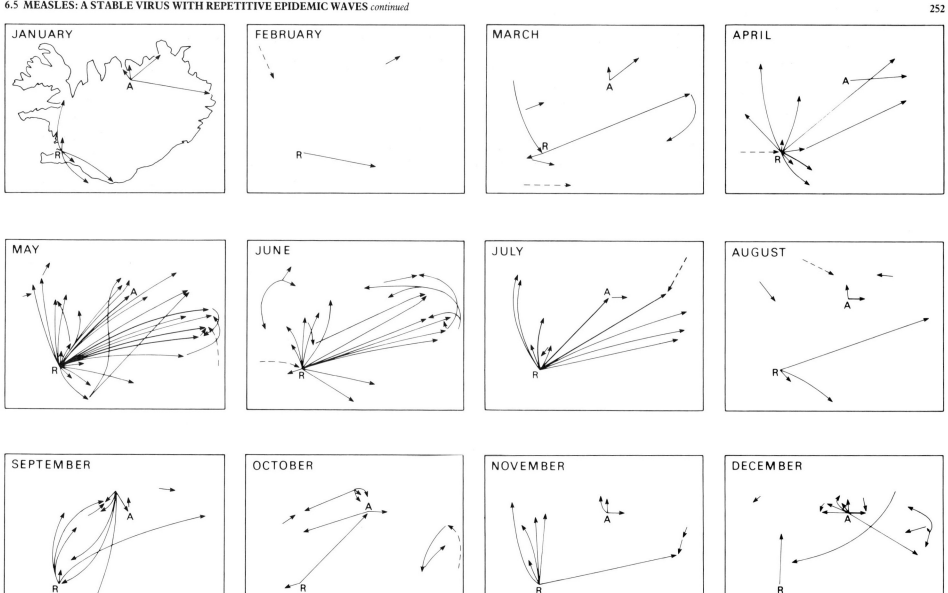

Figure 6.5 (I) Movements of index cases noted in physicians' records since 1896 arranged by month

When we examine the detailed history of any major epidemic, many of these features can be found. Thus in diagram (H), proportional circles have been used to map the numbers of cases of measles reported in each medical district for the various months of Wave VIII (November 1946 to June 1947). The open circles are used to denote places which reported measles cases in a preceding month but not in the month in question. Like most of the epidemic waves studied, this one started in the capital, Reykjavík, in November. By December, the disease had reached Akureyri, the largest settlement in Iceland outside the Reykjavík region, and to places in the eastern fjords. Localized spread round these centres took place in subsequent months, for example in the Reykjavík area in January and February. Together, these hierarchical and contagious elements resulted in the wholesale dissemination of the disease throughout Iceland by the middle of 1947.

Seasonality The movements of the index cases can be mapped in a different way, on a monthly basis, to permit examination of the seasonal pattern of disease diffusion. This is done in diagram (I). In northern temperate latitudes, measles epidemics, like most infectious childhood diseases, commonly have a winter peak. In startling contrast, however, in Iceland the May and June flowering of epidemics is most marked. We need to bear in mind that most of the movements of index cases recorded relate to the pre-1945 period. Thus we find in *Heilbrigðisskýrslur* that medical officers associate this peak with two facts namely, the improved communications between districts after the spring thaw, which permitted greater spatial mobility, and the occurrence of the major communal activity of haymaking in June. In fact the seasonal pattern, as shown in Figures 4.5(D) and (E), is more subtle than the maps in (I)

imply for, in the pre-1939 period, there were two epidemic peaks of roughly equal intensity – the summer one and also the mid-winter one found in other western countries. Nor has the pattern been stable through time. In the post-1945 period, the summer peak has gradually disappeared as Iceland's isolation from the rest of the world has been eliminated by airline travel.

Modelling the spread of measles waves

While study of the movement of index cases gives intuitive insights into the ways epidemics spread, more formal modelling demands closer analysis of the times-series behaviour of regions and a return to quantitative evidence. Comparison of diagrams (A) and (D) shows that throughout the twentieth century, Iceland as a whole has displayed Type II behaviour in terms of the Bartlett model. But if we consider individual Icelandic communities, then a more complex pattern emerges. Reykjavík itself, its hinterland, and the four outlying regional centres of Ísafjörður, Akureyri, Seyðisfjörður and Egilsstaðir all conform to the general Type II form. One offshore island, Flatey, missed half of Iceland's epidemics, while substantial parts of the remote northwest peninsula and northern coast missed out on two or more waves. As a broad generalization, a district with a population of 2,000 or more appears to have been caught up in all the island's measles epidemics. Below that threshold, it occasionally escaped; its chances depended heavily on location, with remoteness playing a major protective role.

Epidemic size and frequency Since both the size and the relative accessibility of the various communities which make up the Icelandic population have been changing over the last eighty years, it is important to determine how far

the epidemic waves have responded to these changes. If we plot the waves for the whole of Iceland [diagram (J)] between 1896 and 1945 in terms of the size of epidemics (number of cases reported) and spacing between epidemics (time in years between epidemics), and compare them

Early epidemic waves 1896-1945

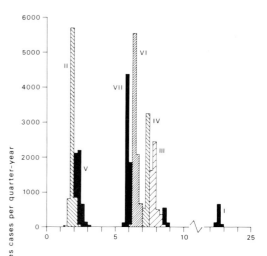

Post-war epidemic waves 1946-1982

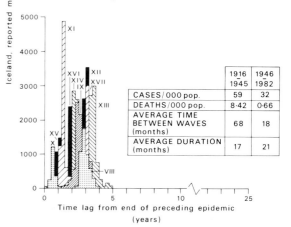

Figure 6.5 (J) Contrasts in time intervals between epidemics for the earlier and later measles waves in Iceland, 1896–1982

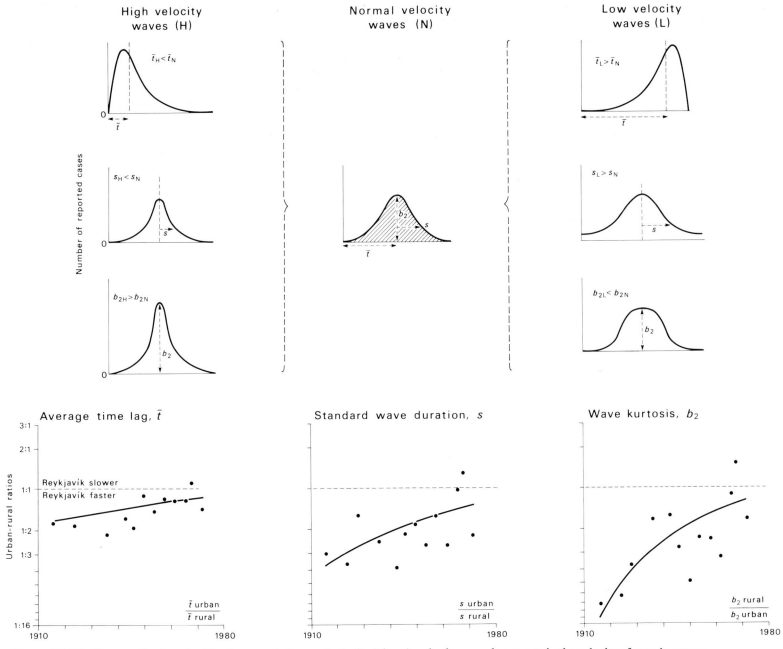

Figure 6.5 (K) Characterization of epidemic waves in terms of velocity (above) and urban–rural contrasts in the velocity of measles waves within Iceland, 1910–1980 (below)

with the same characteristics for the waves between 1945 and 1975, certain sharp changes are evident. As in (D), the waves are distinguished by roman numerals. Irregular waves separated by generally long time intervals are replaced after 1945 by more regular waves at shorter intervals. Only seven waves arrived in the first fifty years, and these fell into three groups. Two occurred after gaps of around two years, four with gaps of six to eight years, and one after a gap of over twenty years. In the post-1945 period, the nine waves followed hard upon each other after gaps of two to four years. The occasional virus contact allowed by sea transport was replaced by continual virus bombardment once international air transport promoted Keflavík into a regular transatlantic staging post. Air passenger traffic to Iceland has increased fifteen-fold in the thirty years from 1945 to 1975.

Epidemic velocity In the same way as Iceland has become more closely tied to the virus reservoir areas of Europe and, until recently, North America, the outlying parts of the country have become more integrated with the national capital. This linkage is shown by comparing the velocity of epidemic waves passing through Reykjavík with that for the rest of the island [diagram (K)]. Velocity is an elusive characteristic to measure. Given the essentially unimodal shapes of the histograms of reported cases against time shown in (D) and (J), the statistical measures of the mean time to infection, $\bar{t}$, standard deviation, s and peakedness, b_2, may be used (Cliff and Haggett, 1981). As shown in the upper part of diagram (K), a 'fast' wave will have a short average time, $\bar{t}$, from its start to peak infection, be of short duration, s, and be sharply peaked (b_2). A 'slow' wave will have the reverse characteristics.

For the Iceland epidemics, the values obtained

for the measures have been plotted as a ratio (urban value divided by rural value). Over the sixty-year period covered in (K), all the ratios move towards unity and point to a decreasing contrast between the rural and urban parts of the island. The graphs suggest that this has been achieved both by a decreasing velocity for waves moving through Reykjavík and an acceleration in the velocity of waves moving through the rest of Iceland.

There are grounds for arguing that the first trend is due partly to particularly successful public health measures in the Reykjavík area. The number of qualified doctors per thousand population was much higher there than in the rest of the country for most of the study period; between 1916 and 1972, it rose from 1.0 to 2.6 in Reykjavík, while moving only from 0.7 to 0.8 in the rest of Iceland.

If the control of measles within urban Iceland was improving, then the ability of the measles virus to be transferred rapidly around rural Iceland by index cases was being enhanced. Transport innovations and the increased mixing of infectives and susceptibles play a major role in understanding the rural trend. Today, Iceland has a complete round-the-island road network and the most heavily used (in passenger miles per thousand residents) domestic airline system in Europe. The ambulatory school system in which a teacher visited outlying farms for a few weeks each term, characteristic of the pre-1945 period, has been largely replaced by boarding schools in which children from isolated farms spend weeks in residential accommodation. The vulnerable school-age population in today's rural areas is thus more concentrated and more accessible than in earlier decades to the measles virus brought in from other parts of Iceland.

Epidemic forecasts Converting a general understanding of an epidemic spread process into a

testable model with forecasting capability has long been a central epidemiological goal. Bailey (1975) reviews the wide range of approaches, both deterministic and stochastic, used by researchers over the past century and this work is considered in detail in Figure 7.4. However, in essence most recognize, for a single area, the basic idea encapsulated in diagram (A), in which the future number of new infectives in a population is generated by the mixing of susceptibles (those at risk) with existing infectives (those already carrying the virus). The rate of mixing is controlled by a parameter. When suitably modified to allow for the clinical history of the disease, vaccination rates and recovery rates, reasonable approximations to epidemic wave trains can be generated.

In the case of Iceland, we can use our geographical knowledge of the contact system between areas implied by the movements of index cases shown in (G) to augment the basic model in two ways. First, a single, country-wide version can be replaced by one disaggregated into a series of local-area models. Each of these can incorporate the particular mixing parameter appropriate to the social structure of the local community being characterized. Second, these local models can then be linked to allow an exchange of susceptibles and infectives between adjacent areas. Clearly, what we mean by 'adjacent' will depend critically on the spatial contact between places and the form of the vector maps of index cases already illustrated. Given the present contact structures within Iceland, we can regard Reykjavík, in epidemiological terms, as a near-neighbour of all other Icelandic communities, even though they may be geographically remote.

The detailed structure of an appropriate forecasting model is considered at length in Cliff, Haggett, Ord and Versey (1981). The results obtained suggest that forecasting future

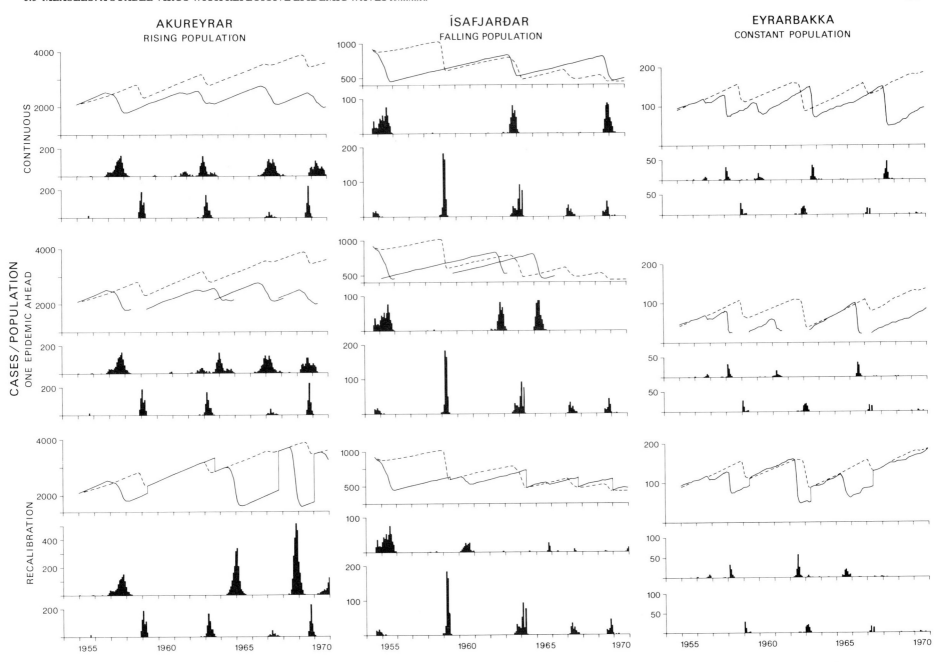

Figure 6.5 (L) *Ex-post* forecasts of measles epidemics and susceptible population sizes in three Icelandic medical districts for three different forecasting strategies

epidemic maps is no less difficult than forecasting the weather in mid-latitudes. Nevertheless, given the introduction of the virus into Iceland we can say something of its probable rate and direction of propagation. Diagram (L) shows the *ex-post* forecasts generated by the model for three Icelandic medical districts whose populations rose, fell and were steady over the period, 1945–70. The number of measles cases actually reported is drawn as the bottom line of histograms for each medical district. The corresponding forecasts appear as the histograms immediately above them. The pecked lines represent the susceptible populations estimated from demographic data. The solid lines record the susceptible populations projected by the model. The 'continuous' forecasts were obtained by running the model on continuously for a fifteen-year period from 1955. The 'one epidemic ahead' forecasts were calculated by projecting the time of the next epidemic and then restarting the model at that time with the same parameter values. This prevents errors cumulating. In the 'recalibration' forecasts, the demographic estimates of the susceptible population were used to update the model after each epidemic. In all instances, epidemic size is over-estimated. However, if we look at our ability to forecast the *times* of recurrences accurately, reasonable results are obtained. The continuous and one epidemic ahead forecasts seem to work equally well for a rising population total; recalibration produces the best forecasts with constant and falling population levels.

The significance of these forecasts is obvious. If it becomes possible to predict where and when epidemics are likely to occur then, given sufficient advance warning, medical care and vaccination can be made available on a regional basis to permit the chains of infection to be interrupted and epidemics controlled.

Conclusion

Burnet's vision of ultimate extinction of the measles virus from the planet rests on a global vaccination programme reducing the sizes of the geographically distributed populations at risk to some level at which the chains of infections cannot be maintained. In terms of the Bartlett model, this means systematically reducing the wave order of different communities from I to II, and from II to III, eventually bringing the Type III waves into phase so that the fade out of all the remaining active areas coincides. In this task, forecasting models of the sort outlined above have a role to play in guiding the efficient organization of the eradication programme.

There is an immense gap between theory and practice, and not a few dangers in the added risks arising from raising the age of measles attacks in only partially vaccinated populations. If the geographical reconstruction of the ways in which diseases move through human populations is to aid in the design of efficient containment programmes, then islands may remain uniquely valuable for studying virus movements. The research possibilities for island biogeography which Charles Darwin saw nearly 150 years ago remain to be fully exploited.

Sources and Further Reading

The material and diagrams on the geography of measles epidemics in Iceland are drawn from A.D. Cliff, P. Haggett, J.K. Ord and G.R. Versey (1981), *Spatial Diffusion: An Historical Geography of Epidemics in an Island Community*, Cambridge: Cambridge University Press. This is summarized in A.D. Cliff and P. Haggett (1984), 'Island epidemics', *Scientific American*, 250, pp.110–17. Icelandic epidemiological data are published in *Heilbrigðisskýrslur* (Public Health in Iceland), available for all years or groups of years from the Office of the Director of Public Health, Reykjavík. Demographic data are published in *Mannfjöldaskýrslur* (Population and Vital Statistics), published decennially by the Statistical Bureau of Iceland, Reykjavík.

Authoritative accounts of measles epidemiology are given in F.L. Black (1984), 'Measles', in *Viral Infections of Humans: Epidemiology and Control*, second edition, edited by A.S. Evans, New York: Plenum, pp.397–418, and in Sir Macfarlane Burnet and D.O. White (1972), *Natural History of Infectious Disease*, fourth edition, Cambridge: Cambridge University Press.

The relationship between community size and endemicity of measles is considered in two seminal articles, namely, M.S. Bartlett (1957), 'Measles periodicity and community size', *Journal of the Royal Statistical Society A*, 120, pp.48–70, and F.L. Black (1966), 'Measles endemicity in insular populations: critical community size and its evolutionary implication', *Journal of Theoretical Biology*, 11, pp.207–11. Ways of measuring the velocity with which epidemics of infectious disease move through a community are discussed in A.D. Cliff and P. Haggett (1982), 'Measuring the velocity of epidemic waves', *International Journal of Epidemiology*, 11, pp.82–9. The basic reference on mathematical models of disease spread is N.T.J. Bailey (1975), *The Mathematical Theory of Infectious Diseases and its Applications*, London: Griffin.

CHAPTER SEVEN
FUTURE MAPS

Figure over   A three-dimensional computer printout of estimates of the fox population in Switzerland, based on hunting statistics for 1974 to 1975. The foreground shows the alpine region with relatively low overall density. The central and northern parts of the country show variable densities above the critical level of 0.3 per sq km, below which rabies tends to die out

Source   F. Steck and A. Wandeler (1980) 'Epidemiology of fox rabies in Europe', *Epidemiologic Reviews* 2, pp.71–96, Figure 9, p.88. The computer program was developed by H. Burri at the Federal Office of Statistics, Berne, Switzerland.

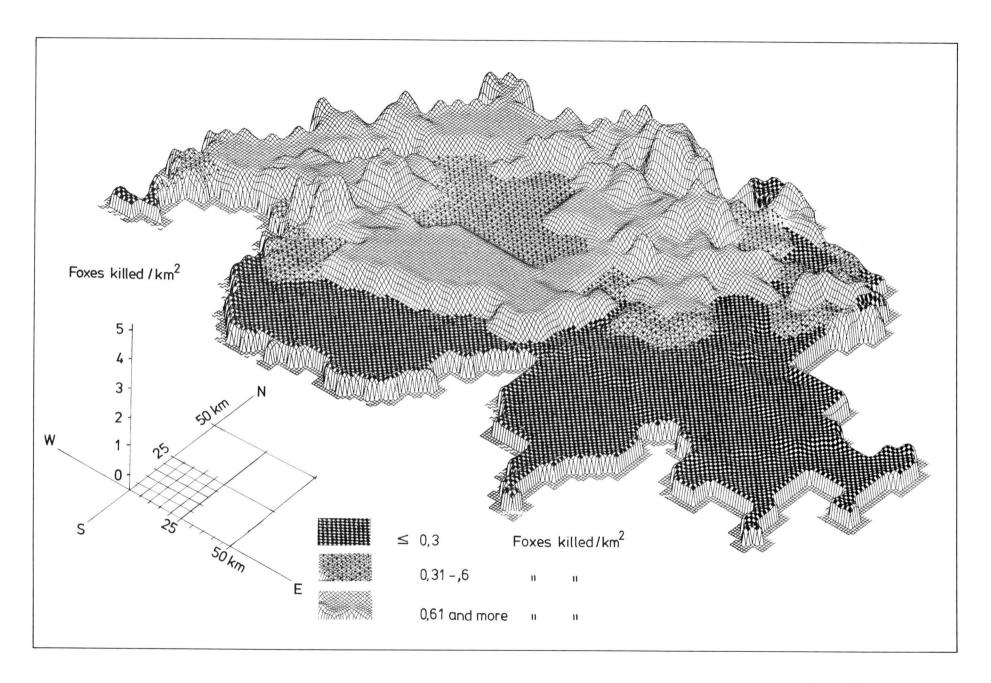

Foxes killed / km^2

N

50 km

25

W

0

S

25

50 km

E

5
4
3
2
1
0

≤ 0,3   Foxes killed / km^2

0,31 -,6   "   "

0,61 and more   "   "

ERZ BV, BERN/BERNE 25.2.1980

FUTURE MAPS

INTRODUCTION

This Atlas began with an analysis of cholera in John Snow's London of 1849–54. More than a century later, many aspects of medical mapping have altered in ways unsuspected by Snow, and the process of change is an accelerating one.

In this brief final chapter, we examine some of the areas in which this change is taking place. Thus Figures 7.1, 7.2 and 7.3 look at the revolution in cartography, mapping and map transformations wrought by computer-based technology. We then conclude the Atlas with Figures 7.4 and 7.5, in which computer-based forecasting models are used as a means of projecting future epidemic maps and of devising optimal patterns for the geographical location of future health care facilities.

All of the plates in this final chapter depend for their results upon high-speed data processing, and so it is appropriate that we start with computer-based cartography.

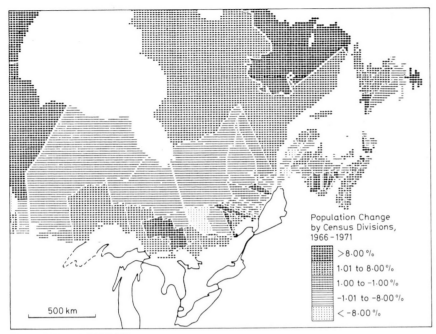

Figure 7.1 (A) SYMAP

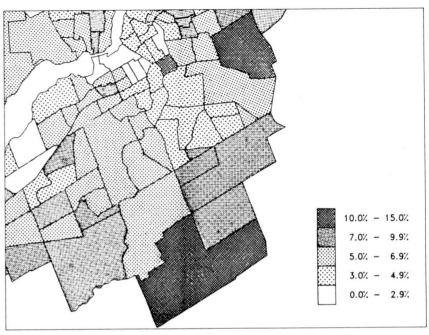

Figure 7.1 (C) GIMMS

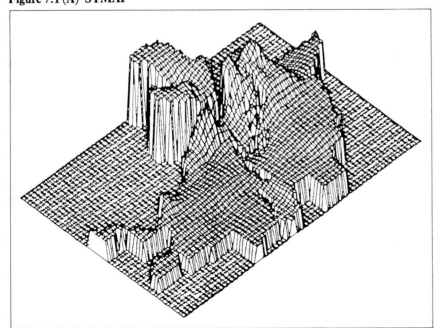

Figure 7.1 (B) PREVU

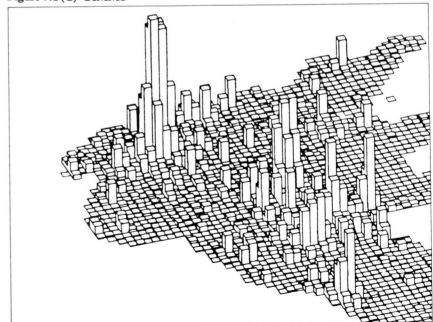

Figure 7.1 (D) DURHAM

7.1 COMPUTERS AND MAPPING

Cartographers began to explore the power of computing in the early 1950s and now find themselves in the middle of an information technology revolution. Storage and processing powers are doubling almost annually while the real costs of hardware are falling. An entirely new technology has been invented and many operations that were formerly executed painstakingly by hand are now carried out more rapidly and more accurately by machine. There used to be a substantial time lag between technological development and its full-scale implementation in cartography, but that time lag is being steadily reduced.

Computer-assisted mapping involves developments in three components of any computer system – hardware, software, and data file structuring – and each of these is reviewed in turn. Finally we look at how maps are entered into and retrieved from a computer system.

Hardware and software

The hardware configuration of a standard computer system consists of four elements namely, a central processor unit (CPU), data input devices, external storage devices (such as floppy disks, magnetic tapes and hard disks) and data output devices; as shown, appropriate linkages are required to communicate between the four elements.

Input devices → Central processor → Output devices
↑ ↓
External storage devices

Computer systems are commonly classified into three groups on the basis of increasing CPU power. These groups are small-capacity *micro-computers*, medium-capacity *minicomputers* and high-capacity *mainframes*.

Software describes the programs and routines required to make the computer perform useful tasks for the cartographer. In mapping software, each cartographic task is broken into its separate components to create a step by step logical structure called an *algorithm*. Mapping packages have to be tailored to the particular architecture, speed and file-handling capacity of the computer system. Thus the ODYSSEY package developed at Harvard for very sophisticated mapping processes is tailored to a mainframe, SAS-MAP to medium capacity minicomputers and MICRO-MAP to desktop microcomputers. Each mapping package tends to be continuously modified and published in successive revisions (commonly denoted by roman numerals as in (MICROMAP II) and, historically, such packages tend to migrate down from larger to smaller machines as the software become more flexible and the hardware becomes more powerful.

Spatial data files

Changes in the volume of data and the ability to handle it quickly and efficiently represent the greatest explosion of all. As described in Figure 2.2, not only is disease data being produced in increasing quantities by the statistical reporting agencies of each country, but it is becoming available in computer readable form. To make such data of value in mapping, it has to be *geocoded*; that is, given some locational reference point and built into a locational reference system at either a global or a national level (cf. Figure 3.1). Coding may run down through a spatial hierarchy so that, at the lowest level, the addresses of individual patients or the locations of a street accident can be pinpointed (see Figures 3.16, 3.17 and 5.5).

If properly geocoded, the digital data base of disease data can be integrated with conventional cartographic information. Such cartographic data is linear when used to reproduce physical features on a map such as coastlines and the boundaries of administrative areas. These features are commonly required to create a map base for disease plotting and, because they are capable of vector representation, they can be readily translated into digital form. The United States National Cartographic Center at the United States Geological Survey in Reston, Virginia, is one centre where this massive conversion task is being undertaken. The implication is that both epidemiological data and environmental data can be brought into a common digital format.

Graphic input from maps

In addition to locational data files, geographical information can be directly entered into the computer from the map. This can be done in two ways. The first is by vector digitizing, in which lines on the map are followed by a manual or electromechanical device to give their spatial coordinates at appropriate sampling intervals. Such digital line graphs (DGL) are widely used by national mapping agencies. For example, the United States Geological Survey is currently encoding its 1/24,000 topographic sheets using this system. The slow process of manual digitizing can be speeded up if semi-automatic line followers, such as those developed by Laser-Scan at Cambridge, are employed.

An alternative approach to vector digitizing is raster digitizing. This method uses scanning lines, as in a television set, to decompose a spatial image into a matrix of discrete picture elements (called pixels). Vast amounts of data are generated, but the method is non-selective and its resolution depends upon the number of rasters. Thus a scan of a 48cm by 60cm map at 25 microns yields over 400 million pixels (Robinson, *et al.*, 1984, p.419). Subsequent manual editing is needed to recover the original vector elements such as boundaries.

Digitizing allows one of the problems discussed in Chapter 2 to be overcome. For example, each line segment making up the polygons of boundaries of the medical districts of Iceland (see Figure 2.11) may be digitized and dated; each piece of medical information can be associated with its appropriate *hreppur*. Then, at any given date, an appropriate map may be constructed from the combined spatial (boundary) and non-spatial (epidemiological) information and compared with a map for any other time period. Billions of pieces of information can thus be handled very efficiently in ways unforeseen a decade ago.

Graphic output as maps

Actual output of maps for direct viewing and interpretation takes two main forms. One group of devices generate *hard-copy* maps on printers and plotters. The simplest, and historically the earliest, method was to use the ordinary typewriter characters of a line printer; map (A) shows an example of population characteristics by census divisions in eastern Canada produced by the SYMAP system developed at the Harvard Laboratory for Computer Graphics in the 1960s.

Line printers were supplemented with a succession of ever faster and more complex dot printers (matrix, electrostatic, laser, and ink-jet) which can generate both monochrome and colour maps. Map (C) gives an example of an early dot-matrix choropleth map of the percentage of the population aged 5 and under in Ottawa–Hull, produced by using the GIMMS mapping package.

Another class of hard-copy printers consists of vector plotters (such as CALCOMP) which produce a map by linework with pens and ink; again, monochrome or colours can be used. The maps in (B) produced by the PREVU system and in (D) by the DURHAM system were printed in this way.

A second kind of output is *soft-copy* (or ephemeral), in which the map is displayed the screen of a computer terminal. Map production by this form of electronic display has several advantages over hard-copy output. Mapping is so fast that it becomes interactive in the sense that maps can be called up onto the screen, inspected, modified at the keyboard or by use of a *mouse* device, and accepted or rejected. Since only one out of many maps will eventually be converted into hard copy, the cost of mapping is much lower. For example, the PREVU system in map (C) allows a spatial distribution to be viewed from several angles and its vertical and horizontal scales modified. Other systems provide facilities for zooming in on part of the map to display it in more detail, generalizing it using filter functions as described in Figures 1.10–1.12, as well as providing more complex image and colour enhancements.

The general approach in mapping has been to move from hard copy to interactive soft copy; or, in computer terms, towards random access maps where the spatial data file can be rapidly manipulated and interrogated to produce one or two potential maps on an epidemiological question of interest from the many possible maps contained within the disk store. The term, *geographical information system* (GIS), is given to such a data base.

The output from a GIS is commonly used as input to other computer-based statistical and mathematical models, and we consider some in the succeeding figures.

Sources and Further Reading

The four examples of computer-produced maps are taken from D.R.F. Taylor, editor (1980), *Progress in Contemporary Cartography*, vol. 1, *The Computer in Contemporary Cartography*, New York: John Wiley, pp.203, 204, 210 and 215.

The applications of computers to mapping are considered in M.S. Monmonier (1982), *Computer-Assisted Cartography: Principles and Prospects*, Englewood Cliffs, NJ: Prentice Hall; J.R. Carter (1984), *Computer Mapping*, Washington, DC: Association of American Geographers; and in D.R.F. Taylor, editor (1980), *Progress in Contemporary Cartography*, vol. 1, *The Computer in Contemporary Cartography*, New York: John Wiley. The increasingly important role of graphics in information presentation and analysis is considered in E.R. Tufte (1983), *The Visual Display of Quantitative Information*, Cheshire, Conn.: Graphics Press.

The specific applications of computers to medical mapping are reviewed in National Center for Health Statistics (1979), *Proceedings of the 1976 Workshop on Automated Cartography and Epidemiology*, Publication No. PHS-79-1254, Hyattsville, Md: US Department of Health, Education and Welfare, and R.T. Aageenbrug, editor (1979), *Auto-Carto IV: Applications in Health and Environment*, Falls Church, Va.: American Congress on Surveying and Mapping. Computer cartography has an impenetrable jargon of technical terms; for some basic definitions see D.T. Edson and J. Denegre, editors (1980), *Glossary of Terms in Computer Assisted Cartography*, third edition, Falls Church, Va.: American Congress on Surveying and Mapping. The potential value of geographical information systems is reviewed in the Department of Environment's (1987) report on *Handling Geographic Information*, London: HMSO.

7.2 MULTIDIMENSIONAL SCALING I: GLOBAL LEVEL

Map-scaling problems

One particular set of mapping methods which have been fundamentally changed by the advent of high-speed computers are those for the transformation of conventional maps into other metrics. In this diagram, the principles involved in such transformations are outlined and illustrated by mapping the countries of the Pacific Basin into configurations which reflect their accessibility in time-space and frequency-of-contact space by international and domestic airline carriers. The implications of the hemispheric linkages so defined for the observed incidence of measles in some Pacific island groups in the post-war period are then outlined.

The computational procedures involved are complex because the transformations to be discussed involve mapping a non-planar set of similarities between areas onto a 2-dimensional map with a minimum degree of *stress*. This aspect of the methodology is considered in the next figure.

Multidimensional scaling (MDS)

When a conventional map of a portion of the earth's surface is drawn, some distortion inevitably results in translating a curved segment of the globe onto a flat (2-dimensional) piece of paper. The particular *map projection* used will determine the nature and extent of the distortion introduced but, subject to this proviso, all the map projections in common use attempt to ensure that the locations of points on the map reflect their relative positions on the globe.

An alternative way of examining spatial structure is to use *multidimensional scaling*, MDS, (Kendall, 1971, 1975; Kruskal and Wish, 1978). This technique enables a map to be constructed in which the positions of the points on the map correspond not to their (scaled) geographical locations on the globe but to their degree of similarity on some variable collected for them. So, for example, points may be mapped from geographical space into a 'disease space'; then places which display similar behaviour in terms of, say, the frequency and attack rates for an infectious disease are located close to each other on the MDS map even though they may be far removed geographically. The greater the degree of similarity between the places on the variable measured, the closer together the places will be in the MDS space. Conversely points which are dissimilar on the variable measured will be widely separated in the MDS space, irrespective of their geographical location on the globe.

Transformations to other metrics are possible. For example, we might wish to map geographical space into a travel cost space. Then places which are 'near' to each other in travel cost characteristics will be located in close proximity on the MDS map; places with very different characteristics will be widely separated.

The Pacific basin in time-space

Diagram (A) uses *isochrones* (lines joining places of equal time) to plot, for 1975, the relative time accessibility by scheduled airline carriers of 25 places in the Pacific basin. The place names associated with the identity numbers are listed with the map. The isochrones have been standardized so that 100 denotes average accessibility; values less than 100 indicate superior accessibility and values greater than 100 (stippled) demarcate the relatively less accessible parts of the basin. The diagram shows that a large part of the central Pacific centred on the Trust Territories of the Pacific (18) is up to 20 percent more inaccessible than average while, from French Polynesia (4) eastwards to the Americas, accessibility falls by a factor of almost two.

The area covered by the maps in (B) is delimited by the box on (A). The maps indicate why the zone of inaccessibility in the central Pacific exists. The left-hand map uses flow lines (cf. Figure 3.3) to show the linkages in seats per week provided by international carriers such as Qantas and Pan American between various centres in 1975; the right-hand map gives the same information for 1981. Not only have route capacities multiplied but the amount of overflying of the Pacific, bypassing local centres, has increased. For example, the maps suggest that Fiji (3) had less stop-over traffic in 1981 than in 1975 and so in that sense had become less accessible.

To produce the map shown in (C), MDS has been used to transform the conventional geographical map (A) into a time metric; the relatively accessible places on (A) are now plotted in close proximity on (C), while the relatively inaccessible places have been moved apart. The effect is to push North America and the Far East closer together than they are on a conventional map because of the frequent flights from Tokyo (21) to San Francisco (23). The inaccessible portion of the central Pacific basin apparent in (A) is now mapped as two outposts, one to the north (note the new position of 18, the Trust Territories) and one to the south (13, Papua New Guinea is no longer located to the north of Australia but has been relocated in the south).

Accessibility and measles epidemics

As discussed in Figure 4.7(E), measles is a communicable disease relying on person-to-person

Figure 7.2 (A) Relative time accessibility in 1975 by scheduled airline carriers between 25 centres in the Pacific basin

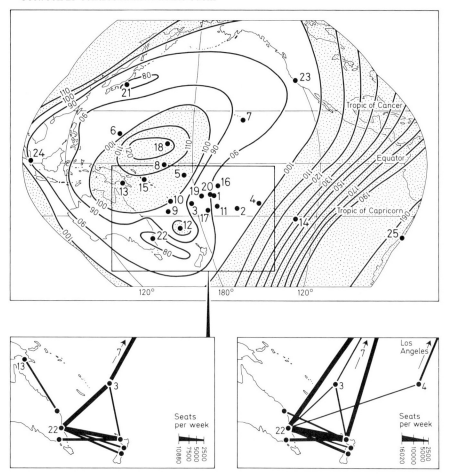

Figure 7.2 (B) Route capacities by international carriers in seats per week, 1975 (left) and 1981 (right), within the southwest Pacific

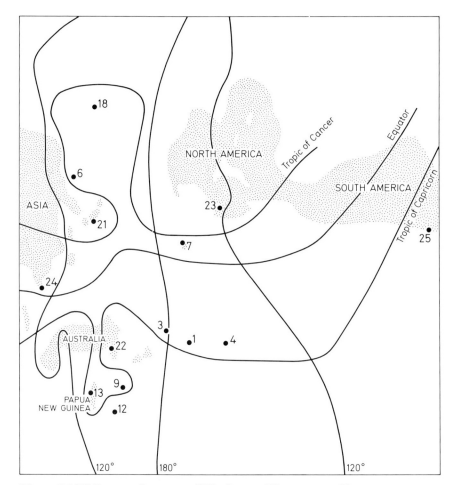

Figure 7.2 (C) Data on time accessibility in map (A) recomputed by multidimensional scaling (MDS) to give a time-space map

Key to Figures (A) – (D)

1 American Samoa; 2 Cook Islands; 3 Fiji; 4 French Polynesia; 5 Kiribati and Tuvalu; 6 Guam; 7 Hawaii; 8 Nauru; 9 New Caledonia; 10 Vanuatu; 11 Niue; 12 Norfolk Island; 13 Papua New Guinea; 14 Pitcairn; 15 Solomon Islands; 16 Tokelau; 17 Tonga; 19 Wallis and Futuna; 20 Western Samoa; 21 Tokyo; 22 Sydney; 23 San Francisco; 24 Singapore; 25 Santiago.

transmission for its survival. If we study the time-series of reported cases of measles per thousand population in the various Pacific island groups located within the box on map (A), we might expect the similarity of their time-series, both in terms of disease intensity and phasing of epidemic episodes, to increase directly with degree of contact. Diagram (D) illustrates this.

To establish the level of similarity between the island-groups in terms of the behaviour of their time-series of measles incidence, cross-correlation analysis (see Figure 5.11) was applied to data for the period, 1953–67. For each island system, vectors have been drawn on the left-hand map of (D) pointing to the island system whose time-series had the biggest cross-correlation with it within 12 months of lag 0. The time lag at which the maximum cross-correlation occurred is indicated by the line type.

Inspection of the map suggests two geographically discrete sub-systems, each with its own distinctive cross-correlation structure. The first, in the western Pacific, consists of New Caledonia (9), Vanuatu (10), the Solomons (15) and the Trust Territories of the Pacific (18). Here leads and lags for the point of maximum cross-correlation ranged up to two months. The second is in the eastern Pacific and includes American Samoa (1), the Cook Islands (2), Fiji (3), Kiribati and Tuvalu (5), Tonga (17) and Western Samoa (20), with leads and lags of up to five months. Outside these two regional sub-systems, and with little statistical association with them, lie French Polynesia (4) and Guam (6), while Hawaii (7) is weakly linked to the eastern Pacific sub-system.

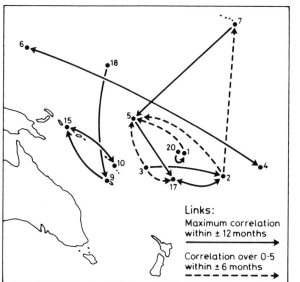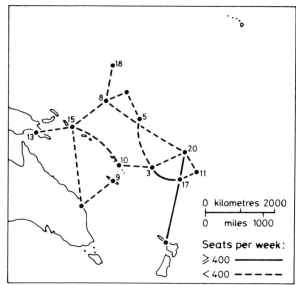

Figure 7.2 (D) Association between epidemic measles behaviour, 1953–1967 (left), and inter-island linkages in seats per week, 1975, (right) by domestic airlines within the southwest Pacific

The right-hand map of (D) plots the local linkages between the island-groups as measured by route capacity in seats per week provided in 1975 by domestic airline carriers. As noted above, the international carriers increasingly overfly the region. The vectors on the airline map show the same broad contact sub-systems as the cross-correlation bonds. The main links between the two sub-systems occur (a) via a lengthy route along their northern perimeters through Kiribati and Tuvalu (5) and Nauru (8) and (b) between Fiji (3) and Vanuatu (10).

The analysis thus indicates the importance of viewing the relationships between places in terms of the metric (such as time or cost, for example) which is most appropriate for the problem being tackled. The plotting of places in terms of accessibility metrics like time and cost distances is particularly valuable when communicable diseases are being studied and may frequently provide a fresh perspective on the disease patterns occurring.

Sources and Further Reading

See under Figure 7.3.

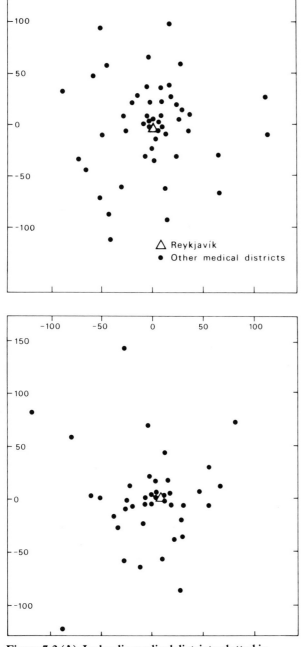

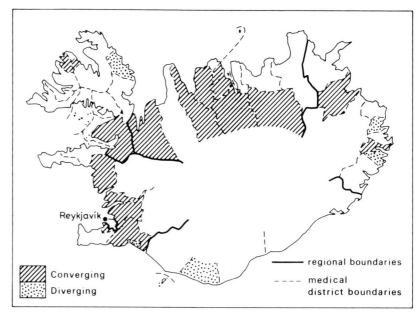

Figure 7.3 (B) Districts converging on or diverging from the capital city, Reykjavík, in terms of the MDS maps, 1945–1952, 1953–1960, 1961–1968 and 1969–1970

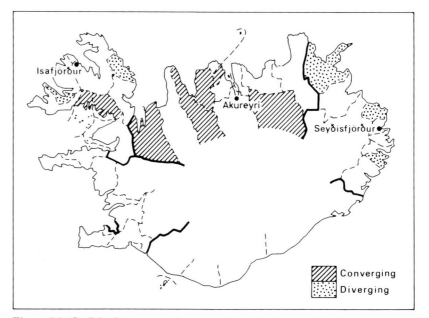

Figure 7.3 (A) Icelandic medical districts plotted in MDS space in terms of influenza behaviour 1945–1952 (above) and 1969–1970 (below)

Figure 7.3 (C) Districts converging on or diverging from regional centres (named) in terms of the MDS maps, 1945–1952, 1953–1960, 1961–1968 and 1969–1970

7.3 MULTIDIMENSIONAL SCALING II: LOCAL LEVEL

In the previous figure, multidimensional scaling (MDS) was used at a macro-geographical scale to transform the locations of a series of places in the Pacific basin from a conventional map projection into an accessibility space. In this space, the relative locations of places were determined by their comparative accessibility as measured by travel times and airline route capacities, rather than by their geographical separation. In the present diagram, we explore an alternative metric at a local geographical scale by transforming the medical districts of Iceland into a 'disease incidence' space. The example is used to exemplify the computational procedures involved in the technique which are outlined in a technical appendix.

Iceland as a multidimensional scaling structure

To illustrate the method, we examine the degree of similarity of the 50 medical districts of Iceland on monthly influenza incidence in four time periods from 1945 to 1970 namely: 1945–52, 1953–60, 1961–68 and 1969–70. For a description of influenza as a disease and its epidemiology, see section 6.4. Using this metric, the relative locations of medical districts will reflect their degree of similarity on influenza incidence; the greater the similarity, the closer together the districts will be in the MDS space.

Diagram (A) shows the locations of the medical districts in the MDS spaces for 1945–52 and 1969–70. 1945–52 covers the period when the H1N1 strain of the influenza A virus was in circulation; 1969–70 was dominated by the H3N2 strain. The locations of the districts are given as a point pattern, with Reykjavík marked by a triangle. The plots show Reykjavík at the centre of the space and that districts are clustered more closely around Reykjavík in the later time period than they are in the earlier. This implies that medical districts have, over time, become more like the capital, Reykjavík, in the incidence of influenza, a result which cross-checks with Figure 6.5(K) where medical districts were shown to have become more like the capital in terms of rate of propagation of measles epidemics.

To examine the extent to which (1) medical districts have 'converged on' Reykjavík in terms of influenza incidence, and (2) medical districts have similarly converged on their nearest regional centres, diagrams (B) and (C) have been prepared. Those medical districts which, over the period from 1945 to 1970, either moved consistently nearer to (converging) or consistently farther from (diverging) Reykjavík in terms of their point locations in the four MDS spaces, are marked on map (B). This confirms that most medical districts in the west and north of the country have moved closer to Reykjavík over time in influenza behaviour. Only the remote districts in the fjord areas of northwest and eastern Iceland and on the south coast, where outwash from a permanent icecap makes road communication with Reykjavík difficult, do not exhibit such a trend.

Map (C) examines the behaviour of medical districts with respect to their regional capitals (named) in each of the regions delimited by the solid lines. In the north, there is a fairly consistent convergence of medical districts on Akureyri, the largest city in Iceland outside the Reykjavík region. In the east, medical districts have become increasingly dissimilar to Seyðisfjörður. Overall, the two maps imply an increased bonding of medical districts to the large cities in terms of their influenza time-series, a trend which almost certainly reflects the growing internal cohesiveness of Iceland in the post-1945 period brought about by the development of an extensive airline network (cf. section 6.5).

Sources and Further Reading

In Figure 7.2, map (B) is based on unpublished work by Dr P. Forer of the University of Canterbury, Christchurch, New Zealand. The changing air traffic flows in Figure 7.2 (C) are constructed from maps in M. Taylor and C.C. Kissling (1983), 'Resource dependence, power networks and the airline systems of the South Pacific', *Regional Studies*, 17, pp.237–50.

In Figure 7.3 the MDS maps of Iceland are redrawn from A.D. Cliff, P. Haggett and J.K. Ord (1986), *Spatial Aspects of Influenza Epidemics*, London: Pion, pp.185–94. The Icelandic epidemiological data used are as described in Figure 3.10 of this Atlas.

Multidimensional scaling as a mapping method is described in D.G. Kendall (1975), 'The recovery of structure from fragmentary information', *Philosophical Transactions of the Royal Society of London A*, 279, pp.547–82, and D.G. Kendall (1971), 'Construction of maps from odd bits of information', *Nature*, 231, pp.158–9. Geographical applications are considered in R.G. Golledge and G. Rushton (1972), *Multidimensional Scaling: Review and Geographical Applications*, Technical Paper No. 10, Washington, DC: Association of American Geographers, Commission on College Geography, and in A.C. Gatrell (1981), 'Multidimensional scaling', in *Quantitative Geography*, edited by N. Wrigley and R.J. Bennett, London: Routledge and Kegan Paul, pp. 151–63.

Standard accounts of the different algorithms which can be used in scaling are given in J.B. Kruskal (1964), 'Multidimensional scaling', *Psychometrika*, 29, pp.1–42, and J.B. Kruskal and M. Wish (1978), *Multidimensional Scaling*, Beverly Hills, Ca.: Sage.

The epidemiological effects of changing spatial relationships are considered in A.D. Cliff and P. Haggett (1985), *The Spread of Measles in Fiji and the Pacific: Spatial Components in the Transmission of Epidemic Waves through Island Communities*, Publication HG18, Canberra: Australian National University, Research School of Pacific Studies, Department of Human Geography. The impact of air travel on epidemiological processes is considered by H.E. Whittingham (1967), 'Impact of air travel on epidemiology', *British Journal of Clinical Practice*, 2, pp.409–15, and by P. Dorolle (1968), 'Old plagues in the jet age: international aspects of present and future control of communicable disease', *British Medical Journal*, 4, pp.789–92. See also R.H. Black (1956), 'The epidemiology of malaria in the southwest Pacific: changes associated with increasing European contact', *Oceania*, 27, pp.725–31; and N. McArthur (1967), *Island Populations in the Pacific*, Canberra: Australian National University Press. Map transformations at the scale of the Pacific involve complex problems in map projections; see D.H. Maling (1973), *Coordinate Systems and Map Projections*, London: George Philip.

Technical appendix

To conduct the MDS analysis described in Figure 7.3, the time-series of reported cases of influenza for each of the 50 medical districts were reduced to a binary form by recording 1 if cases were reported in a given month and 0 otherwise. The source of data was *Heilbrigðisskýrslur* (Public Health in Iceland), 1945–70. The time-series were then split into four parts corresponding to the year blocks 1945–52, 1953–60, 1961–68 and 1969–70. This gave three 50(districts) × 96 (months) and one 50 × 24 binary matrices, $\mathbf{A}$, say. That is, if $\mathbf{A} = \{a_{ij}\}$, $a_{ij} = 1$ if cases were reported in medical district i in month t and $a_{ij} = 0$ otherwise.

Now define $\mathbf{B} = \mathbf{A}\mathbf{A}^{\mathrm{T}}$. Then $\mathbf{B}$ is a symmetric matrix and has as its ijth element, b_{ij}, the number of months in a given block of years in which there were reported cases of influenza in medical districts i and j. The matrix $\mathbf{B}$ is a similarity matrix reflecting the similarity between medical districts in terms of their incidence of influenza. From $\mathbf{B}$ a matrix $\mathbf{D}$ ($= \{\delta_{ij}\}$) of dissimilarities ($\delta_{ij} = K - b_{ij}$ for some constant K) can be obtained. This matrix of dissimilarities serves as the basis for the MDS procedure.

Broadly stated, the problem of MDS is to find a configuration of n points in m-dimensional space such that the interpoint distances in the configuration reflect the experimental dissimilarities of the n objects (points). This may be viewed as a problem of statistical fitting. The dissimilarities are fixed given quantities and we wish to find the m-dimensional configuration of objects whose inter-object distances 'fit them best'. The ultimate locations of the points in the configuration are selected to preserve the rank ordering of the relative distances of the experimental dissimilarities. Thus the final distance metric may be regarded as a monotone transformation of the rank ordering.

By adopting as our central goal the requirement of a monotonic relationship between the observed dissimilarities and the distances in the configuration, the accuracy of a proposed solution can be judged by the degree to which this condition is approached. For a proposed configuration, we perform a monotonic regression of distance upon dissimilarity and use the residual sum of squares, suitably Normalized, as a quantitative measure of fit, known as the stress. The configuration we seek is that with minimum stress.

The interpretability of the coordinates is of obvious importance so our analysis is carried out in two dimensions ($m = 2$). Denote the n points in the configuration by $x_1 \ldots x_n$ and let $x_i = [x_{i1}, x_{i2}]^T$, where the second subscript denotes the space dimension. Let d_{ij} be the (euclidean) distance between the points x_i and x_j. Then we define the stress, S, of the fixed configuration $x_1 \ldots x_n$ to be

$$S_{(x_1, \ldots x_n)} = \underset{d_{ij} \text{ satisfying } M}{\text{minimum}} \left[\sum_{i<j} (d_{ij} - \hat{d}_{ij})^2 / \sum_{i<j} d_{ij}^2 \right]$$

where M is the monotonicity condition. The exact form of M depends on how we deal with ties in the dissimilarities. Commonly, M is the condition

whenever $\delta_{ij} < \delta_{rs}$ then $\hat{d}_{ij} \le \hat{d}_{rs}$,

and whenever $\delta_{ij} = \delta_{rs}$ then $\hat{d}_{ij} = \hat{d}_{rs}$.

The configuration with minimum stress is found iteratively and compuational details are given in Kruskal (1964). At each stage of the iterative procedure, the monotone regression to find the $\{\hat{d}_{ij}\}$ from the fixed known values $\{d_{ij}\}$ of the distances in the current configuration is also computed to yield the plots shown in Figure 7.3 (A). Although the technical details have been discussed in the context of the Icelandic samples, the same procedures have been followed in Figure 7.2 with the Pacific data.

7.4 MAPPING AND FORECASTING

One important role played by modern high-speed computers in mapping is in the solution of the complex models required to forecast future maps of disease incidence. As shown in Figure 3.1 and Chapter 5, such models must incorporate information on space-time interactions if reasonable projections are to be produced. The resulting models can rarely be solved analytically, and approximations have to be obtained using computer-based simulation techniques. In this diagram one such model is described and illustrated by generating *ex-post* forecasts of some measles epidemics for selected medical districts of Iceland.

Nature of process models

In attempting to model and to forecast the likely time and space paths which will be followed by an infectious epidemic disease as it moves through a geographically distributed population, one of two basic strategies may be followed. In the first, described earlier in Figure 5.18, a model is built around the assumption that past levels of cases of the disease provide the key to the case levels which may be expected in the future. Such models are relatively undemanding of data and rely for their precision upon a fairly simple structure and accurate identification of the space-time dependencies among areas illustrated in Figure 3.1(C).

In the second, considered in this figure, a model of the process whereby the disease is passed from one person to the next is built, taking into account features like the infectious period of the disease and the sizes and locations of the populations at risk.

The Hamer–Soper model

The classic model of epidemic disease transmission from person-to-person was developed as a result of work by Hamer (1906) and Soper (1929) on measles and it has become known as the Hamer–Soper model. The essential elements are illustrated in diagram (A). At any time t we assume that the total population in the region can be divided into three classes namely: the population at risk or susceptible population of size S_t, the infected population of size I_t and the recovered population of size R_t. The recovered population is taken to be composed of people who have had the disease but who can no longer pass it on to others because of recovery, isolation on appearance of overt symptoms, or death.

As shown in diagram (A), the model operates at a given time, t, by allowing four types of transition.

(a) New cases of the disease are generated by contact between susceptibles and infectives to yield the time-series of infectives shown for area i. The same process in a set of areas i, j, k . . . yields a map of infectives at t. Projected into the future, this mechanism generates time-series forecasts of numbers of infectives at $(t + 1)$, $(t + 2)$ . . . and forecast maps.

The rate of contact between susceptibles and infectives is referred to as the infection rate. It reflects the degree of mixing by local movements between susceptibles and infectives.

(b) An infective is removed from circulation and enters the recovered population at some recovery rate.

(c) Susceptibles are 'born' at some birth rate. This renews the stock of susceptibles by (literally) births and in-migration of susceptibles from other areas to offset the reduction in S which occurs through transition (a).

(d) The susceptible stock may also be depleted by leakage through vaccinations, at some vaccination rate, to the recovered population.

The equations required to run the model are given in the technical appendix. In general terms, starting sizes are determined for the S, I and R populations. Random variables are used to fix both the waiting time to the next transition and the type of transition [(a) – (d)] which will occur. The event happens, the population stocks (S, I and R) are updated and the process is repeated.

Application to Iceland

Diagram (B) shows an application of the model to measles epidemics in four medical districts of Iceland between 1954 and 1970 (Cliff, Haggett, Ord and Versey, 1981, pp. 159–70). The model was calibrated on data relating to the period 1945–53 and then run forward from 1954–70 to generate *ex-post* forecasts. On the charts relating to each of the four districts, the pecked line gives the S population estimated from demographic data while the solid line plots the estimates of S from the model. The lowest line of histograms records the number of measles cases which actually occurred while the upper line of histograms shows the number of cases (I) estimated by the model.

It is evident that reasonable projections have been obtained both in terms of the phasing of epidemics and their magnitude. The wave trains of epidemics in Reykjavíkur and Akureyrar are modelled as effectively as the once-in-16-years

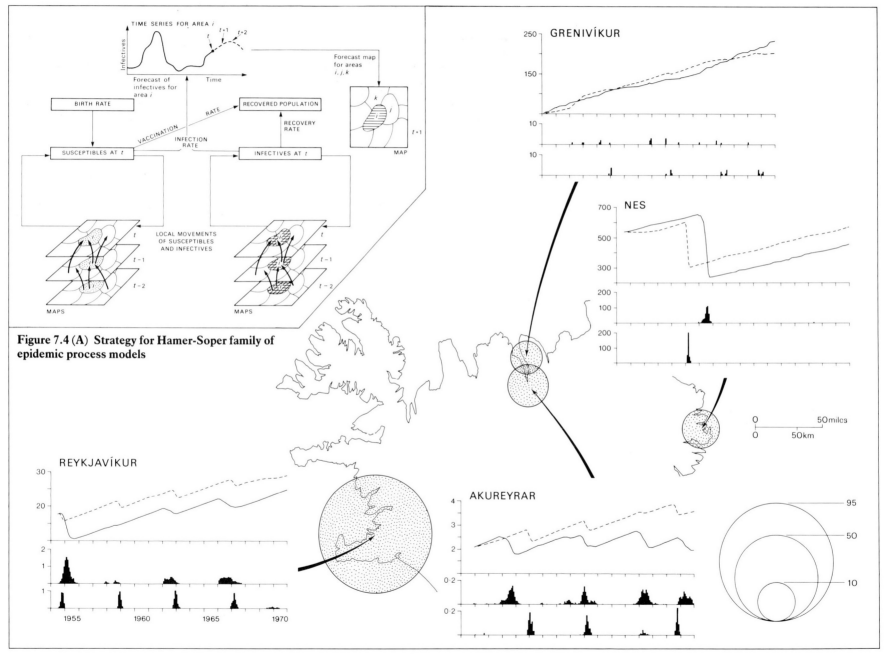

Figure 7.4 (A) Strategy for Hamer-Soper family of epidemic process models

Figure 7.4 (B) Application of Hamer–Soper model to measles epidemics in four Icelandic medical districts

outbreak in Nes, and the 16 years with no epidemic in Grenivikur.

The modelling of the size of the S population is less successful, generally being underestimated.

Sources and Further Reading

The diagrams are based on work reported extensively in A.D. Cliff, P. Haggett, J.K. Ord and G.R. Versey (1981), *Spatial Diffusion: an Historical Geography of Epidemics in an Island Community*, Cambridge: Cambridge University Press, pp.159–83.

The early attempts to model epidemic processes go back to the start of this century; see W.H. Hamer (1906), 'Epidemic diseases in England', *Lancet*, 1, pp.733–9, and H.E. Soper (1929), 'Interpretation of periodicity in disease prevalence', *Journal of the Royal Statistical Society A*, 92, pp.34–73. The Hamer–Soper model provides the basis of threshold theorems which give the conditions under which a minor outbreak will burgeon. Mathematical details appear in W.O. Kermack and A.G. McKendrick (1927), 'Contributions to the mathematical theory of epidemics, I', *Proceedings of the Royal Society A*, 115, pp.700–21. Some of the more elementary models are summarized in P. Haggett (1975), 'Simple epidemics in human populations: some geographical aspects of the Hamer–Soper diffusion models', in *Processes in Physical and Human Geography: Bristol Essays*, edited by R.F. Peel, M.D.I. Chisholm and P. Haggett, London: Heinemann, pp.371–91, while more advanced models are considered in N.T.J. Bailey (1981), 'Spatial models in epidemiology', *Lecture Notes on Biomathematics*, 38, pp.233–61.

Alternative models are the chain binomial outlined in A.D. Cliff and J.K. Ord (1978), 'Forecasting the progress of an epidemic', in *Towards the Dynamic Analysis of Spatial Systems*, edited by R.L. Martin, N.J. Thrift and R.J. Bennett, London: Pion, pp.191–204, and time-series formulations described in A.D. Cliff, P. Haggett and J.K. Ord (1983), 'Forecasting epidemic pathways for measles in Iceland: the use of simultaneous equation and logic models', *Ecology of Disease*, 2, pp.377–96.

Technical appendix

Formalization of transitions Transitions (a) – (d) in the main text are normally tabulated as in Table 7.4.1. The infection rate is denoted by β, the recovery rate by μ, the birth rate by ν and the vaccination rate by ϵ. The table implies that the infection and recovery rates are proportional to the sizes of the S and I populations, while the birth and vaccination rates are constant. All transitions are assumed to be independent and to depend only on the present state of the population, so that the probability density of time between any pair of successive transitions is

$$r \exp(-rt) \quad \text{where} \quad r = \sum_{i=1}^{4} r_i, \qquad (7.4.1)$$

and r_i denotes the rate at which transition i occurs. The probability that the next transition is of type i is

$$r_i/r, \, i = 1,2,3,4. \qquad (7.4.2)$$

The model is generally fitted using Monte Carlo techniques. An exponential random variable is thus used to fix the waiting time to the next transition and a uniform random variable to select the type of transition.

Operation of the model An infective is isolated after an average period of $1/\mu$ days. While he is infectious he causes new infections at the rate of S per day. If we ignore changes in S, one infective infects an average of $\beta S/\mu$ ($= \kappa$ say) susceptibles before he recovers. When $\kappa \leq 1$ we would expect a small epidemic to die out. However, when $\kappa > 1$ a small epidemic will spark off a major outbreak although as the epidemic spreads S will fall and $\beta S/\mu$ can become less than unity. Thus the general pattern will be for the S population to build up [transition type (c)] to around the critical population size $S = \mu/\beta$ when an epidemic will spread until the S population falls sufficiently for the epidemic phase to pass.

In large communities, if a disease is endemic, the period between epidemic peaks is approximately $\mu/\beta\nu$, the mean time for the birth of μ/β susceptibles. In smaller communities where there is fade out the period is longer because, once the critical S population size is reached, there is a delay until the disease is reintroduced from outside.

It is the Hamer–Soper model which provides the theoretical underpinnings for the Kendall waves discussed in

Figure 5.6, as well as for Bartlett's ideas on critical community size for measles endemicity outlined in Figure 6.5(A). The model was also used to generate the forecasts of measles in Iceland illustrated in Figure 6.5(L).

Further developments The basic model defined in Table 7.4.1 is capable of many extensions. For example, geographical interactions between regions can be handled by defining transitions like those given in Table 7.4.1 for each region. Additional transitions could be created to handle out-migration of the population, while the infection parameter might be made time dependent to allow for decreasing temporal infectivity of a disease.

Table 7.4.1 *Transition types and rates*

Type of transition	Rate
(a) $S \to S-1; I \to I+1; R \to R$	βIS
(b) $S \to S; I \to I-1; R \to R+1$	μI
(c) $S \to S+1; I \to I; R \to R$	ν
(d) $S \to S-1; I \to I; R \to R+1$	ϵ

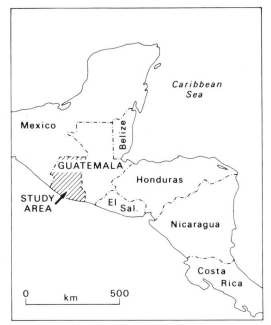

Figure 7.5 (A) Study area in southwest Guatemala

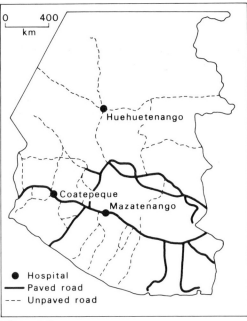

Figure 7.5 (B) Road system

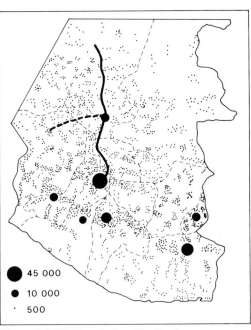

Figure 7.5 (C) Population distribution

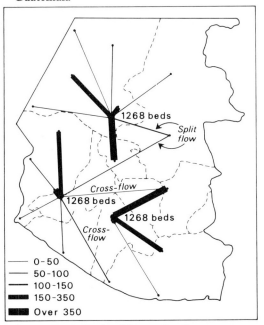

Figure 7.5 (D) Optimal flows of patients to hospitals (equal bed capacity)

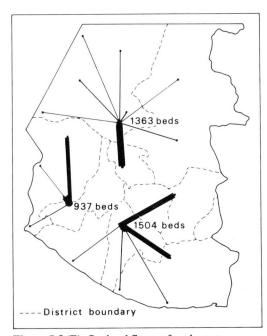

Figure 7.5 (E) Optimal flows of patients to hospitals (variable bed capacity)

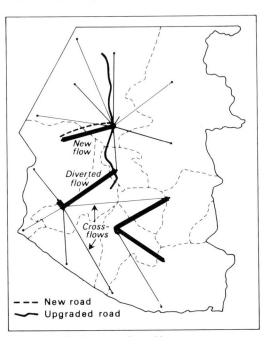

Figure 7.5 (F) Impact of road improvements on optimum flows in (D)

7.5 MAPPING AND OPTIMIZATION

So far in this Atlas we have focused upon the geographical patterns produced by the incidence of disease, and we have not considered the public health implications of sickness through the need for new hospitals, more doctors and so on: that would require a separate atlas. But, given the uneven distribution of disease both in space and time, we conclude with a public health example which also underlines the role that computers might play.

Locational decisions on the placement of capital intensive buildings and equipment are critical to the efficient operation of health care services, and several models exist which enable optimal locational patterns to be obtained. They address the questions of 'where and when should a new hospital be built?' or 'should a new wing be added to this hospital or to that?'.

Given the huge costs of such projects and scarce financial resources, accurate future maps of the best way of allocating these resources are badly needed.

As was the case in the previous figure, the available models are computationally burdensome without high-capacity computing power, and their routine application to issues of the sort described has been a function of the growing availability of these machines and their associated software. In this final figure of the Atlas we explore one of the simplest of such models, the so-called *transportation problem*, and illustrate its use by considering the problem of hospital location and capacities in the developing country of Guatemala.

The basic allocation problem

Given an existing set of hospitals in a region, the initial problem faced by administrators is how best to allocate patients to the hospitals under their control. In part the allocations will reflect the availability of specialized medical facilities in certain hospitals. However, for routine visits not requiring these facilities, such as out-patient trips then, from the patient's point of view, the allocation is best made to minimize journey times (or costs or distances travelled). In general, this suggests that patients should attend the hospital nearest to their home.

While this may be optimal from the patient's viewpoint it may not be optimal for the set of hospitals under the control of a single authority. The capacities of hospitals and the geographical distribution of patients may vary so much that a policy of sending patients to the nearest hospital might result in some hospitals being over-used and others being under-used.

The assignment procedure therefore has to be examined as a system problem covering all hospitals and all patients simultaneously if an overall optimum is to be achieved. The allocation problem is made more complex if the transportation system (the linkages) whereby patients travel from home to hospital is itself subject to change. For example, the provision of a new road in a particular area may drastically reduce travel costs and times making a nearby hospital more accessible than before.

Southwest Guatemala

The issues raised are explored in this series of diagrams which examine the allocation of patients to hospitals in southwest Guatemala both before and after hypothetical changes in the bed capacities of the various hospitals and improvements to the road network. The example is based upon a study by Gould and Leinbach (1966).

The location of the study area appears in map (A). Map (B) shows the area at a larger geographical scale. The three hospitals are located at Huehuetenango, Coatepeque and Mazatenango. The existing road system by which patients travel in from the surrounding rural areas to the hospitals for treatment is also marked. Two categories of road exist, paved and unpaved. Map (C) gives the geographical distribution of the population to be served by the hospitals. There are seven large towns with populations in excess of 10,000 while the remaining population is rural and scattered in small villages throughout the region. District boundaries are shown by the pecked lines. (C) also plots the location of proposed new and upgraded roads.

An optimal allocation pattern

Details of the transportation problem model used by Gould and Leinbach are provided in the technical appendix. The model produces a patient-allocation pattern which minimizes the cost over the entire system of moving patients to hospitals. Cost may be measured in any metric such as money, time, distance travelled and so on. The pattern of movements is called the optimal configuration and the model is normative. The differences between the normative and the patient movements actually occurring therefore provide a measure of the efficiency of the current allocation pattern and suggest where changes might be made.

Map (D) illustrates a solution to the allocation problem given the road network shown in (B) and equal bed capacities (1268) at the three hospitals. The vector widths are proportional to the flows of patients. Because of the constraints on beds and the large populations to be served in some districts, difficult patient-journeys result. For example in the northeast district, a split flow is marked where patients cannot attend the local hospital at Huehuetenango but face a 600 km journey across country to Coatepeque. Similar capacity constraints at Mazatenango force cross flows away from the nearest hospital to Coatepeque.

Impact of changed bed totals

In (E), we assume that the bed capacities at the hospitals can be changed. The total number of beds in the system is unaltered at 3804, but they have been distributed among the hospitals in a different configuration which reflects certain diagnostic signals (shadow prices) generated by the model. Given these revised capacities, the optimal allocation eliminates the split flow and cross-flows apparent in (D) and patients are allocated to the geographically nearest hospital.

Impact of highway improvements

In (F), optimal allocations have been produced by the model assuming that (a) the hospital bed capacities given in (D) exist and (b) the new and upgraded roads mapped in (C) have been built. Again changes are evident compared with the allocation shown in (D). The new road gives the western part of the study area access to Huehuetenango and results in the diversion to that hospital of a major flow of patients currently attending Coatepeque. To prevent bed capacity at Huehuetenango being exceeded, patients in the centre of the study area are diverted from Huehuetenanago to Coatapeque using the upgraded road in that area. However, because of the restrictions on bed capacities the cross-flows noted in (D) have returned.

Implications

The power of these programming models lies in their ability to generate patterns of flows which would result from a variety of capital investment scenarios in both hospital capacities and the road network. Consequences can be explored before a commitment to invest is made. This leads to more efficient use of scarce resources which is particularly valuable in developing countries. In the present example, maps (E) and (F) demonstrate that some combination of investment both in the road network and in changed bed capacities would produce an allocation of patients to hospitals which minimizes travel and therefore increase the access of patients to medical care. It emphasizes the extent to which the problems of health, transport cost, network structure and the locations and capacities of hospitals are all tightly interwoven.

Conclusion

The resolution of these problems would occupy several volumes. We conclude the present Atlas with the hope that the examples provided have illustrated the way in which mapping methods can improve our understanding of disease processes and encourage closer collaboration between geographers, medical scientists and, in the spirit of this final figure, those responsible for investment decisions in heath care provision. If such increased collaboration occurs, then the Atlas will have achieved one of its purposes.

Sources and Further Reading

The maps of Guatemala are redrawn from P.R. Gould and T.R. Leinbach (1966), 'An approach to the geographic assignment of hospital services', *Tijdschrift voor Economische en Sociale Geografie*, 57, pp.203–6. For a similar study in the United States see R. Morrill (1959), 'Highways and services: the case of physicians' care', in *Studies of Highway Development and Geographic Change*, edited by W.L. Garrison, B.J.L. Berry, D.F. Marble, J.F. Nystuen and R.L. Morrill, Seattle: University of Washington Press, pp.229–76.

The optimization methods used are summarized in P. Haggett, A.D. Cliff and A.E. Frey (1977), *Locational Analysis in Human Geography*, second edition, London: Edward Arnold, pp.491–516. General questions of optimal allocation of medical services are considered in B.H. Massam (1975), *Location and Space in Social Administration*, London: Edward Arnold. See also D.R. Phillips (1986), 'The demand for and utilization of health services', in *Medical Geography: Progress and Prospect*, edited by M. Pacione, London: Croom Helm, pp.200–47.

Technical appendix

To formulate the transportation problem we make the following definitions. Let i denote the typical area generating patients (the catchment area) who are to be allocated to the typical hospital j. Let x_{ij} denote the number of patients moved from catchment area i to hospital j at the per unit transport cost c_{ij}. Then the cost of moving all the patients from i to j will be $c_{ij}x_{ij}$, and the total costs over an entire set of n catchment areas and m hospitals will be

$$\sum_{i=1}^{n} \sum_{i=1}^{m} c_{ij}x_{ij}. \qquad (7.5.1)$$

Let S_i indicate the total number of patients to be moved from catchment area i and let D_j denote the capacity (in number of beds) of the jth hospital.

The linear programming transportation problem may then be written as

$$\text{Minimise } Z = \sum_{i=1}^{n} \sum_{j=1}^{m} c_{ij}x_{ij}, \qquad (7.5.2)$$

subject to

$$\sum_{j=1}^{m} x_{ij} \leq S_i, i = 1, 2, \ldots, n, \qquad (7.5.3)$$

$$\sum_{i=1}^{n} x_{ij} \geq D_j, j = 1, 2, \ldots, m, \qquad (7.5.4)$$

and

$$x_{ij} \geq 0, i = 1, 2, \ldots, n; \ j = 1, 2, \ldots, m. \qquad (7.5.5)$$

Thus objective function of the model expressed in (7.5.2) seeks to allocate patients from catchment areas to hospitals in a least–cost manner to the system as a whole, but subject to the constraints that the number of patients allocated from area i to hospital j must not exceed the number in i seeking beds [constraint (7.5.3)] and all beds in each hospital j are taken [constraint (7.5.4)].

Many refinements of the basic model exist. These are discussed in Haggett, Cliff and Frey (1977, pp.491–509), where an appropriate procedure for fitting the model is given.

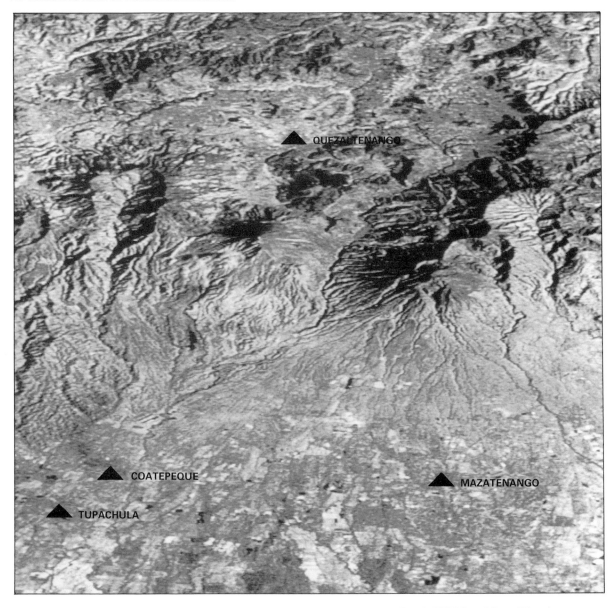

Figure 7.5 (G) **Multi-spectral scanner image of southwest Guatemala from data in NASA archives. The sites indicated are, from left to right, Tupachula, Coatepeque, Quezaltenango and Mazatenango**

DATA SOURCES, ATLASES AND REFERENCES

DATA SOURCES, ATLASES AND REFERENCES

The list that follows is divided into three parts. The first section lists the main sources of statistical data used in compiling the Atlas. It does not attempt to present a representative coverage of sources of disease statistics; these are fully described in the standard accounts [see Alderson (1974) and Alderson and Dowie (1979)]. Likewise, the second section is selective, giving a list of the main disease atlases to which reference is made in the text: a useful guide to such atlases is given in Howe (1986). Finally, the third part lists references to printed works, alphabetically by author, and includes the atlases referred to in section 2. Numbers in brackets after references indicate the sections of the Atlas in which the item is cited.

1 SELECTED SOURCES OF DATA

International

League of Nations (Health Section), Geneva. *Weekly Epidemiological Record*, 1925–47 (Vol. 1–23); *Quarterly Bulletin*, 1925–39.
United Nations Statistical Office, New York. *Demographic Yearbook*, 1948–; *Statistical Yearbook*, 1948–.
World Health Organization, Geneva. *WHO Weekly Epidemiological Record*, 1947– (Vol. 23–); *WHO Weekly Epidemiological and Vital Statistics Report*, 1947–67 (Vol. 1–20), monthly; continued as *World Health Statistics Report*, 1968– (Vol. 21–), monthly; *WHO World Health Statistics Annual*, 1947–.

Regional

Nordic Statistical Secretariat, Nordic Council, Stockholm. *Yearbook of Nordic Statistics*, 1970–.
Pan American Health Organization, Washington, DC. *Weekly Epidemiological Report*, 1945–; *Annual Report of the Director*, 1945–.
South Pacific Commission, Noumea. *South Pacific Health Service: Inspector General's Annual Report*, 1946–59; *Annual Epidemiological Report*, 1960–.

National

Iceland

Hagstofa Íslands [Statistical Bureau of Iceland], Reykjavík. *Mannfjöldaskýrslur* [Population and Vital Statistics], 1911–, decennial; *Tölfraeðihandbók* [Statistical Abstract of Iceland], 1911–, irregular.
Landlæknisemblaettið [Office of the Director of Public Health], Reykjavík. *Skýrslur um Heilbrigði Manna á Íslandi*, [Report on Public Health in Iceland], 1881–1900, irregular; *Skýrslur um Heilsufar og Heilbrigðismálefni á Íslandi*. [Report on the State of Sanitation and Public Health in Iceland], 1901–10, irregular; *Heilbrigðisskýrslur*. [Public Health in Iceland], 1911–25, irregular; 1926–, annual.

United Kingdom

Communicable Diseases Surveillance Centre, Public Health Laboratory Service, Colindale. *Communicable Disease Report*, 1978–, weekly; *CDR Monthly Tabulations*, 1977–.
Houses of Parliament, Westminster. British Parliamentary Papers: Great Britain Parliamentary Papers 1850, XXI: *Report of the General Board of Health on the Epidemic Cholera of 1848 and 1849*; Great Britain Parliamentary Papers 1850, XXII: *Report by the General Board of Health on the Supply of Water to the Metropolis*; Great Britain Parliamentary Papers 1854–5, XXI: *Report and Appendix to Report of the Committee for Scientific Inquiries in Relation to the Cholera-Epidemic of 1854*.
Office of Population Censuses and Surveys, London. *Registrar General's Weekly Return*, 1898–1974; *OPCS Weekly Monitor*, 1974.

United States

Centers for Disease Control, Atlanta. *Morbidity and Mortality Weekly Report*, 1952–; *Reported Incidence of Notifiable Diseases in the United States*, 1958–, annual; *Special Surveillance Reports*, 1958–, irregular.
Department of Commerce, Washington, DC. *Arrivals and Departures by Selected Ports*, 1975–, annual; *Analysis of International Travel to the United States*, 1975–, annual.
Department of Transportation, Washington, DC. *International Travel Statistics*, 1970–, annual.
National Center for Vital Statistics. *US Vital and Health Statistics Series*, 1975–, monthly.

Local archives

Epidemiological Research Centre, Cirencester. Records of infectious diseases from the epidemiological records of Dr R.E. Hope-Simpson, 1946–76.

National Archives, Suva, Fiji. Methodist Missionary Society Archives. *Fiji Argus*, Levuka, Fiji, 1875; *Fiji Times*, Levuka, Fiji, 1875.

2   SELECTED ATLASES OF DISEASE DISTRIBUTIONS

World

American Geographical Society (1950–5). Sheets of the 'Atlas of Diseases'. *Geographical Review*, 40, pp.648–9; 41, pp.272–3, 638–9; 42, pp.98–101, 282–3, 628–30; 43, pp.89–90, 253–5, 404; 44, pp.133–6, 408–10, 583–4; 45, pp.416, 572.

Howe, G.M., ed. (1986). *Global Geocancerology: A World Geography of Human Cancers*. Edinburgh: Churchill Livingstone.

Rodenwaldt, E. and H.J. Jusatz (1952–61). *World Atlas of Epidemic Diseases*, vol. 1–3. Hamburg: Falk.

Zeiss, H., ed. (1941–5). *Seuchen Atlas*. Gotha: Jutus Perthes (Hermann Haack Geographisch-Kartographische Ansatt).

Africa

Hall, S.A. and B.W. Langlands (1975). *Atlas of Disease Distribution in Uganda*. Nairobi: East Africa Publishers.

Americas

Canadian Ministry of Supply and Services (1980). *Mortality Atlas of Cancer*. Hull, Quebec: Canadian Government Publications Centre.

Mason, T.J., F.W. McKay Jr, R. Hoover, W.J. Bia and J.F. Fraumeni Jr (1975). *Atlas of Cancer Mortality for United States Counties, 1950–69*, National Institutes of Health, Publication No. 75–780. Washington, DC: Government Printing Office.

Mason, T.J., J.F. Fraumeni Jr, R. Hoover and W.J. Blot (1981). *An Atlas of Mortality from Selected Diseases*, National Institutes of Health, Publication No. 81–2397. Washington, DC: Government Printing Office.

Asia

Chen, K.-P., H.-Y. Wu, C.-C. Yen and Y.-J. Cheng (1979). *Colour Atlas of Cancer Mortality by Administrative and Other Classified Districts in Taiwan Area, 1968–78*, Special Publication No. 3. Taiwan: National Science Council.

Chinese Academy of Medical Sciences (1981). *Atlas of Cancer Mortality in the People's Republic of China*. Shanghai: China Map Press, pp.77–8, 85–6.

Daiwa Health Foundation (1980). *Atlas of Cardiovascular Disease for Cities, Towns and Villages in Japan, 1969–74*. Tokyo: Daiwa Health Foundation.

Segi, M. (1977). *Atlas of Cancer Mortality for Japan by Cities and Counties, 1969–76*. Tokyo: Daiwa Health Foundation.

Europe

Becker, N., R. Frentzel-Beyme and G. Wagner (1984). *Krebsatlas der Bundesrepublik Deutschland*, 2nd edn. Berlin: Springer Verlag.

Central Bureau voor Statistick (1980). *Atlas of Cancer Mortality in the Netherlands 1969–1978*. The Hague: Netherlands Bureau of Statistics.

Frenzel-Beyme, R., R. Leuter and G. Wiebett (1979). *Cancer Atlas of the Federal Republic of Germany*. Berlin: Springer Verlag.

Gardner, M.J., P.D. Winter, C.P. Taylor and E.D. Acheson (1983). *Atlas of Cancer Mortality in England and Wales, 1968–1978*. Chichester: John Wiley.

Gardner, M.J., P.D. Winter and D.J.P. Barker (1984). *Atlas of Mortality from Selected Diseases in England and Wales 1968–78*. Chichester: John Wiley.

Howe, G.M., ed. (1970). *National Atlas of Disease Mortality in the United Kingdom*, 2nd edn. London: Royal Geographical Society.

Kemp, I., P. Boyle, M. Smans and C. Muir (1985). *Atlas of Cancer in Scotland, 1975–1980: Incidence and Epidemiological Perspective*, International Agency for Research on Cancer (IARC), Scientific Publication No. 72. Oxford: Oxford University Press.

Ryckeboer, R., J. Jamssens and J. Thiers (1983). *Atlas de la mortalité par cancer en Belgique, 1969–76*. Brussels: Institut d'Hygiène et d'Épidémiologie.

Oceania

Borman, B. (1982). *A Cancer Mortality Atlas of New Zealand*, Special Report No. 63. Wellington: New Zealand Department of Health.

Borman, B. and S. Leitaua (1984). *A General Mortality Atlas of New Zealand*, Special Report No. 71. Wellington: New Zealand Department of Health.

3 REFERENCES

Aaby, P. (1988). 'Measles mortality'. *Review of Infectious Diseases*, 10, pp.451–91. [3.3]

Aageenbrug, R.T., ed. (1979). *Auto-Carto IV. Applications in Health and Environment*. Falls Church, Va.: American Congress on Surveying and Mapping. [7.1]

Abraham, B. (1981). 'Missing observations in time series'. *Communications in Statistics A*, 10, pp.1643–53. [2.10]

Acheson, R.M., ed. (1965). *International Comparability in Epidemiology*. Washington, DC: Milbank Memorial Foundation. [2.1, 2.3]

Ackerknecht, E.H. (1965). *History and Geography of the Most Important Diseases*. New York: Hafner. [1.1]

Alderson, M. (1974). *Central Government Routine Health Statistics*. Vol. 2, No. 3, *Reviews of United Kingdom Statistical Sources*, ed. W.F. Maunder. London: Heinemann for Royal Statistical Society and Social Science Research Council. [2.2]

Alderson, M. (1981). *International Mortality Statistics*. London: Macmillan. [2.1]

Alderson, M. and R. Dowie (1979). *Health Surveys and Related Studies*. Vol. 9, No. 16, *Reviews of United Kingdom Statistical Sources*, ed. W.F. Maunder. Oxford: Pergamon for Royal Statistical Society and Social Science Research Council. [2.2]

American Geographical Society (1950–5). Sheets of the 'Atlas of Diseases'. *Geographical Review*, 40, pp.648–9; 41, pp.272–3, 638–9; 42, pp.98–101, 282–3, 628–30; 43, pp.89–90, 253–5, 404; 44, pp.133–6, 408–10, 583–4; 45, pp.416, 572. [3.1]

Anderson, D.O. (1968). 'Geographic variations in deaths due to emphysema and bronchitis in Canada'. *Canadian Medical Association Journal*, 98, pp.231–41. [3.11–3.12]

Anderson, R.M. and R.M. May (1982). 'Vaccination against rubella and measles: quantitative investigations of different policies'. *Journal of Hygiene (London)*, 90, pp.259–235. [4.9]

ApSimon, H. and J. Wilson (1986). 'Tracking the cloud from Chernobyl'. *New Scientist*, 17 July 1986, pp.42–5. [5.3]

ApSimon, H.M., J.J.N. Wilson, S. Guirguis and P.A. Stott (1987). 'Assessment of the Chernobyl release in the immediate aftermath of the accident', *Nuclear Energy*, 26, pp.259–301. [5.3]

Armstrong, B. (1980). 'The epidemiology of cancer in the People's Republic of China'. *International Journal of Epidemiology*, 4, pp.305–15. [3.7]

Armstrong, R.W. (1969). 'Standardized class intervals and rate computation in statistical maps of mortality'. *Annals of the Association of American Geographers*, 59, 382–90. [1.6]

Armstrong, R.W., M. Kannan Kutty and S.K. Dharmalingham (1974). 'Incidence of nasopharyngeal carcinoma in Malaysia, with special reference to the state of Selangor'. *British Journal of Cancer*, 30, pp.86–94. [3.7]

Bacharach, M. (1970). *Biproportional Matrices and Input–Output Change*. Cambridge: Cambridge University Press. [5.17]

Bachi, R. (1963). 'Standard distance measures and related methods for spatial analysis'. *Regional Science Association, Papers and Proceedings*, 10, pp.83–132. [1.15]

Bailey, N.T.J. (1975). *The Mathematical Theory of Infectious Diseases and Its Application*. London: Griffin. [5.6, 6.5]

Bailey, N.T.J. (1981). 'Spatial models in epidemiology'. *Lecture Notes on Biomathematics*, 38, pp.233–61. [7.4]

Barham, S.Y. and F.D.J. Dunstan (1983). 'Missing values in time series'. In *Time Series Analysis: Theory and Practice*, vol. 2, ed. O.D. Anderson. Amsterdam: North-Holland. [2.10]

Bartlett, M.S. (1957). 'Measles periodicity and community size'. *Journal of the Royal Statistical Society A*, 120, pp.48–70. [6.5]

Baroyan, O.V., L.A. Genchikov, L.A. Rvachev and V.A. Shashkov (1969). 'An attempt at large-scale influenza epidemic modelling by means of a computer'. *Bulletin of the International Epidemiological Association*, 18, pp.22–31. [6.4]

Baroyan, O.V., L.A. Rvachev and Y.G. Ivannikov (1977). *Modelling and Prediction of Influenza Epidemics in the USSR*. Moscow: Gamaleia Institute of Epidemiology and Microbiology. [6.4]

Basu, R.N., Z. Jezek and N.A. Ward (1979). *The Eradicatin of Smallpox from India*. Geneva: World Health Organization. [6.3]

Benenson, A.B. (1984). 'Smallpox'. In *Viral Infections of Humans: Epidemiology and Control*, 2nd edn, ed. A.S. Evans. New York, NY: Plenum, pp.541–68. [6.3]

Benjamin, B. (1968). *Health and Vital Statistics*. London: Allen and Unwin. [2.7, 5.1]

Benjamin, B., ed. (1980). *Medical Records*, 2nd edn. London: Heinemann. [2.2]

Bennett, R.J. (1979). *Spatial Time Series: Analysis, Forecasting and Control*. London: Pion. [4.3]

Bentley, C.A. (1916). *Report on Malaria, Part 1*. Calcutta. [3.5]

Berry, R.J. (1982). 'The leukaemias'. In *Epidemiology of Diseases*, ed. D.L. Miller and R.D.T. Farmer. Oxford: Blackwell Scientific, pp.146–51. [3.8]

Berry, R.J. (1982). 'Carcinoma of the bladder'. In *Epidemiology of Diseases*, ed. D.L. Miller and R.D.T. Farmer. Oxford: Blackwell Scientific, pp.266–72. [3.6]

Black, D. (Chairman of the Independent Advisory Group) (1984). *Investigation of the Possible Increased Incidence of Cancer in West Cumbria*. London: Her Majesty's Stationery Office. [3.8]

Black, F.L. (1966). 'Measles endemicity in insular populations: critical community size and its evolutionary implication'. *Journal of Theoretical Biology*, 11, pp.207–11. [2.3, 6.5]

Black, F.L. (1984). 'Measles'. In *Viral Infections of Humans: Epidemiology and Control*, 2nd edn, ed. A.S. Evans. New York, NY: Plenum, pp.397–418. [3.3, 6.5]

Black, R.H. (1956). 'The epidemiology of malaria in the southwest Pacific: changes associated with increasing European contact'. *Oceania*, 27, pp.725–31. [7.3]

Blot, W.J. and J.F. Fraumeni (1978). 'Geographic patterns of bladder cancer in the United States'. *Journal of the National Cancer Institute*, 61, pp.1017–23. [3.6]

Blumenstock, D.I. (1953). 'The reliability factor in the drawing of isarithms'. *Annals of the Association of American Geographers*, 43, pp.289–304. [1.10]

Box, G.E.P. and G.M. Jenkins (1976). *Time Series Analysis: Forecasting and Control*, rev. edn. San Francisco, Ca.: Holden-Day. [5.18]

Brimblecombe, P. (1987). *The Big Smoke: A History of Air Pollution in London since Medieval Times*. London: Methuen. [3.12]

Brockington, F. (1975). *World Health*, 3rd edn. Edinburgh: Churchill Livingstone. [2.1, 2.3]

Buchanan, C. (1963). *Traffic in Towns*. London: Her Majesty's Stationery Office. [3.17]

Burkitt, D. (1962). 'Determining the climatic limitations of a children's cancer common in Africa'. *British Medical Journal*, 2, pp.1019–23. [5.16]

Burnet, Sir Macfarlane and D.O. White (1972). *Natural History of Infectious Disease*, 4th edn. Cambridge: Cambridge University Press. [4.7, 6.5]

Canadian Ministry of Supply and Services (1980). *Mortality Atlas of Cancer*. Hull, Quebec: Canadian Government Publications Centre. [3.6]

Carter, J.R. (1984). *Computer Mapping*. Washington, DC: Association of American Geographers. [7.1]

Castner, H.W. and A.H. Robinson (1969). *Dot Area Symbols in Cartography: The Influence of Pattern on Their Perception*, Technical Monograph No. CA–4. Washington, DC: American Congress on Surveying and Mapping. [1.3]

Central Bureau voor Statistick (1980). *Atlas of Cancer Mortality in the Netherlands 1969–1978*. The Hague: Netherlands Bureau of Statistics. [3.6]

Centers for Disease Control (1986). 'Premature mortality in the United States: public health issues in the use of potential life lost'. *Morbidity and Mortality Weekly Report*, 35, suppl. 2, pp.1–11. [2.5]

Chang, J.-H. (1968). 'Rainfall in the tropical southwest Pacific'. *Geographical Review*, 58, pp.142–4. [4.6]

Chang, K.-T. (1978). 'Measurement scales in cartography'. *American Cartographer*, 5, pp. 57–64. [1.2]

Chatfield, C. (1980). *The Analysis of Time Series: An Introduction*, 2nd edn. London: Chapman and Hall. [4.1, 4.2, 4.3, 5.12]

Chen, K.-P., H.-Y. Wu, C.-C. Yen and Y.-J. Cheng (1979). *Colour Atlas of Cancer Mortality by Administrative and Other Classified Districts in Taiwan Area, 1968–78*, Special Publication No. 3. Taiwan: National Science Council. [3.6]

Chinese Academy of Medical Sciences (1981). *Atlas of Cancer Mortality in the People's Republic of China*. Shanghai: China Map Press, pp.77–8, 85–6. [3.7]

Choi, K. and S.B. Thacker (1981). 'An evaluation of influenza mortality surveillance, 1962–79. Pt. 1: Time-series forecasts of expected pneumonia and influenza deaths. Pt. 2: Percentage of pneumonia and influenza deaths as an indicator of influenza activity'. *American Journal of Epidemiology*, 113, pp.215–26, 227–35. [2.4]

Chorley, R.J. and P. Haggett (1965). 'Trend-surface mapping in geographical research'. *Transactions of the Institute of British Geographers*, 37, pp.47–67. [1.12]

Choynowski, M. (1959). 'Maps based upon probabilities'. *Journal of the American Statistical Association*, 54, pp.385–8. [1.7, 3.2]

Clemow, F.G. (1903). *The Geography of Disease*. Cambridge: Cambridge University Press. [1.1]

Cleveland, W.P. and G.C. Tiao (1976). 'Decomposition of seasonal time series: a model for the Census X-11 program'. *Journal of the American Statistical Association*, 77, pp.581–7. [4.2]

Cliff, A.D. and P. Haggett (1980). 'Geographical aspects of epidemic diffusion in closed communities'. In *Statistical Applications in the Spatial Sciences*, ed. N. Wrigley. London: Pion, pp.5–44. [4.7]

Cliff, A.D. and P. Haggett, (1981). 'Graph theory'. In *Quantitative Geography*, ed. N. Wrigley and R.J. Bennett. London: Routledge and Kegan Paul, pp.225–34. [1.9]

Cliff, A.D. and P. Haggett, (1981). 'Mapping respiratory disease'. In *Scientific Foundations of Respiratory Medicine*, ed. J.G. Scadding, G. Cumming and W.M. Thurlbeck. London: Heinemann. [3.2, 3.11–12]

Cliff, A.D. and P. Haggett, (1981). 'Measuring

the velocity of epidemic waves'. *International Journal of Epidemiology*, 11, pp.82–9. [5.9, 6.5]

Cliff, A.D. and P. Haggett, (1984). 'Island epidemics'. *Scientific American*, 250, pp.110–17. [6.5]

Cliff, A.D. and P. Haggett, (1985). *The Spread of Measles in Fiji and the Pacific: Spatial Components in the Transmission of Epidemic Waves through Island Communities*, Publication HG18. Canberra: Australian National University, Research School of Pacific Studies, Department of Human Geography. [2.10, 4.5, 4.6, 4.9, 5.4, 5.11, 7.3]

Cliff, A.D., P. Haggett and R. Graham (1983). 'Reconstruction of diffusion processes at different geographical scales'. *Journal of Historical Geography*, 9, pp.29–46. [5.5]

Cliff, A.D., P. Haggett and J.K. Ord (1983). 'Forecasting epidemic pathways for measles in Iceland: the use of simultaneous equation and logic models'. *Ecology of Disease*, 2, pp.377–96. [7.4]

Cliff, A.D., P. Haggett and J.K. Ord (1986). *Spatial Aspects of Influenza Epidemics*. London: Pion. [2.4, 2.12, 5.15, 6.4, 7.3]

Cliff, A.D., P. Haggett, J.K. Ord and G.R. Versey (1981), *Spatial Diffusion: An Historical Geography of Epidemics in an Island Community*. Cambridge: Cambridge University Press. [2.3, 2.11, 2.12, 3.1, 4.5, 4.7, 5.5, 5.8, 5.10, 5.11, 5.15, 5.17, 5.18, 6.5, 7.4]

Cliff, A.D., P. Haggett, J.K. Ord, K.A. Bassett and R.B. Davies (1975). *Elements of Spatial Structure: A Quantitative Approach*. Cambridge: Cambridge University Press. [5.14]

Cliff, A.D. and J.K. Ord (1973). *Spatial Autocorrelation*. London: Pion. [1.9]

Cliff, A.D. and J.K. Ord (1978). 'Forecasting the progress of an epidemic'. In *Towards the Dynamic Analysis of Spatial Systems*, ed. R.L. Martin, N.J. Thrift and R.J. Bennett. London: Pion, pp.191–204. [7.4]

Cliff, A.D. and J.K. Ord (1981). *Spatial Processes: Models and Applications*. London: Pion. [1.9, 1.11, 3.11–12, 4.8, 5.16]

Colley, J.R.T. (1982). 'Chronic non-specific lung disease (CNSLD) and asthma'. In *Epidemiology of Diseases*, ed. D.L. Miller and R.D.T. Farmer. Oxford: Blackwell Scientific, pp.163–75. [3.11–12]

Cook, P. and D. Burkitt (1970). *An Epidemiological Study of Seven Malignant Tumours in East Africa*. London: Medical Research Council. [5.16]

Cook-Mozaffari, P.J., F.L. Ashwood, T. Vincent, D. Forman and M. Alderson (1987). *Cancer Incidence and Mortality in the Vicinity of Nuclear Installations, England and Wales 1959–80*, Office of Population Censuses and Surveys, Studies on Medical and Population Subjects, Publication No. 51. London: Her Majesty's Stationery Office. [3.8]

Cooney, M.K., C.E. Hall and J.P. Fox (1970). 'The Seattle Virus Watch Program. Pt. 1: Infection and illness experience of Virus Watch Families during a community-wide epidemic of echovirus 30 aseptic meningitis'. *American Journal of Public Health*, 60, pp.1456–65. [2.2]

Court-Brown, W.M., F.W. Spiers, R. Doll, B.J. Duffy and M.J. McHugh (1960). 'Geographical variations in leukaemia mortality relation to background radiation and other factors'. *British Medical Journal*, 1, pp.1753–9. [3.8]

Craft, A.W., S. Openshaw and J.M. Birch (1985). 'Childhood cancer in the Northern Region, 1968–82: incidence in small geographical areas'. *Journal of Epidemiology and Community Health*, 39, pp.53–7. [3.8]

Creighton, C. (1894, 1965). *History of Epidemics in Britain*. Vol. 2, *1666–1893*, 2nd edn with additional material by D.E.C. Eversley, E.A.

Underwood and L. Overrall. London: Cass. [1.1]

Cresswell, W.L. and P. Froggart (1963). *The Causation of Bus Driver Accidents: An Epidemiological Study*. London: Oxford University Press. [3.17]

Cryer, J.D. (1986). *Time Series Analysis*. Boston, Mass.: Duxbury Press. [Preface, 4.1–4.3]

Cuff, D.J. and M.T. Mattson (1982). *Thematic Maps: Their Design and Production*. New York, NY: Methuen. [1.5]

Daiwa Health Foundation (1980). *Atlas of Cardiovascular Disease for Cities, Towns and Villages in Japan, 1969–74*. Tokyo: Daiwa Health Foundation. [3.10]

Dempsey, M. (1947). 'Decline in tuberculosis death rate fails to tell entire story'. *American Review of Tuberculosis*, 56, pp.157–64. [2.5]

Department of the Environment (1987). *Handling Geographic Information*. London: Her Majesty's Stationery Office. [7.1]

Detels, R., J.A. Brody, J. McNew and A.H. Edgar (1973). 'Further epidemiological studies of subacute sclerosing panencephalitis'. *Lancet*, 2, pp.11–14. [4.9]

Dickinson, G.C. (1963). *Statistical Mapping and the Presentation of Statistics*. London: Edward Arnold. [1.2]

Dixon, C.W. (1962). *Smallpox*. London: Churchill Livingstone. [6.3]

Doll, R. (1959). *Methods of Geographical Pathology*. Oxford: Oxford University Press. [3.1]

Doll, R., ed. (1980). *The Geography of Diseases*. London: Churchill Livingstone. [3.1]

Doll, R. (1983). Forward. In *Atlas of Cancer Mortality in England and Wales 1968–1978*, ed. M.J. Gardner, P.D. Winter, C.P. Taylor and E.D. Acheson. Chichester: John Wiley. [3.6]

Doll, R. and R. Peto (1981). *The Causes of Cancer*. Oxford: Oxford University Press. [3.6]

Doll, R., C. Muir and J. Waterhouse (1970). *Cancer Incidence on Five Continents*, vol. 2. Geneva: World Health Organization. [3.6]

Dorolle, P. (1968). 'Old plagues in the jet age: international aspects of present and future control of communicable disease'. *British Medical Journal*, 4, pp.789–92. [7.3]

Downie, A.W. (1970). 'Smallpox'. In *Infectious Agents and Host Reactions*, ed. S. Mudd. Philadelphia, Pa.: Saunders, pp.487–518. [6.3]

Draper, N.R. and H. Smith (1981). *Applied Regression Analysis*, 2nd edn. New York, NY: Wiley. [1.14]

Dutt, A.K., C.B. Monroe, H.M. Dutta and B. Prince (1987). 'Geographic patterns of AIDS in the United States'. *Geographical Review*, 77, pp.456–71 [6.2]

Earickson, R. (1970). *The Spatial Behaviour of Hospital Patients. A Behavioural Approach to Spatial Interaction in Metropolitan Chicago*. University of Chicago, Department of Geography Research Papers No. 124. Chicago, Ill.: University of Chicago Press. [3.5]

Edson, D.T. and J. Denegre, ed. (1980). *Glossary of Terms in Computer Assisted Cartography*, 3rd edn. Falls Church, Va.: American Congress on Surveying and Mapping. [7.1]

Elveback, L.R., J.P. Fox, E. Ackerman, A. Langworthy, M. Boyd and L. Gatewood (1976). 'An influenza simulation model for immunization studies'. *American Journal of Epidemiology*, 103, pp.152–65. [6.4]

Evans, A.S. (1984). *Viral infections of Humans*, 2nd edn. New York, NY: Plenum. [2.2]

Evans, A.S. and J.C. Niederman (1984). 'Epstein-Barr virus'. In *Viral Infections of Humans: Epidemiology and Control*, 2nd edn, ed. A.S. Evans. London: Plenum, pp.209–33. [3.7]

Farmer, R.D.T., A. Nixon and J. Connolly (1982). 'Accidents'. In *Epidemiology of Dis-eases*, ed. D.L. Miller and R.D.T Farmer. Oxford: Blackwell Scientific, pp.369–86. [3.15]

Fenner, F. (1977). 'The eradication of smallpox'. *Progress in Medical Virology*, 23, pp.1–21. [6.3]

Fenner, F. (1986). 'The eradication of infectious diseases'. *Supplement to SAMJ*, 11 October 1986, pp.35–9. [4.9]

Fenner, F., D.A. Henderson, I. Arita, Z. Jesek and I.D. Ladnyi (1988). *Smallpox and Its Eradication*. Geneva: World Health Organization. [6.3]

Fine, P.E.M. (1982). 'Applications of mathematical models to the epidemiology: a critique'. In *Influenza Models: Prospects for Development and Use*, ed. P. Selby. Lancaster, Pa.: MTP Press, pp.15–85. [6.4]

Fisher, H.T. (1982). *Mapping Information: The Graphic Display of Quantitative Information*. Cambridge, Mass.: Abt Books. [1.2]

Flannery, J.J. (1971). 'The relative effectiveness of some graduated point symbols in the presentation of quantitative data'. *The Canadian Cartographer*, 8, pp.96–109. [1.3]

Fletcher, C. and R. Peto (1976). *The Natural History of Chronic Bronchitis and Emphysema*. Oxford: Oxford University Press. [3.11–12]

Forster, F. (1966). 'Use of a demographic base map for the presentation of areal data in epidemiology'. *British Journal of Preventive and Social Medicine*, 20, pp.156–71. [1.18]

Fraser, K.B. and S.J. Martin (1978). *Measles Virus and its Biology*. London: Academic Press. [3.3]

Frenzel-Beyme, R., R. Leuter and G. Wiebett (1979). *Cancer Atlas of the Federal Republic of Germany*. Berlin: Springer Verlag. [3.6]

Friðriksdóttir, E.A. and Ó. Ólafsson (1987). *Rannsókn á 7562 slysum byggð á gögnum Slysadeildar Borgarspítalans árið 1979* (An analysis of 7562 home accidents in the Greater Reykjavík Area, 1979), Special Publication No. 2 of *Heilbrigðisskýrslur* (Public Health in Iceland), Reykjavík: Office of the Director General of Public Health. [3.15]

Gardner, M.J., P.D. Winter and E.D. Acheson (1982). 'Variations in cancer mortality among local authority areas in England and Wales: relations with environmental factors and search for causes.' *British Medical Journal*, 284, pp.784–7. [3.6]

Gardner, M.J., P.D. Winter, C.P. Taylor and E.D. Acheson (1983). *Atlas of Cancer Mortality in England and Wales 1968–1978*. Chichester: John Wiley. [3.6]

Gardner, M.J., P.D. Winter and D.J.P. Barker (1984). *Atlas of Mortality from Selected Diseases in England and Wales 1968–78*. Chichester: John Wiley. [3.10, 3.11–12, 3.17]

Gatrell, A.C. (1981). 'Multidimensional scaling'. In *Quantitative Geography*, ed. N. Wrigley and R.J. Bennett. London: Routledge and Kegan Paul, pp.151–63. [7.2]

Gilg, A.W. (1973). 'A study in agricultural disease diffusion: the case of the 1970–71 fowl-pest epidemic'. *Transactions of the Institute of British Geographers*, 59, pp.77–97. [5.6]

Gillis, C.R. (1977). 'Malignant neoplasms'. In *World Geography of Human Diseases*, ed. G.M. Howe. London: Academic Press, pp.507–34. [3.6]

Glick, B.J. (1982). 'The spatial organization of cancer mortality'. *Annals of the Association of American Geographers*, 72, pp.471–81. [3.6, 5.14]

Golledge, R.G. and G. Rushton (1972). *Multidimensional Scaling: Review and Geographical Applications*, Commission on College Geography, Technical Paper No. 10. Washington, DC: Association of American Geographers, Commission on College Geography. [7.2]

Gottmann, J.M. (1981). *Time Series Analysis*. Cambridge: Cambridge University Press.

[4.1, 4.2, 4.3]

Gould, P.R. (1970). 'Is *Statistix Inferens* the geographical name for a wild goose?' *Economic Geography*, suppl., 46, pp.439–48. [5, Intro.]

Gould, P.R. and T.R. Leinbach (1966). 'An approach to the geographical assignment of hospital services'. *Tijdschrift voor Economische en Sociale Geographie*, 57, pp.203–6. [7.5]

Granger, C.W.J. (1969) 'Spatial data and time-series analysis'. In *London Papers in Regional Science*. Vol. 1, *Studies in Regional Science*, ed. A.J. Scott. London: Pion, pp.1–24. [5.12]

Griffiths, D.A. (1973). 'The effects of measles vaccination on the incidence of measles in the community'. *Journal of the Royal Statistical Society A*, 136, pp.441–9. [4.9]

Gzundman, E., G. Kzueger, E. Gzundman, G.R.F. Kzueger and D. Ablashi, ed. (1981). *Nasopharyngeal Carcinoma*. Stuttgart: Gustav Fischer Verlag. [3.7]

Haberman, S.J. (1973). 'The analysis of residuals in cross-classified tables'. *Biometrics*, 29, pp.205–20. [1.8]

Haggett, P. (1972). 'Contagious processes in a planar graph: an epidemiological application'. In *Medical Geography: Techniques and Field Studies*, ed. N.D. McGlashan. London: Methuen, pp.307–24. [5.2, 5.14]

Haggett, P. (1975). 'Simple epidemics in human populations: some geographical aspects of the Hamer–Soper diffusion models'. In *Processes in Physical and Human Geography: Bristol Essays*, ed. R.F. Peel, M.D.I. Chisholm and P. Haggett. London: Heinemann, pp.371–91. [7.4]

Haggett, P. (1976). 'Hybridizing alternative models of an epidemic diffusion process'. *Economic Geography*, 52, pp.136–46. [5.13]

Haggett, P. (1978). 'Regional and local components in elementary space-time models of contagious processes'. In *Timing Space and Spacing Time*, vol. 3, ed. T. Carlstein, D.

Parkes and N.J. Thrift. London: Edward Arnold. [5.13]

Haggett, P., A.D. Cliff and A.E. Frey (1977). *Locational Analysis in Human Geography*, 2nd edn. London: Edward Arnold. [1.12, 1.13, 1.16, 3.1, 3.4, 5.12, 5.18, 7.5]

Hall, E.J. (1984). *Radiation and Life*. Oxford: Pergamon. [5.3]

Hall, S.A. and B.W. Langlands (1975). *Atlas of Disease Distribution in Uganda*. Nairobi: East Africa Publishers. [5.16]

Halsey, N.A., J.F. Modlin and J.T. Jabbour (1978). 'Subacute sclerosing panencephalitis (SSPE): an epidemiological review'. In *Persistent Viruses*, ed. J.G. Stevens, G.J. Todoro and C.F. Fox. ICN–UCLA Symposia on Molecular and Cellular Biology, vol. 11. New York, NY: Academic Press, pp.101–14. [4.9]

Hamer, W.H. (1906). 'Epidemic diseases in England'. *Lancet*, 1, pp.733–9. [7.4]

Harvey, L.A. and D. St. Leger-Gordon (1953). *Dartmoor*. London: Collins. [3.9]

Henderson, D.A. (1974). 'Importation of smallpox into Europe'. *WHO Chronicle*, 28, pp.428–30. [6.3]

Hepple, L.W. (1981). 'Spatial and temporal analysis: time series analysis'. In *Quantitative Geography*, ed. N. Wrigley and R.J. Bennett. London: Routledge and Kegan Paul, pp. 92–6. [4.1]

Higgins, I.T.T. (1973). 'The epidemiology of chronic respiratory disease'. *Preventive Medicine*, 2, pp.14–33. [3.11–12]

Hill, I.D. and M.C. Pike, (1976). *Chi-squared Integral (S15). Collected ACM Algorithms, 299.1.2*. New York: Association of Computing Machinery. [3.8]

Hinman, A.R., A.D. Brandling-Bennett and P.I. Nieburg (1979). 'The opportunity and obligation to eliminate measles from the United States'. *Journal of the American Medical Association*, 242, pp.1157–62. [3.3, 4.9]

Hinman, A.R., A.D. Brandling-Bennett, R.H. Bernier, C.D. Kirby and D.L. Eddins (1980). 'Current features of measles in the United States: feasibility of measles elimination'. *Epidemiologic Reviews*, 2, pp.153–70. [4.9]

Hinman, A.R., W.A. Orenstein, A.B. Bloch, K.J. Bart, D.L. Eddins, R.W. Amler and C.D. Kirby (1982). 'Impact of measles in the United States'. Paper to International Symposium on Measles Immunization, Washington, DC, March 1982. [4.9]

Hinman, E.H. (1966). *World Eradication of Infectious Diseases*. Springfield, Ill.: Thomas. [6.3]

Hirsch, A. (1883). *Handbook of Geographical and Historical Pathology*, vol. 1–3, trans. Charles Creighton (*Handbuch der historische-geographische Pathologie*, 2nd German edn. 1864). London: The New Sydenham Society. [5.4]

Hopkins, D.R. (1983). *Princes and Peasants: Smallpox in History*. Chicago, Ill.: Chicago University Press. [6.3]

Howe, G.M., ed. (1970). *National Atlas of Disease Mortality in the United Kingdom*, 2nd edn. London: Royal Geographical Society. [2.7, 3.2, 3.11–12]

Howe, G.M. (1972). *Man, Environment and Disease in Britain: A Medical Geography of Britain through the Ages*. New York: Barnes and Noble. [1.1]

Howe, G.M. (1979). 'Mortality from selected malignant neoplasms in the British Isles: the spatial perspective'. *Geographical Journal*, 145, 401–15. [3.6]

Howe, G.M. (1986a). 'Disease mapping'. In *Medical Geography: Progress and Prospect*, ed. M. Pacione. London: Croom Helm. [1.2]

Howe, G.M., ed. (1986b) *Global Cancerology: A World Geography of Human Cancers*. Edinburgh: Churchill Livingstone. [3.6]

Howe, G.M., L. Burgess and P. Gatenby (1977).

'Cardiovascular disease'. In *World Geography of Human Diseases*, ed. G.M. Howe. London: Academic Press, pp.431–76. [3.10]

Hsu, M.L. and A.H. Robinson (1970). *The Fidelity of Isopleth Maps: An Experimental Study*. Minneapolis: University of Minnesota Press. [1.10]

Hubert, L.J., R.G. Golledge, C.M. Constanzo and G.D. Richardson (1981). 'Assessing homogeneity in cross-classified proximity data'. *Geographical Analysis*, 13, pp.38–50. [5.16]

Hunter, J.M. (1956). 'River blindness in Nangodi, northern Ghana: a hypothesis of cyclical advance and retreat'. *Geographical Review*, 56, 398–416. [Preface]

Hunter, J.M. and J.C. Young (1971). 'Diffusion of influenza in England and Wales'. *Annals of the Association of American Geographers*, 61, pp.637–53. [1.18, 6.4]

Ichimaru, M., T. Ichimaru and J.L. Belsky (1978). 'Incidence of leukaemia among bomb survivors belonging to a fixed cohort in Hiroshima and Nagasaki, 1950–71. Radiation dose, years after exposure, age at exposure and type of leukaemia'. *Japanese Journal of Radiation Research*, 19, pp.262–82, 391–407. [3.8]

International Atomic Energy Agency Report (1986). Facts about low-level radiation. Vienna: IAEA. [3.9]

International Commission on Radiological Protection (in press). *Lung Cancer Risk from Environmental Exposure to Radon Daughters*, ICRP Publication No. 50. Oxford: Pergamon Press. [3.9]

Janerich, D.T., R.G. Skalko and I.H. Porter (1974). *Congenital Defects*. New York, NY: Academic Press. [3.14]

Janerich, D.T. and A.P. Polednak (1983). 'Epidemiology of birth defects'. *Epidemiologic Reviews*, 5, pp.16–37. [3.14]

Jenkins, G.M. and D.G. Watts (1968). *Spectral Analysis and its Applications*. San Francisco, Ca.: Holden-Day. [5.12]

Jenks, G.F. and M.R. Coulson (1963). 'Class intervals for statistical maps'. *International Yearbook of Cartography*, 3, pp.119–34. [1.6]

Jenner, E. (1798). *An Inquiry into the Causes and Effects of the Variolae Vacciniae, a Disease Discovered in Some of the Western Counties of England, Particularly Gloucestershire, and Known by the Name of Cowpox*. London: Sampson Low. [6.3]

Joarder, A.K., D. Tarantola and J. Tulloch (1980). *The Eradication of Smallpox from Bangladesh*. New Delhi: WHO Regional Publications. [6.3]

Jusatz, H. (1977). 'Cholera'. In *A World Geography of Human Diseases*, ed. G.M. Howe. London: Academic Press, pp.131–43. [1.1]

Kahn, C. (1963). 'History of smallpox and its prevention'. *American Journal of Diseases of Children*, 106, pp.597–609. [6.3]

Källen, A., P. Arcuri and J.D. Murray (1985). 'A simple model for the spatial spread and control of rabies'. *Journal of Theoretical Biology*, 116, pp.377–93. [5.7]

Kearns, G. (1985). *Urban Epidemics and Historical Geography: Cholera in London, 1848–9*, Publication No. 16, Research Paper Series of the Historical Geography Research Group of the Institute of British Geographers. Norwich: Geo Books. [1.1]

Keates, J.S. (1982). *Understanding Maps*. London: Longman. [1.2]

Kendall, D.G. (1957). 'La propagation d'une épidémie ou d'un bruit dans une population limitée'. *Publications of the Institute of Statistics, University of Paris*, 6, pp.307–31. [5.6]

Kendall, D.G. (1971). 'Construction of maps from odd bits of information'. *Nature*, 231, pp.158–9. [7.2]

Kendall, D.G. (1975). 'The recovery of structure from fragmentary information'. *Philosophical Transactions of the Royal Society of London A*, 279, pp.547–82. [7.2]

Kendall, M.G. (1973). *Time Series*. London: Griffin. [4.2]

Kermack, W.O. and A.G. McKendrick (1927). 'Contributions to the mathematical theory of epidemics, I'. *Proceedings of the Royal Society A*, 115, pp.700–21. [7.4]

Keyfitz, N. and W. Flieger (1968). *World Population: An Analysis of Vital Data*. Chicago, Ill.: University of Chicago Press. [2.12]

Kilbourne, E.D. (1973). 'The molecular epidemiology of influenza'. *Journal of Infectious Diseases*, 127, pp.478–87. [6.4]

Kilbourne, E.D., ed. (1975). *The Influenza Viruses and Influenza*. New York, NY: Academic Press. [6.4]

Koch, R. (1987). 'The anatomy of a virus', *New Scientist*, 26 March, pp.46–51 [6.2]

Kopec, R.J. (1963). 'An alternative method for the construction of Thiessen polygons'. *Professional Geographer*, 15, pp.24–6. [1.16]

Knox, E.G. (1964). 'Epidemiology of childhood leukaemia in Northumberland and Durham'. *British Journal of Preventative and Social Medicine*, 18, pp.17–24. [3.8]

Knox, E.G. (1964). 'The detection of space-time interactions'. *Applied Statistics*, 13, pp.25–9. [5.16]

Knox, E.G. (1986). 'A transmission model for AIDS'. *European Journal of Epidemiology*, 2, pp.165–77. [6.2]

Krumbein, W.C. (1955). 'Experimental design in the earth sciences'. *Transactions of the American Geophysical Union*, 36, pp.1–11. [1.13]

Kruskal, J.B. (1964). 'Multidimensional scaling'. *Psychometrika*, 29, pp.1–42. [7.2]

Kruskal, J.B. and M. Wish (1978). *Multidimensional Scaling*. Beverly Hills, Ca.: Sage. [7.2]

Kuhn, H.W. and R.E. Kuenne (1962). 'An efficient algorithm for the numerical solution of the generalised Weber problem in spatial economics'. *Journal of Regional Science*, 4, pp.21–33. [5.10]

Kupka, K. (1978). 'International classification of diseases, ninth revision'. *WHO Chronicle*, 32, pp.219–25. [2.1]

Lam, N.S. (1983). 'Spatial interpolation methods: a review'. *American Cartographer*, 10, pp.129–49. [1.10]

Langmuir, A.D. (1963). 'The surveillance of communicable diseases of national importance'. *New England Journal of Medicine*, 268, pp.182–92. [2.2]

Learmonth, A.T.A. (1957). 'Some regional contrasts in the regional geography of malaria in India and Pakistan'. *Transactions of the Institute of British Geographers*, 23, pp.37–59. [3.5]

Learmonth, A.T.A. (1977). 'Malaria'. In *A World Geography of Human Diseases*, ed. G.M. Howe. London: Academic Press, pp.61–108. [3.5]

Learmonth, A.T.A. and M.N. Pal (1959). 'A method for plotting two variables on the same map using isopleths'. *Erdkunde*, 13, pp.145–50. [1.10]

Lenoir, G.M., G.T. O'Connor and C.L.M. Olweny, ed. (1985). *Burkitt's Lymphoma: A Human Cancer Model*, International Agency for Research on Cancer (IARC), Scientific Publication No. 60. Oxford: Oxford University Press. [5.16]

McArthur, N. (1967). *Island Populations in the Pacific*. Canberra: Australian National University Press. [2.10, 4.6, 5.4, 5.11, 7.3]

MacDonald, D.W. (1980). *Rabies and Wildlife. A Biologist's Perspective*. Oxford: Oxford University Press. [5.7]

MacDougall, E.B. (1976). *Computer Programming for Spatial Problems*. London: Edward Arnold. [1.10]

McGlashan, N.D. and N.K. Chick (1974). 'Assessing spatial variations in mortality: ischaemic heart disease in Tasmania'. *Australian Geographical Studies*, 12, pp.190–206. [3.10]

McHarry, J., ed. (1985). *Report of the First National Conference on the Health Effects of Low Level Radiation*. Lydney, Glos.: Severnside Campaign Against Radiation. [3.8]

Mackay, J.R. (1953). 'The alternative choice in isopleth interpolation'. *Professional Geographer*, 5, pp.2–4. [1.10]

McNicol, M.W. (1982). 'Tuberculosis'. In *Epidemiology of Diseases*, ed. D.L. Miller and R.D.T. Farmer. Oxford: Blackwell Scientific, pp.31–9. [3.2]

Maling, D.H. (1973). *Coordinate Systems and Map Projections*. London: George Philip. [1.4, 7.3]

Mann, J. (1987). AIDS in Africa. *New Scientist*, 1553, 26 March, pp.40–3 [6.2]

Mantel, N. (1967). 'The detection of disease clustering and a generalised regression approach'. *Cancer Research*, 27, pp.209–20. [5.16]

Marble, D.F., ed. (1980). *Computer Software for Spatial Data Handling*. Washington, DC: US Geological Survey. [1.10]

Mardia, K.V. (1972). *Statistics of Directional Data*. London: Academic Press. [4.5]

Marier, R. (1977). 'The reporting of communicable diseases'. *American Journal of Epidemiology*, 105, pp.587–90. [2.2]

Mason, T.J., F.W. McKay Jr, R. Hoover, W.J. Blot and J.F. Fraumeni Jr (1975). *Atlas of Cancer Mortality for United States Counties, 1950–69*, National Institutes of Health, Publication No. 75–780. Washington, DC: Government Printing Office. [3.6]

Mason, T.J., J.F. Fraumeni Jr, R. Hoover and W.J. Blot (1981). *An Atlas of Mortality from Selected Diseases*, National Institutes of Health, Publication No. 81–2397. Washington, DC: Government Printing Office. [3.6]

Massam, B.H. (1975). *Location and Space in Social Administration*. London: Edward Arnold. [7.5]

Matanoski, G.M. and E.A. Elliott (1981). 'Bladder cancer epidemiology'. *Epidemiologic Reviews*, 3, pp.203–29. [3.6]

May, J.M. (1959). *Ecology of Human Disease*. New York: MD Publications. [1.2, 3.1]

May, R. (1976). 'Models for single populations'. In *Theoretical Ecology: Principles and Applications*, ed. R. May. Oxford: Basil Blackwell, pp.4–25. [5.9]

May, R. and R.M. Anderson (1987). 'Transmission dynamics of HIV infection'. *Nature*, 326, pp.137–42. [6.2]

Mayer, J.D. (1981). 'Geographical clues about multiple sclerosis'. *Annals of the Association of American Geographers*, 71, pp.28–39. [4.9]

Meade, M.S. (1983). 'Cardiovascular disease in Savannah, Georgia'. In *Geographical Aspects of Health: Essays in Honour of Andrew Learmonth*, ed. N.D. McGlashan and J.R. Blunden. London: Academic Press, pp.175–96. [3.10]

Miller, K.L. and J.S. Kahn (1962). *Statistical Analysis in the Geological Sciences*. New York, NY: John Wiley. [1.12]

Moellering, H. (1974). *The Journey to Death: A Spatial Analysis of Fatal Traffic Crashes in Michigan, 1969*, Michigan Geographical Publication No. 13. Ann Arbor: Department of Geography, University of Michigan. [3.16]

Moellering, H. and W.R. Tobler (1972). 'Geographical variances'. *Geographical Analysis*, 4, pp.34–50. [1.11]

Mollison, D. (1977). 'Spatial contact models for ecological and epidemic spread'. *Journal of the Royal Statistical Society B*, 39, pp.283–326. [5.7]

Monkhouse, F.J. and H.R. Wilkinson (1971).

Maps and Diagrams: Their Compilation and Construction, 3rd edn. London: Methuen. [1.2, 2.6, 4.5]

Monmonier, M.S. (1974). 'Measures of pattern complexity for choropleth maps'. *American Cartographer*, 1, pp.59–69. [1.6]

Monmonier, M.S. (1982). *Computer-Assisted Cartography: Principles and Prospects*. Englewood Cliffs, NJ: Prentice-Hall. [7.1]

Moran, P.A.P. (1948). 'The interpretation of statistical maps'. *Journal of the Royal Statistical Society B*, 10, pp.243–51. [1.9]

Morrill, R. L. (1959). 'Highways and services: the case of physicians' care'. In *Studies of Highway Development and Geographic Change*, ed. W.L. Garrison, B.J.L. Berry, D.F. Marble, J.F. Nystuen and R.L. Morrill. Seattle: University of Washington Press, pp.229–76. [7.5]

Morrill, R.L. (1970). 'The shape of diffusion in space and time'. *Economic Geography*, 46, pp.259-68. [5.6]

Muller, J., W.C. Wheeler, J.F. Gentlemen, J.F. Suranyi and R.A. Kusiak (1985). 'Study of mortality of Ontario miners'. In *Occupational Radiation Safety in Mining*, vol. 1. Toronto: Canadian Nuclear Association, pp. 335–43. [3.9]

Murray, J.D., E.A. Stanley and D.L. Brown (1986). 'On the spatial spread of rabies among foxes'. *Proceedings of the Royal Society B*, 229, pp.111–50. [5.7]

National Academy of Sciences (1986). *Mobilisation Against AIDS: The Unfinished Story of a Virus*. Cambridge, Mass.: Harvard University Press. [6.2]

National Center for Health Statistics (1979). *Proceedings of the 1976 Workshop on Automated Cartography and Epidemiology*, Publication No. PHS-79-1254. Hyattsville, Md.: US Department of Health, Education and Welfare. [7.1]

National Council on Radiation Protection and Measurements (1984). *Exposures from the Uranium Series with Emphasis on Radon and its Daughters*, NCRP Report No. 77. Washington, DC: Government Printing Office. [3.9]

National Radiological Protection Board (1986). *Living with Radiation*, 3rd edn. London: Her Majesty's Stationery Office. [3.8]

Neft, D.S. (1966). *Statistical Analysis for Areal Distributions*, Monograph Series No. 2. Philadelphia, Pa.: Regional Science Research Institute, University of Pennsylvania. [1.15]

Nordic Statistical Secretariat (1985). *Yearbook of Nordic Statistics 1984*. Stockholm: Nordic Council. [2.12]

Norman, L.G. (1962). *Road Traffic Accidents: Epidemiology, Control and Prevention*. Geneva: World Health Organization. [3.16]

Openshaw, S., A.W. Craft, M. Charlton and J.M. Birch (1988). 'Investigation of leukaemia clusters by use of a geographical analysis machine'. *Lancet*, 1, pp.272–3. [3.8]

Openshaw, S. and P.J. Taylor (1981). 'The modifiable areal unit problem'. In *Quantitative Geography*, ed. N. Wrigley and R.J. Bennett. London: Routledge and Kegan Paul, pp.60–70. [4.8]

O'Riordan, M.C., A.C. James, B.M.R. Green and A.D. Wrixon (1987). *Exposure to Radon Daughters in Dwellings*, Publication No. NRPB-GS6. Chilton, Oxfordshire: National Radiological Protection Board. [3.9]

Orlando, P., G. Gallelli, F. Perdelli, S. de Flora and R. Malcontenti (1986). 'Alimentary restrictions and I-131 in human thyroids'. *Nature*, 324, p.23. [5.3]

Palmer, D.F., W.R. Dowdle, M.T. Coleman and G.C. Schild (1975). *Advanced Laboratory Techniques for Influenza Diagnosis*, Immunology Series No. 6. Atlanta, Ga.: Centers for Disease Control. [2.4]

Peckham, C., R.D.T. Farmer and E.M. Ross (1982). 'Congenital malformations'. In *Epidemiology of Diseases*, ed. D.L. Miller and R.D.T. Farmer. Oxford: Blackwell Scientific, pp.452–66. [3.14]

Pelling, M. (1978). *Cholera, Fever and English Medicine, 1825–1865*. Oxford: Oxford University Press. [1.1]

Peterman, T.A., D.P. Drotman and J.W. Curran (1985). 'Epidemiology of the Acquired Immunodeficiency Syndrome (AIDS)'. *Epidemiologic Reviews*, 7, pp.1–21. [6.2]

Pielou, E.C. (1969). *An Introduction to Mathematical Ecology*. New York, NY: John Wiley/Interscience. [1.16]

Phillips, D.R. (1986). 'The demand for and utilization of health services'. In *Medical Geography: Progress and Prospect*, ed. M. Pacione. London: Croom Helm. [7.5]

Prothero, R.M. (1965). *Migrants and Malaria*. London: Longmans Green. [3.5]

Pyle, G.F. (1971). *Heart Disease, Cancer and Stroke in Chicago*, Department of Geography, University of Chicago, Research Paper No. 134. Chicago, Ill.: University of Chicago Press. [3.10]

Pyle, G.F. (1979). *Applied Medical Geography*. New York, NY: John Wiley. [1.2]

Rhynsberger, D. (1973). 'Analytic delineation of Thiessen polygons'. *Geographical Analysis*, 5, pp.133–44. [1.16]

Ripley, B.D. (1981). *Spatial Statistics*. New York, NY: John Wiley. [1.10–1.12]

Road Research Laboratory (1963). *Research on Road Safety*. London: Her Majesty's Stationery Office. [3.17]

Robinson, A.H. (1982). *Early Thematic Mapping in the History of Cartography*, Chicago: University of Chicago Press, pp.170–82. [Preface]

Robinson, A.H. and B.B. Petchenik (1976). *The Nature of Maps: Essays Towards Understanding Maps and Mapping*. Chicago, Ill.: University of Chicago Press. [1.2]

Robinson, A.H., R.D. Sale, J.L. Morrison and P.C. Muehrcke (1984). *Elements of Cartography*, 5th edn. New York, NY: John Wiley. [Preface, 1.2–1.6, 3.3, 7.1]

Rodenwaldt, E. and H.J. Jusatz (1952–61). *World Atlas of Epidemic Diseases*, vol. 1–3. Hamburg: Falk. [Preface]

Rogers, A. (1974). *Statistical Analysis of Spatial Dispersion*. London: Pion. [1.17]

Rosenberg, C.E. (1962). *The Cholera Years: The United States in 1832, 1849 and 1866*. Chicago: University of Chicago Press. [1.1]

Rutherford, W.H. (1980). *Accident and Emergency Medicine*. Tunbridge Wells: Pitman Medical. [3.15]

Rvachev, L.A. and I.M. Longini (1985). 'A mathematical model for the global spread of influenza'. *Mathematical Biosciences*, 75, pp.3–22. [6.4]

Ryan, B.F., B.L. Joiner and T.A. Ryan (1985). *Minitab Handbook*, 2nd edn. Boston, Mass.: Duxbury Press. [Preface, 1.7, 1.12–1.14]

Ryckeboer, R., J. Jamssens and J. Thiers (1983). *Atlas de la mortalité par cancer en Belgique, 1969–76*. Brussels: Institut d'Hygiène et d'Épidémiologie. [3.6]

Sarkar, J.K., S. Ray and P. Manji (1970). 'Epidemiological and virological studies in the off-season smallpox cases in Calcutta'. *Indian Journal of Medical Research*, 58, pp.829–39. [6.3]

Sayers, B.McA., B.B. Mansourian, T.P. Tan and K. Bogel (1977). 'A pattern-analysis study of a wild-life rabies epizootic'. *Medical Informatics*, 2, pp.11–34. [5.7]

Segi, M. (1977). *Atlas of Cancer Mortality for Japan by Cities and Counties, 1969–76*. Tokyo: Daiwa Health Foundation. [3.6]

Selby, P., ed. (1976). *Influenza: Virus, Vaccines, Strategy*. London: Academic Press. [6.4]

Selby, P. (1981). *Influenza Epidemics Modelling: Prospectus for Prediction and Control*. Geneva:

Sandoz Institute. [6.4]

Senser, D.J., H.B. Dull and A.D. Langmuir (1967). 'Epidemiological basis for the eradication of measles'. *Centers for Disease Control, Public Health Reports*, 82, pp.253–6. [4.9]

Serfling, R.E. (1963). 'Methods for current statistical analysis of excess pneumonia–influenza deaths'. *Centers for Disease Control, Public Health Reports*, 78, pp.494–506. [2.4]

Siegel, S. (1956). *Nonparametric Statistics for the Behavioral Sciences*. New York, NY: McGraw Hill. [1.2]

Siemiatycki, J., G. Brubaker and A. Geser (1980). 'Space-time clustering of Burkitt's lymphomas in East Africa: analysis of recent data and a new look at old data'. *International Journal of Cancer*, 25, pp.197–203. [5.16]

Simmons, J.S., T.F. Whayne, G.W. Anderson and H.W. Horack (1944–54). *Global Epidemiology: A Geography of Disease and Sanitation*, vol. 1–3. Philadelphia, Pa.: Lippincott. [3.1]

Skoda, L. and J.C. Robertson (1972). *Isodemographic Map of Canada*. Ottawa: Lands Directorate, Department of the Environment. [1.18]

Smith, F.B. and M.J. Clark (1986). 'Radionuclide deposition from the Chernobyl cloud'. *Nature*, 322, pp.690–1. [5.3]

Smith, J.W.G. (1976). *Surveillance of Influenza: Report of the Public Health Laboratory Service*. Colindale, London: Epidemiological Research Laboratory. [2.4]

Smith, J.W.G. (1976). 'Vaccination strategy'. In *Influenza: Virus, Vaccines, Strategy*, ed. P. Selby. London: Academic Press, pp.271–94. [6.4]

Smith, P. (1982). 'Spatial and temporal clustering'. In *Cancer Epidemiology and Prevention*, ed. D. Schotenfeld and J.F. Fraumeni. Philadelphia, Pa.: Saunders. [3.8]

Snedecor, G.W. and W.G. Cochran (1980).

Statistical Methods, 7th edn. Ames, Iowa: Iowa State University Press. [1.7, 1.13, 1.14, 2.7]

Snow, J. (1854). *On the Mode of Communication of Cholera*, 2nd edn. London: Churchill Livingstone. [1.1, 1.15]

Sokal, R.R. (1979). 'Ecological parameters inferred from spatial correleograms'. In *Contemporary Quantitative Ecology and Related Econometrics*, ed. G.P. Patil and M.L. Rosenzweig. Fairland, Md.: International Cooperative Publishing House, pp.167–96. [5.14]

Soper, H.E. (1929). 'Interpretation of periodicity in disease prevalence'. *Journal of the Royal Statistical Society A*, 92, pp.34–73. [7.4]

Spink, W.W. (1978). *Infectious Diseases: Prevention and Treatment in the Nineteenth and Twentieth Centuries*. Folkestone, Kent: Dawson for the University of Minnesota Press. [1.1]

Steck, F. and A. Wandeler (1980). 'Epidemiology of fox rabies in Europe'. *Epidemiologic Reviews*, 2, pp.71–96. [5.7]

Stephan, F.F. (1934). 'Sampling errors and the interpretation of social data ordered in time and space'. *Journal of the American Statistical Association*, 29, pp.165–6. [5, Intro.]

Stock, R.F. (1976). *Cholera in Africa: Diffusion of the Disease 1970–75 with Particular Emphasis on West Africa*, African Environmental Special Report No. 3. London: International African Institute. [5.1]

Stocks, P. (1949). *Sickness in the Population of England and Wales in 1944–47: Studies on Medical and Population Subjects, No. 2*. London: Her Majesty's Stationery Office. [2.3]

Stocks, P. and M. Karn (1928). 'A study of the epidemiology of measles'. *Annals of Eugenics*, 3, pp.361–98. [5.2]

Stuart-Harris, C.H. (1965). *Influenza and Other Virus Infections of the Respiratory Tract*, 1st edn. London: Edward Arnold. [6.4]

Stuart-Harris, C.H. and G.C. Schild (1976) *Influenza: The Viruses and the Disease*, 2nd edn. London: Edward Arnold. [6.4]

Stuart-Harris, C.H., G.C. Schild and J.S. Oxford (1985). *Influenza: The Viruses and the Disease*, 3rd edn. London: Edward Arnold. [2.4, 6.4]

Sviatlovsky, E.E. and W.C. Eels (1937). 'The centrographic method and regional analysis'. *Geographical Review*, 27, pp.240–54. [1.15]

Swinscow, T.D.V. (1983). *Statistics at Square One* (articles published in the British Medical Journal), 8th edn. London: British Medical Journal. [1.7, 1.13, 1.14, 2.7]

Taylor, D.R.F., ed. (1980). *Progress in Computer Cartography*, vol. 1. *The Computer in Contemporary Cartography*. New York, NY: John Wiley. [7.1]

Taylor, M. and C.C. Kissling (1983). 'Resource dependence, power networks and the airline systems of the South Pacific'. *Regional Studies*, 17, pp.237–50. [7.2]

Thé, G. de- (1978). 'Epidemiological evidence for causal relationship between Epstein-Barr virus and Burkitt's lymphoma from Ugandan prospective study'. *Nature*, 274, pp.756–61. [5.16]

Thé G. de-, J.H.C. Ho and C. Muir (1984). 'Nasopharyngeal carcinoma'. In *Viral Infections of Humans: Epidemiology and Control*, 2nd edn, ed. A.S. Evans. London: Plenum, pp.621–52. [3.7]

Thé, G. de- and X. Yto, ed. (1978). *Nasopharyngeal Carcinoma: Etiology and Control*. Lyons: International Agency for Research on Cancer. [3.7]

Thomas, R.W. (1981). 'Point pattern analysis'. In *Quantitative Geography*, ed. N. Wrigley and R.J. Bennett. London: Routlege and Kegan Paul, pp.164–76. [1.17]

Tobler, W.R. (1973). 'Choropleth maps without class intervals'. *Geographical Analysis*, 5, pp.262–5, 358–60. [1.6]

Tufte, E.R. (1983). *The Visual Display of Quantitative Information*. Cheshire, Conn.: Graphics Press. [7.1]

Tukey, J.W. (1962). 'The future of data analysis'. *Annals of Mathematical Statistics*, 33, pp.1–67. [1.8]

United Nations Scientific Committee on the Effects of Atomic Radiation (1982). *Ionizing Radiation: Sources and Biological Effects*. New York, NY: United Nations. [3.9, 5.3]

Unwin, D.J. (1975). *An Introduction to Trend-Surface Analysis*, Concepts and Techniques in Modern Geography No. 5. Norwich: Geoabstracts. [1.12]

Wasserman, P. and J. O'Brien (1983). *Statistical Sources: A Subject Guide*, 8th edn. Detroit, Mich.: Gale Research. [2.1]

Waterhouse, J., C. Muir, P. Correa and J. Powell, ed. (1976). *Cancer Incidence on Five Continents*. Lyons: International Agency for Research on Cancer. [3.6]

Wernstedt, F.L. (1972). *World Climatic Data*. Lamont, Pa.: Climatic Data Press. [4.6]

White, R.R. (1972). 'Probability maps of leukaemia mortalities in England and Wales'. In *Medical Geography: Techniques and Field Studies*, ed. N.D. McGlashan. London: Methuen, pp.173–86. [3.8]

Whitehead, H. (1856). *Report on the Outbreak of Cholera to St. James' Vestry, 1855*. London: [1.16]

Whittingham, H.E. (1967). 'Impact of air travel on epidemiology'. *British Journal of Clinical Practice*, 2, pp.409–15. [7.3]

Whittle, P. (1954). 'On stationary processes in the plane'. *Biometrika*, 41, pp.434–49. [1.10]

Wilson, A.G. (1970). *Entropy in Urban and Regional Modelling*. London: Pion. [3.4]

Winterton, M.R. (1980). 'The Soho cholera epidemic 1854'. *History of Medicine*, 7, pp.11–20. [1.16]

Wolfe, R.J. (1982). 'Alaska's great sickness, 1900: an epidemic of measles and influenza in a virgin soil population'. *Proceedings of the American Philosophical Society*, 126, pp.91–121. [5.4]

World Health Organization (1980). *The Global Eradication of Smallpox: Final Report of the Global Commission for the Certification of Smallpox Eradication*. Geneva: WHO Monographs. [6.3]

World Health Organization (1984). 'WHO Expert Committee on Rabies'. *WHO Technical Report Series*, 709. [5.7]

World Health Organization (1986). 'WHO Expert Committee on Malaria: Eighteenth Report'. *WHO Technical Report Series*, 735. [3.5]

Wrixon, A.D. (1987). 'Radiation doses and risks of leukaemia around nuclear sites'. *National Radiological Protection Board, Radiological Protection Bulletin*, 83, pp.6–12. [3.8]

Yekutiel, P. (1980). *Eradication of Infectious Diseases: A Critical Study*. Basel: Karger. [4.9]

Young, J.C. (1977). 'Bronchitis'. In *World Geography of Human Diseases*, ed. G.M. Howe. London: Academic Press, pp.319–37. [3.11–12]

Zeiss, H., ed. (1941–5). *Seuchen Atlas*. Gotha: Jutus Perthes (Hermann Haack Geographisch-Kartographische Ansatt). [Preface]

INDEX

INDEX